About this book

Considerable thought has gone into designing this book to meet the requirements of students who have a limited time in which to assimilate information, yet need to take in a maximum detail without re-reading portions of text or becoming fatigued. Many features of this book have been designed to ease reading and assimilation.

Summary Headings

These headings (bold-faced sentences scattered throughout) provide a summary of the text following them, giving a quick overview of the whole section. These proved so popular with students using our other textbook (*Pathology*) that we used them here.

Figure Legends

The figure legends are, in general, not repetitive of the main text and are designed to be read when referenced from the main text. This serves two purposes: firstly it maintains the flow of information, and secondly it provides a refreshing break from reading the main text. For this reason many of the captions are used as the vehicle to explain complex pieces of information, particularly those relating to three-dimensional structure.

Clinical Boxes (blue)

We have chosen many clinical examples to illustrate the vital role that an understanding of histology will play in subsequent studies of human biology, disease, and clinical practice.

Practical Histology Boxes (green)

Many students give up on microscopy because they feel that they cannot see what they have just read about. The practical histology sections are designed to put histology into a classroom teaching perspective and hopefully lessen the anxiety of the students who feel that they cannot use a microscope.

Advanced Concepts

In these sections (indicated by a star icon) we supply more advanced knowledge than is strictly necessary for an understanding of the basic principles. These sections often contain the results of up-to-date research, including some of the most important elements of progress in cell biology.

Key Facts Boxes

These are indicated by a staggeringly original icon and provide half-a-dozen of the most important Key Facts relating to the subject just covered. They are ideal for pre-examination panic states to get a student's thoughts in line and focused on the most important concepts.

End of Chapter Review Questions

These simple questions in true/false format allow a student to asses both memory and comprehension.

Feedback

Many of the changes in the presentation of this book have been stimulated by the comments on the first edition made by teachers and students who used the book for their courses and personal study. This has proved so successful that we again wish to canvas the comments of the users of this second edition in the hope of further improving it in subsequent editions. We hope that teachers and students will again take this opportunity to have an input into the creation of this valuable teaching resource, and are happy to receive suggestions about any new material and illustrations which could be included.

We can be contacted by letter at the address given but are also happy to receive comments on the Internet/Email.

Email addresses:
James.Lowe@nottingham.ac.uk
Alan.Stevens@nottingham.ac.uk

Acknowledgements

We wish to thank the laboratory staff of the University Department of Histopathology, Queen's Medical Centre, Nottingham, for the skill and patience with which they have produced the sections which we have photographed for this book. In particular we are grateful to Ian and Anne Wilson, Angela Crossman, Janet Plamor, Lianne Ward and David McQuire for paraffin sections, Neil Hand for acrylic resin sections and for the immunocytochemical preparations of the pancreatic islets, Ken Morrell and his team for immunocytochemical preparations, and Janet Palmer for enzyme histochemical preparations. We owe a particular vote of thanks to Trevor Gray who has spent many hours searching out suitable material for transmission and scanning electron microscopy, and is responsible for all of the electron micrographs in this book, as well as the thin epoxy resin sections.

Bill Brackenbury photographed all the gross specimens, and also provided us with many of the very low magnification photomicrographs. Isabella Streeter kindly word-processed much of the new textual material and legends for the new illustrations.

Many professional colleagues at Queen's Medical Centre and elsewhere contributed suitable tissue for processing and subsequent photomicrography. Dr. J. Wendy Blundell provided the arteriograms for Chapter 15 and, with Dr. Ian Leach, supplied material and photomicrographs for Chapter 9. Dr. Peter Furness kindly allowed us to use one of his electron micrographs showing the polyanionic sites in the glomerulus. Dr. Jane Zuccollo provided us with material relating to human fetal and neonatal histology, and Dr. Mark Stephens supplied us with a rare slide of an early human implantation site. Dr. Mark Wilkinson provided material for Chapter 10 and Jocelyn Germaine of the London Hospital kindly made available some of the material used in the section on teeth in Chapter 11. Dr. David Clark gave valuable help and advice in the preparation of Chapter 7 and Dr. Barbara Bain kindly allowed us to use a transparency of a large granular lymphocyte in Chapter 8. Dr. George Lindop some years ago supplied us with a transparency showing the localisation of renin in the human glomerulus; we were unable to find room for it in the first edition, but it now is illustrated as Figure 15.29b. Professor L. Michaels generously allowed us to use his transparency of the human organ of Corti (Fig. 19.5b).

We would like to thank all of the staff of Times Mirror International Publishers who have been involved in the preparation of this second edition. Special thanks to Louise Cook, the Development Editor, for keeping us as nearly under control as can be expected, and also for the Belgain beer; to Elaine Graham and Louise Crowe, the Project Managers, for managing to squeeze our quart into a pint pot without getting cross; to Gudrun Hughes, Production Controller, who controlled things; and to Pete Wilder, Lynda Payne, Greg Smith, Richard Prime, Marie McNestry, Mark Willey, Tim Read, Rob Curran, and James Lauder who are responsible for all the pretty, arty, illustrational stuff without which this book would be almost drab. Thanks also to Roger Ashton-Griffiths and Ellen Sarewitz who checked our text for idiocies and typographical errors.

Finally, we are grateful to Dianne Zack, our lovely publisher, for her sustained enthusiasm and energy, for the numerous faxes she sent us (when we were flagging) to tell us how brilliant we were, and how scintillating the book was going to be. Not only that, but she also assiduously translated our English writings into American! We still think that 'Oesophagus' looks prettier than 'Esophagus' but are not inclined to argue.

And, of course, we still adore Fiona Foley.

Dedication

This book is dedicated to the winemakers of:

Chateau de Marchesseau. Lalande de Pomerol (Bordeaux)

CVNE Imperial Rioja Gran Reserva (Spain)

Chateau Leoville Barton (Bordeaux)

Robert Mondavi Cabernet Sauvignon (California)

and

a staggeringly good **Barolo** which carried us through a crisis so deep
that we forgot to note the year and producer
(but it may have been a riserva from Fontanafredda).

Contents

1. Histology: Don't Switch Off!

INTRODUCTION

Histology is central to biological and medical science.

Histology is the study of the microscopic structure of biological material and the ways in which individual components are structurally and functionally related. It is central to biological and medical science since it stands at the cross-roads between biochemistry, molecular biology and physiology on the one side, and disease processes and their effects on the other.

Samples of human biological material can be obtained from many areas of the body by quick safe techniques (Fig. 1.1), using instruments such as:

- scalpels for directly accessible tissues such as the skin, mouth, nose etc.;
- needles into solid organs;
- endoscopic tubes into the alimentary tract or body cavities;
- special flexible cannulae along blood vessels.

Knowledge of normal histologic appearances is essential if abnormal diseased structures are to be recognized, and to comprehend how abnormal biochemical and physiologic processes result in disease.

This is an exciting period in histology, for we are now able to explore the physiologic and molecular basis of biological structures through the development of techniques that allow us to examine the chemical makeup of living tissues down the microscope. It is now becoming clear why various biological structures are shaped and arranged as they are.

Histology was once an empirical subject.

The study of histology began with the development of simple light microscopes and techniques for preparing thin slices of biological material to make them suitable for examination. Despite their simple equipment, and somewhat inadequately prepared material, early histologists learned a surprising amount about the structure of biological material. Such studies led Virchow to propound his cellular theory of the structure of living organisms that established the cell as the basic building block of most biological material. Each cell was considered as an individual unit surrounded by a wall called the cell membrane and containing within it all of the machinery for its function. In those early years a vocabulary of histology was developed, based on light microscopic analysis of cells and accompanied by a limited understanding of cell physiology and function.

Collections of cells having similar morphologic characteristics were described as forming tissues. These were originally subdivided into four types:

- epithelial tissues, or cells which cover surfaces, line body cavities or form solid glands such as salivary glands;
- muscular tissues, or cells with contractile properties;
- nervous tissues referred to cells forming the brain, spinal cord, and nerves.
- connective tissue, or cells that produce an extracellular matrix and serve to link or support other specialized tissues by forming tendons, bones or fatty tissue.

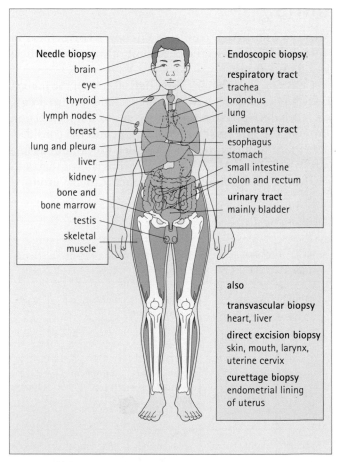

Fig. 1.1 Histology in diagnostic medicine.
It is now possible to obtain small samples from many areas of the body by various techniques. Histological examination of such samples is an increasingly important and direct way of diagnosing disease.

Modern histology is a precise science.

Modern investigative techniques have revolutionized our understanding of cells. The techniques of electron microscopy, cloning of cells in culture, protein sequencing and molecular genetics have also given unprecedented insight into the working of cells.

While improvements in knowledge and understanding have been matched in other sciences by the rapid emergence of new vocabularies, this has not always been the case in histology. For many years the terms and classifications that originated from early histologic studies were retained. With every new discovery about the structure of living material, attempts were made to force the new information into an old, often inappropriate classification of cells and tissues.

Fortunately, this rigid histologic system is now giving way to a more exciting and functional approach based on our understanding of cell biology.

CELLS ARE BASIC FUNCTIONAL UNITS

Modern knowledge confirms Virchow's correctness in describing the cell as the basic unit of structure of most living organisms.

Cells vary considerably. Although all cells in the human body are ultimately derived from a single fertilized egg, each cell develops structural attributes to suit its function through the process of differentiation, and is a considerably more sophisticated and complex unit than was formerly suspected. Molecular biology has shown that cells of diverse morphologic appearance can be grouped together because of common functional attributes or interactions.

Some cells are adaptable. It has also become apparent that even in the adult there are populations of highly adaptable, uncommitted cells, which can modify both their structure and functional activity to adapt to changing environmental demands. This facility is of vital importance in adaptation to internal or external stress, and is commonly seen in disease processes (e.g. replacement of damaged heart muscle by strong fibrous tissue following a heart attack).

The general structural and biological properties of cells are discussed in Chapter 2, and many of their specialized functional attributes in Chapters 3, 4 and 5.

Cells are now classified according to function.

It is now possible to classify cells into groups based on their main function. The groupings which will be used in this book are: epithelial cells, supporting cells, contractile cells, nerve cells, germ cells, blood cells, immune cells, and hormone secreting cells (Fig. 1.2). It is important, however, to recognize that a cell may have several functions and be a member of more than one cell group. For example:

- many of the hormone-producing cells are also epithelial in type, being tightly bound together by specialized junctions to form a gland;
- many immune cells are also blood cells;
- some support cells are also contractile.

The structural and functional specializations delineating each type of cell group are broadly outlined in Chapters 3, 4 and 5, and discussed in more detail throughout the book.

Cell group	Epithelial cells	Support cells	Contractile cells	Nerve cells	Germ cells	Blood cells	Immune cells	Hormone-secreting cells
Example	gut and blood vessel lining, covering skin	fibrous support tissue, cartilage, bone	muscle	brain	spermatozoa, ova	circulating red and white cells	lymphoid tissues (nodes and spleen)	thyroid and adrenal
Function	barrier, absorption, secretion	organize and maintain body structure	movement	direct cell communication	reproduction	oxygen transport, defence	defence	indirect cell communication
Special features	tightly bound together by cell junctions (see Chapter 3)	produce and interact with extracellular matrix material (see Chapter 4)	filamentous proteins cause contraction (see Chapter 5)	release chemical messengers onto surface of other cells (see Chapter 6)	half normal chromosome complement (see Chapters 16 and 17)	proteins bind oxygen, proteins destroy bacteria (see Chapter 7)	recognize and destroy foreign material (see Chapter 8)	secrete chemical messengers (see Chapter 14)

Fig. 1.2 Modern functional cell classification.

Tissues are functional arrangements of cells.

A tissue is an assembly of cells arranged in a specific organized fashion. In some cases the cells are all of the same structure forming **simple tissues**. For example fat cells forming adipose tissue. However, most apparently distinct tissues contain a mixture of cells with different functions, which may be termed **compound tissues** (Fig. 1.3). For example, 'nervous tissue' contains nerve cells (neurons), support cells (astrocytes), immune cells (microglia) and epithelial cells (ependyma).

The concept of simple and compound tissues is useful in descriptive histology, but for brevity the unqualified term tissue is used to imply either type.

Connective tissue is a term which underemphasizes its highly specialized role.

The one exception to the acceptable use of the term tissue is the old expression 'connective tissue'. This was used to describe a wide range of living material containing cells associated with a dominant extracellular matrix component. In theory, its function was to act as a supporting stroma, serving more highly specialized cell types.

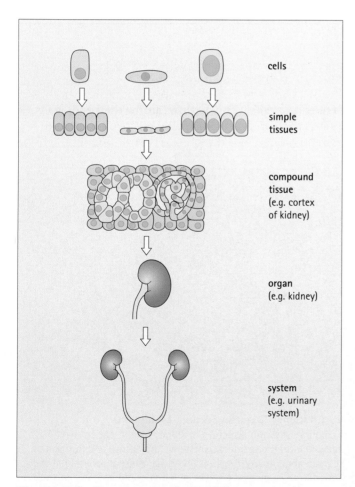

Fig. 1.3 Cells, tissues, organs and systems.

The original group of 'connective tissues' included cell/matrix combinations such as bone, cartilage, tendon, fibrous tissue, adipose tissue, bone marrow and blood. It has also been traditional to use the term 'loose areolar connective tissue' to describe tissue that is partly made up of support cells that produce an extracellular matrix, but also contains cells belonging to the immune system (e.g. lymphocytes and macrophages), nerve cells and blood vessels.

In this book, the term 'connective tissue' has been avoided because it underemphasizes the structural organization involved in this group of highly developed tissues. Instead, the concept of support cells is used, which emphasizes the importance of interactions between extracellular matrix and cells.

Support cells and their specializations are discussed in Chapter 4, while bone, tendons and ligaments are discussed in Chapter 13.

Tissues form organs and systems.

An organ, for example, the heart, liver or kidney, is an anatomically distinct group of tissues, usually of several types, which perform specific functions.

The term 'system' can be used to:
- describe cells with a similar function but widely distributed in several anatomic sites;
- describe a group of organs which have similar or related functional roles.

The specialized hormone-producing cells scattered in the gut and lung (diffuse endocrine system) cannot be an organ as they do not form an anatomically distinct mass, whereas the tongue, esophagus, stomach, intestines, exocrine pancreas and rectum are components of the alimentary system, and the kidney, pelvicalyceal system, ureters and bladder are part of the urinary system.

The relationships between cells, tissues, organs and systems are shown in Figure. 1.3.

HISTOLOGY IN OTHER DISCIPLINES

Cell histology is aligned to cell biology.

The most common way to study cells is by light microscopy. Tissues are mounted on glass slides as thin preparations, stained with appropriate dyes, illuminated by light and viewed using glass lenses. The analysis of the fine structure of cells by light microscopy is referred to as **cytology**.

There is a limit to the detail that can be resolved using light microscopy, with very small structures within cells being invisible. Until recently the only way to look at the fine intracellular detail of individual cells was by using electron microscopy, which greatly increases resolution allowing the subcellular composition of cells to be defined.

These techniques are now complemented by the increasing use of immunohistochemical methods.

Antibodies are applied to specific cell constituents to visualize details within cells at the light microscopic level that are not visible by other techniques. For example, the location of specific proteins or subcellular components can now be defined in light microscopic preparations.

It is also now possible to demonstrate specific DNA and RNA sequences by the technique of *in situ* hybridization, thereby gaining fundamental insight into the molecular mechanisms of cells.

A clear understanding of the fine structure and molecular organization of cells greatly improves comprehension of biochemical and physiologic processes. This overlap between structure, physiology, biochemistry and genetics is now embraced by the term **cell biology**.

Systems histology is aligned to anatomy.

Study of the arrangement of different tissues at the microscopic level (systems histology) gives insight into the structure and function of organs and systems. This type of study is an extension of anatomy, and is often termed microscopic anatomy for this reason.

The study of systems histology is an important component of human biology and in most curricula is taught alongside normal anatomy.

Histology is essential for understanding pathology.

Pathology (understanding disease processes) accounts for nearly half of the study required by medical practitioners irrespective of their specialization, and from its earliest beginnings has always been intimately linked to a study of systems histology and microanatomy. In most curricula, however, pathology is taught at a later stage than histology, so that by the time students are studying diseases they have forgotten normal histology. This is unfortunate as most disease processes are associated with histologic abnormalities. In modern medicine a histologic diagnosis is the mainstay of clinical practice. This is illustrated in the box below.

HISTOLOGY IN DISEASE DIAGNOSIS

A 20-year-old student develops kidney failure and the cause is not apparent from blood tests or radiology. The renal physician therefore removes a piece of kidney via a needle so that the diagnosis can be made by histological examination. Special staining methods highlight subtle structural abnormalities by light microscopy (Fig.1.4), while electron microscopy provides valuable information about abnormalities at a subcellular level. On the basis of the abnormalities which are revealed an accurate histologic diagnosis is made and the renal physician can institute appropriate treatment. Clinical management of this patient requires knowledge of the microanatomy of the kidney. Assessment of progress, and the effectiveness of treatment are monitored by repeated biopsy.

A 15-year-old girl has swollen lymph nodes in her neck. A surgeon removes one so that it can be examined histologically, and microscopy reveals that the swelling is caused by a form of cancer. The classification of tumors is determined by histology, and accurate histologic assessment of tumors is the cornerstone of modern cancer treatment. The treatment given to the girl depends on the histologic type of the tumor (i.e. whether it is derived from muscle, lymphoid cells or endocrine cells). This is answered by the histologic reports which, in describing cellular morphology and differentiation, reveal the precise type of tumor.

Fig. 1.4 Kidney (paraffin section, MSB stain).
Micrograph showing a section of kidney from a patient with kidney failure. The special stain shows the nature and location of the main abnormality, destruction of the afferent arteriole of the glomerulus by a disease process called fibrinoid necrosis (arrow).

TECHNIQUES USED IN HISTOLOGY AND CELL BIOLOGY

Light microscopy using wax-embedded sections is the main technique used in histology.

Routine light microscopy uses thin sections of tissue to study cell morphology. Resolution of structures by light microscopy is of the order of 0.2 μm, but in routine practice with paraffin sections this is seldom better than 0.6 μm. Sections are usually obtained as follows:

- tissue is immersed in a preservative solution (fixative), which cross-links or precipitates proteins and prevents degradation;
- tissue is embedded in a firm medium for cutting into thin sections;
- tissue is cut into sections (conventionally 5-8 μm thick) on a microtome.

The wax-impregnated sections are mounted on a glass microscope slide and the wax removed with an organic solvent before the section is rehydrated through increasing dilutions of alcohol in water. When fully rehydrated the sections are stained with any of a number of stains, some of which are outlined below. In routine laboratory practice it generally takes 24 hours to produce a wax section for histology.

In some cases it is necessary to look at fresh tissues which have not been exposed to protein cross-linking in fixation. In this situation tissue is made firm enough to cut by freezing, a technique referred to as preparing a frozen section.

Frozen Sections

The process of fixation and embedding of biological material in paraffin and other media (see page 7) may destroy certain components, particularly enzymes and some antigenic sites. If frozen water is used as the supporting medium, these are better preserved and can be demonstrated by suitable techniques. Fresh (unfixed) material is rapidly frozen to –150°C to –170°C by immersion in, for example, liquid nitrogen, so that it hardens to a solid mass due to freezing of tissue water. Thin sections (5–10 μm) are then cut on a special microtome housed in a refrigerated cabinet (a cryostat), and stained without exposure to alcohol or other organic solvents.

Frozen sections are used to demonstrate the cellular localization of enzymes and soluble lipids, and in the identification of substances using immunofluorescent and immunocytochemical methods.

Further use is made of frozen sections in diagnostic histopathology, when an urgent tissue diagnosis is required of, say, a suspected tumor, while the patient is still on the operating table. In skilled hands, a frozen section of a sample of human tissue stained with hematoxylin and eosin (H&E) can be prepared and examined under the microscope within five minutes of its removal from the body. In this way a rapid and accurate histologic diagnosis can be established while the patient is in the operating theater, enabling the appropriate surgical room procedure to be performed.

Paraffin Embedding

Paraffin embedding is the standard method of preparing thin sections of biological material for histologic examination by light microscopy. It is cheap, comparatively simple and lends itself to automation.

The sample is fixed, usually in an aqueous formalin-based fixative solution, and then progressively **dehydrated** by passage through a series of alcohol solutions (e.g. 60%, 70%, 90%, 100%) until all water (intrinsic tissue water and fixative water) has been removed, and the specimen is thoroughly permeated by absolute alcohol. The alcohol is then replaced by an organic solvent which is miscible both with alcohol and with molten liquid paraffin wax (alcohol is not miscible with paraffin wax). The resulting specimen is immersed in paraffin wax at a temperature just above the melting point of the wax, which is solid at normal working room temperature. When the biologic material is thoroughly permeated by the molten wax it is allowed to cool so that the wax solidifies. The wax acts as a physical support to the sample, allowing thin sections (2–7 μm) to be cut without deformation of the cellular structure and architecture.

Tissue staining is used to see fine detail in cells.
Cells are virtually colorless and so sections need to be stained for light microscopy. A distinction is made between routine and special staining methods. Routine methods use dyes similar to those used in the textile industry to stain tissue components different colors. Special staining techniques, termed histochemistry, can be used to identify specific chemical or enzyme components in cells.

Hematoxylin and eosin (H&E)

The combination of the two dyes, hematoxylin (purple/black) and eosin (red), is the most useful stain for the examination of biological material; is simple to perform, reliable, inexpensive and informative. Cell nuclei stain purple/black (depending on section thickness and the formulation of hematoxylin used), and most components of the cell cytoplasm stain pink/red. Most of the micrographs in this book are stained with H&E, particularly in the Practical Histology sections.

Van Gieson method

The simple Van Gieson method stains collagen pinkish–red and muscle yellow (see Fig. 10.20); it is commonly used in combination with a stain for elastic fibers. The elastic Van Gieson (EVG) stain is valuable for demonstrating and differentiating the common support cell fibers, particularly elastic fibers, which stain brown–black, and collagen fibers which stain pinkish–red; muscle is stained yellow (see Fig. 10.20).

Trichrome methods

The trichrome methods employ a mixture of three dyes to stain different components in different colors. There are many trichrome methods, and they can be used to demonstrate general architecture, to emphasize support fibers, or to distinguish support fibers from muscle fibers. An important use of a trichrome method is the demonstration of the cellular, osteoid and mineralized components of bone in undecalcified bone embedded in acrylic resin (see Figs 13.15a & 13.17b).

Silver methods

Under appropriate conditions, certain biological components, both within cells and in intercellular materials, reduce silver nitrate to form black deposits of metallic silver at the site of chemical reduction. By modifying the conditions of the silver nitrate solution used, these methods can be used to demonstrate a wide range of structures, including reticulin fibers (see Fig. 4.5).

Periodic Acid-Schiff (PAS) method

The widely used PAS method has many applications, particularly in the demonstration of various carbohydrates, either alone (e.g. glycogen) or combined with other molecules such as proteins (e.g. glycoproteins), which are stained magenta. It can therefore be used to delineate basement membranes (see Fig 4.11a) and some neutral mucins secreted by various secretory epithelial cells. The mucous cells of the stomach are strongly PAS positive.

Alcian blue method

The alcian blue dye method is used mainly to demonstrate acidic mucins secreted by some epithelial cells (see Fig. 11.44b), and can be combined with the PAS reaction to distinguish between acidic and neutral epithelial mucins. Through control of pH or other variables in the staining solution, the alcian blue method can be used to demonstrate the extracellular glycosaminoglycan matrix (see Fig. 4.13d) of support cells.

May-Grünwald-Giemsa method

The use of the May-Grünwald-Giemsa method is confined mainly to the examination of smear preparations of blood and bone marrow cells. Most of the micrographs in Chapter 7 show red and white blood cells stained by this method.

Myelin methods

Several staining techniques can be used to demonstrate normal myelin. The dye solochrome cyanin is frequently used to demonstrate myelin in paraffin sections (see Fig. 6.24b). Other methods use modified hematoxylin or osmium tetroxide.

High–resolution light microscopy can be performed with tissue embedded in resin.

Resolution of structures by light microscopy using paraffin sections is seldom better than 0.6 μm, the resolution being limited by the thickness of the section which is rarely thinner than 3 μm. Much better resolution can be obtained by using thinner sections, about 0.5–2 μm, but these cannot be achieved consistently with wax as the embedding medium and using a standard microtome. The use of acrylic and epoxy resins as embedding media allows thinner tissue sections to be cut

Resin-embedded sections are used increasingly in histology, and examples will be provided in this book where appropriate.

Transmission electron microscopy allows resolution of detailed subcellular structures.

Use of an electron beam instead of light allows resolution of structures as small as 1 nm in well-prepared tissues.

Tissue preparation for electron microscopy demands the use of special fixation of very small (less than 2 mm) tissue fragments, the most common fixative containing glutaraldehyde. Osmium tetroxide is also used as a combined fixative and stain because of its ability to stabilize lipid components and to render them electron-dense. In addition, because specimens are subjected to an electron beam in a vacuum, they need to be embedded in a robust material, the most common being epoxy resin.

Acrylic resin embedding

Certain acrylic resins are used in a similar way to paraffin wax as embedding media. When set, they are harder than paraffin wax and offer more support to the tissue than wax. They have two main advantages over paraffin wax for light microscopy:

• with the use of a special microtome, much thinner sections (i.e. 1–2 μm thick) can be obtained than with paraffin wax, giving greater resolution with the light microscope, and enabling much more detail to be seen

• they cause very little tissue shrinkage and enable good quality sections of very hard material to be cut, and are therefore used in the histological examination of mineralized bone (see Figs 13.15a & 13.17b)

Epoxy resin embedding

Epoxy resins are the hardest supporting media for biologic material. With special sectioning machines, sections as thin as 0.5–1 μm can be cut for high resolution light microscopy, and ultra-thin sections can be prepared for transmission electron microscopy.

The transmission electronmicrographs in this book

have been prepared from ultra-thin epoxy resin sections. These resins are resistant to the damaging effects of the electron beam in the electron microscope, and continue to support the biological material, whereas other embedding media volatilize in the electron beam.

Most of the staining methods used with paraffin and acrylic resin sections are unable to penetrate epoxy resins. Fortunately, the stain toluidine blue is an exception, and differentially stains biological components in various shades of blue. The greatest cellular detail obtainable by light microscopy is by the use of 0.5–1 μm epoxy resin sections stained with toluidine blue (see Figs 15.6b and 15.6c).

Toluidine blue stain

Toluidine blue is used to demonstrate cells and fibers in very thin epoxy resin sections. Toluidine blue is one of the very few dyes which will penetrate the dense epoxy resin to stain the tissue section. It gives considerable cellular detail, staining the various components of the cells and fibers in the shades of blue in a way that represents their relative electron density; hence the resulting blue picture closely resembles a low power electronmicrograph but is blue instead of black.

Sections for electron microscopy are typically 0.1 μm thick (ultra-thin sections) to allow good resolution and prevent scattering of electrons. They are stained for electron microscopy by immersion in a solution containing a heavy metal (uranium or lead).

Electron microscopy allows the study of subcellular morphology and is used routinely for morphological study.

Scanning electron microscopy allows resolution of three-dimensional subcellular structures.

Scanning electron microscopy uses solid pieces of tissue rather than sections and allows the perception of three-dimensional views of the surface of cells or tissues (Fig.1.5).

A small piece of fixed tissue is dried and coated in gold. An electron beam then scans the specimen and electrons produced from the surface are used to reconstruct a fine three-dimensional representation of the surface (see Figs 7.2b, 7.14b, 11.11, 11.12 & 11.39d).

If living cells are frozen and then fractured there is a tendency for the fractures to open cells along membranes and distinct planes, which can then be studied using the electron microscope. This technique of cryofracture provides information about the surface features of cell membranes.

Histochemistry allows detection of specific chemical groups in tissues.

Certain dyes have an affinity for specific chemical groups in molecules and these are used to identify and localize specific chemical substances in histologic preparations.

Polysaccharides such as glycogen can be detected by a staining method called the Periodic Acid-Schiff (PAS) technique. Periodic acid is applied to sections to oxidize glycogen glucose residues to aldehydes. Schiff reagent (a

Fig. 1.5 Kidney (scanning electronmicrograph).
This scanning electron micrograph shows the components of the cortex of the kidney, which are largely glomeruli (G) and tubules (T). At higher magnification more surface details are evident (see Fig. 15.11).

colorless bleached dye called fuchsin) is applied; it reacts with the aldehydes to produce purple fuchsin, (see Fig. 4.11).

Lipids can be detected by dyes which are fat-soluble. As lipids are dissolved out of paraffin-processed material, their detection is only possible if sections are prepared by freezing and cutting on a cryostat, then immersed in lipid-soluble dyes such as Sudan Black or Oil Red O.

Enzyme histochemical techniques identify and localize the sites of activity of particular enzymes.

To look at the tissue distribution of specific enzymes, sections of fresh tissue prepared on a cryostat are placed in an incubating solution containing the specific substrate for the enzyme or group of enzymes to be demonstrated, together with any necessary cofactors or inhibitors. The enzyme in the tissue reacts with the substrate to form an insoluble primary reaction product. This is then visualized by its reaction with a visualizing agent, which may be included with the incubating medium or applied as a separate second step.

This technique can be used to show the localization of a vast number of enzymes including acid and alkaline phosphatases, dehydrogenases and ATPases, and is routinely used to detect abnormalities in certain diseased tissue, particularly muscle (see Fig. 13.4).

Since most biological enzyme systems are labile, they may be destroyed by fixation and tissue processing; thus most enzyme histochemical methods are carried out on frozen sections.

Autoradiography is a powerful technique for studying cell functions.

If tissues are provided with radioactively labeled metabolites, cells which take up the metabolite can be detected by dipping sections in a photographic emulsion and allowing the radioactivity to create silver grains in the emulsion.

If radiolabeled thymidine (a DNA component) is incorporated, the autoradiograph will show cells that are actively dividing.

Immunocytochemistry uses antibodies to localize specific proteins in tissue sections.

Immunocytochemistry is one of the most important innovations in histology. Antibodies to specific cell molecules are used to detect their presence in tissue sections. Polyclonal antibodies to a substance are obtained by inoculating an animal (commonly a rabbit or sheep) with the purified protein and then harvesting serum from which a specific antibody can be extracted. Alternatively, monoclonal antibody may be produced by inoculating a mouse and fusing suitable antibody-producing cells with immortal mouse myeloma cells to continually produce antibodies in tissue culture.

2. The Cell

INTRODUCTION

Living cells of all types have certain defining attributes in common. They are composed of smaller elements, termed subcellular structures, which provide the framework for cellular activities.

An important component of the cell is its surrounding wall which consists of a cell membrane. Specialized adaptations of cell membrane surround small particles inside cells termed organelles. The fluid inside the cell, the cytosol, contains many of the essential enzymes and metabolites. The genetic material, in the form of chromosomes, is contained in the nucleus, and energy for cellular activity is largely generated by mitochondria. There is a constant generation of new structural elements within the cell and this takes place in the membrane systems of the endoplasmic reticulum (ER) and Golgi. Equally, cells have to take in substances from outside and break them down using a system of small organelles called lysosomes that contain powerful digestive enzymes. The shape of cells and much of the movement that takes place within cells is organized by an internal scaffolding of proteins known as the cytoskeleton.

The cell cycle of coordinated cell division and growth is achieved by duplication of genetic material (mitosis) and cell contents (cytokinesis).

This chapter describes the main building blocks of cells and the functional relationships which exist between them.

Cells have a common basic structure.

Cells have many common features which are independent of any specialized function (Fig. 2.1):

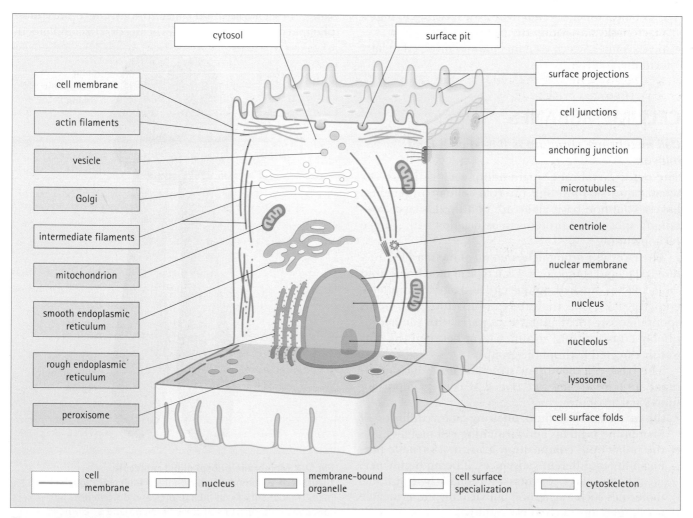

Fig. 2.1 Cell structure.
Diagram to show the main constituents of a cell and their distribution.

- an outer membrane surrounds each cell and separates it from its environment and from other cells;
- they are composed of a solution of proteins, electrolytes and carbohydrates (cytosol), divided up into specialized functional compartments (organelles) by inner membrane systems;
- their shape and fluidity are partly determined by the arrangement of internal filamentous proteins (intermediate filaments, actin and microtubules) which form the cytoskeleton.

Cell membranes delineate several compartments within cells, each with a specialized function.

The main membrane-bound compartments are:
- the nucleus, which contains the cellular DNA;
- mitochondria, which provide energy;
- endoplasmic reticulum (ER), which is involved in biosynthesis of protein and some lipids;
- Golgi, which is involved in processing biosynthetic products for incorporation into the cell or for secretion;
- vesicles, which act as temporary packages of material undergoing transport around the cell;
- lysosomes, which contain hydrolytic enzymes to digest macromolecules within the cell;
- peroxisomes, which contain enzymes involved in fatty acid metabolism.

CELL MEMBRANES

Cell membrane structure is based on a lipid bilayer.

The outer membrane surrounding each cell, and the membranes surrounding internal cellular organelles, have a common basic structure of a lipid bilayer containing specialized proteins in association with surface carbohydrates.

The most important determinant of membrane structure is the lipid component. Each type of membrane lipid molecule has one hydrophilic end and one hydrophobic end (Fig. 2.2); thus they are amphipathic. Such lipids spontaneously form a bilayer in water with the hydrophobic ends forming an inner layer between the outwardly directed hydrophilic groups.

This basic cell membrane structure, into which membrane proteins are inserted (Fig. 2.3), confers important functional attributes:
- the membrane is a fluid, allowing lateral diffusion of membrane proteins and facilitating cell mobility;
- the polar lipid composition leads to a variable permeability to different substances, it being highly permeable to water, oxygen and small hydrophobic molecules such as ethanol, but virtually impermeable to charged ions such as Na^+ and K^+;

- breaks and tears are sealed spontaneously as the polar nature of lipids eliminates free edges where hydrophobic groups would come into contact with the aqueous environment;
- membrane proteins are placed to perform functional roles in processes such as transport, enzymatic activity, cell attachment and cell communication.

There are three major types of membrane lipids: phospholipids, cholesterol and glycolipids.

Lipid forms 50% of the mass of cell membranes.

PHOSPHOLIPIDS make up about 50% of the lipid component and tend to surround membrane proteins, often specifically anchoring proteins with enzyme or transport functions. There are four major phospholipids in the cell membrane:
- phosphatidylcholine;
- sphingomyelin;
- phosphatidylserine;
- phosphatidylethanolamine.

The composition of inner and outer lipid layers is not the same. For example, high concentrations of certain phospholipids in the inner face may be needed to complement

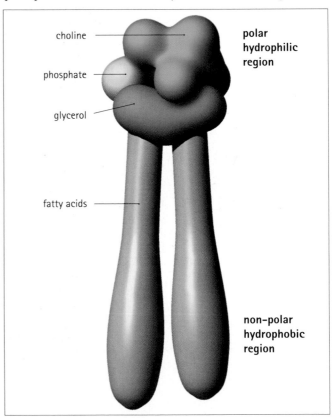

choline

polar hydrophilic region

phosphate

glycerol

fatty acids

non–polar hydrophobic region

Fig. 2.2 Membrane phospholipid molecule.
Diagram of a membrane phospholipid molecule, which is the main component of cell membranes and determines the fundamental properties of the cell membrane as a whole.

the presence of an inner membrane protein because certain proteins need to be linked with specific phospholipids.

CHOLESTEROL in cell membrane limits the movement of adjacent phospholipids and makes the membrane less fluid, and more mechanically stable.

GLYCOLIPIDS are found only in the outer face of cell membranes with their associated sugars exposed to the extracellular space. The functional significance of this is not clear, but glycolipids may be involved in intercellular communication.

One of the most important membrane glycolipids is galactocerebroside, which is a major component of myelin, the fatty insulation layer around nerves (see Chapter 6). Another group of important glycolipids is

the gangliosides, which constitute up to 10% of the lipid in nerve cell membranes.

Membrane proteins carry out most of the specialized functions of cell membranes.

The types of membrane protein encountered vary according to cell type. Membrane proteins:
- attach cytoskeletal filaments to cell membrane;
- attach cells to extracellular matrix (e.g. adhesion molecules);
- transport molecules in or out of cells (e.g. carrier proteins, membrane pump proteins, channel proteins);
- act as receptors for chemical signaling between cells (e.g. hormone receptors);
- possess specific enzymatic activity.

Membrane proteins are able to diffuse laterally over the surface of the cell.

Fig. 2.3 Cell membrane structure.
The cell membrane is composed of a lipid bilayer with phospholipid hydrophobic groups facing inward, and hydrophilic groups facing outward. Protein molecules float within this basic structure with projecting carbohydrate groups being attached to glycolipids or proteins.

Membrane carbohydrates are mostly present on the membrane surfaces which are not in contact with cytosol.

Membranes have associated carbohydrate residues which are mainly confined to the membrane surface which faces away from the cytosol. They are therefore found on the luminal aspect of inner membrane systems as well as on the cell surface, where they have been termed the **glycocalyx**.

Membrane carbohydrates can be demonstrated by staining with lectins, proteins extracted from plants with binding capabilities for specific carbohydrate groups.

TRANSPORT IN AND OUT OF CELLS

Transport of material in or out of a cell takes place by the processes of endocytosis and exocytosis.

Substances may diffuse through cell membranes, or they may be transported by special membrane protein transport systems or channels (e.g. ions). Other material from the extracellular space, as well as surface membrane, may be incorporated into the cell by invagination of the cell surface in a process termed **endocytosis** (Fig. 2.4). The invaginated cell membrane fuses to form an **endocytotic vesicle** or **endosome**, which is a small, sealed, spherical membrane-bound body. The membrane and any material incorporated into such a vesicle can then be processed within the cell.

The terms **pinocytosis** or **potocytosis** are used when cells take up fluid and small molecules to form small vesicles about 50 nm in diameter. The terms **endocytosis** and **phagocytosis** are used when cells ingest large particles to form endosomes more than 250 nm in diameter.

Exocytosis is the reverse of endocytosis, and describes the fusion of a membrane-bound vesicle with the cell surface to discharge its contents into the extracellular space (Fig. 2.4). This mechanism allows secretion of products which have been manufactured by the cell. Fusion of vesicles with the cell membrane also allows new membrane to be incorporated into the cell surface.

There are two types of secretory mechanism. In some cells secretion occurs by a constant fusion of vesicles with surface membrane, termed the **constitutive secretory pathway**. In other cells, fusion of secretory vesicles with the surface has to be triggered by a signal to the cell, termed the **regulated secretory pathway**.

Several proteins have been defined which mediate the processes of membrane fusion. NSF (derived from N-ethylmaleimide sensitive fusion protein) is a water-soluble protein which interacts with proteins called SNAPs (derived from NSF attachment proteins) to form an active fusogenic complex.

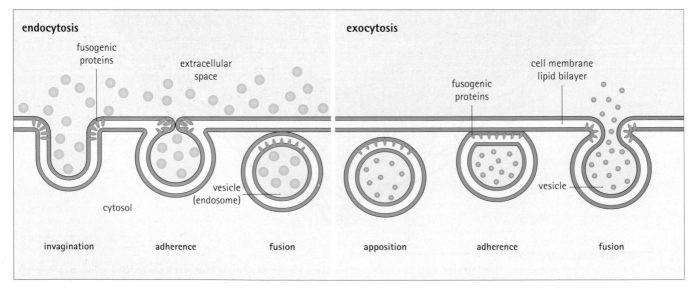

Fig. 2.4 Endocytosis and exocytosis.
It is currently thought that special proteins mediate the process of membrane integration in endocytosis and exocytosis.

The two main vesicles involved in transport of substances into cells are derived from surface membrane invaginations called coated pits and caveoli.

Small invaginations of membrane constantly form at the surface of most cells to ingest extracellular material which is then processed by the cell. The invaginations are drawn down to form vesicles; once the contents have been processed, the vesicle membrane returns to the cell surface.

Clathrin is a protein which braces the coated pit membranes. It forms a hexagonal lattice structure around the outside of the vesicle and accounts for the fuzzy coat seen ultrastructurally. The clathrin scaffolding is broken down by special enzyme systems when the vesicle docks.

Thus, there is a constant shuttle of membrane between cell surface and cell interior (membrane trafficking). These vesicles originate in two main types of specialized areas of cell membrane termed **coated pits** and **caveoli**.

Coated pits are invaginations braced by special membrane-associated proteins and are used to bring material into the cell for further processing (Fig. 2.5). In many instances special receptor proteins are present in the cell membrane which can bind to specific substances outside the cell and draw them inside in a process termed **receptor-mediated endocytosis**. Coated vesicles may also develop from other internal membrane systems inside cells.

Caveoli are invaginations braced by the protein caveolin. Caveoli have three important cellular roles (Fig. 2.6):

- They are used to transport material from the extracellular space on one side to the extracellular space on the other in a process termed **transcytosis**. This happens in cells such as the flat cells which line blood vessels (endothelial cells);
- The surface of caveoli may carry receptor proteins which bind to molecules in the extracellular space. They can concentrate substances from the extracellular space

Fig. 2.5 Ultrastructure and diagrams of coated pit formation.
(a) A coated pit is braced by a coat of protein molecules and bears surface receptors that bind specific extracellular ligands. In most cases the coat protein (visible ultrastructurally as a fuzzy membrane thickening) is **clathrin**, which forms a hexagonal lattice around the pit membrane.
(b)(c)(d) Assembly of the coat protein lattice drives progressive invagination of the pit to form a coated vesicle.
(e) Once internalized, the coat protein is shed and returns to the cell surface to form new coated pits.

This form of transport into cells is termed **receptor–mediated endocytosis** and is a feature of the internalization of iron, low-density lipoprotein and some growth factors.

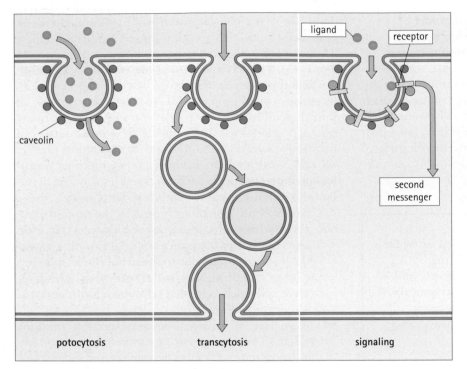

Fig. 2.6 Caveoli
There are three functions of caveoli.

First, receptors on caveoli can concentrate substances from the extracellular space and these can then move into the cytosol. This is termed potocytosis and such caveoli remain as invaginations and do not form vesicles. Secondly, some caveoli form vesicles and internalize material which is then transported across the cell and released from the other side in a process termed transcytosis. Thirdly, some caveoli are the site of concentration of surface receptors which influence intracellular secondary messenger signal systems, thereby making caveoli an important structure in signal transduction.

and transport them into the cell in a process termed **potocytosis**;

- They are also believed to have roles in **intracellular signaling**. The cell membrane associated with caveoli is enriched with many of the cell surface proteins which have function as receptors. Caveoli are believed to allow extracellular events to trigger intracellular secondary cellular messenger systems.

MOVEMENT IN AND OUT OF CELLS

- endocytosis: internalization of material into a cell via endosomes formed from coated pits

- exocytosis: elimination of material from the cell by fusion of vesicles with cell surface membrane and ejection of the vesicle contents

- transcytosis: movement of material from the extracellular space on one side of the cell to the other; mediated by caveoli which pinch off to form vesicles

- potocytosis: concentration and transport of small molecules into the cell; mediated by caveoli which remain at the cell surface

- pinocytosis: internalization of fluid and small molecules into the cell via endosomes

CYTOSOL

The cytosol is the fluid matrix of the cell.

The fluid matrix of the cell contains the following important components:

- much of the machinery involved in protein synthesis, protein degradation and carbohydrate metabolism (it is therefore rich in enzyme systems);
- filamentous proteins that form the cytoskeleton (see page 23);
- some products of metabolism such as glycogen and free lipid, for which it acts as a storage compartment;
- numerous ribosomes, both free in the cytosol and associated with cytosolic surface of rough ER.

Ribosomes are involved in the synthesis of proteins.

Ribosomes synchronize the alignment of both messenger RNA and transport RNA in the production of peptide chains during protein synthesis. Ribosomes are small electron-dense particles, which impart a blue color (basophilic) to the cytoplasm of protein-producing cells on light microscopy (Fig. 2.7). Each ribosome is composed of a small subunit which binds RNA, and a large subunit, which catalyzes the formation of peptide bonds. They are made up of specific ribosomal RNA as well as specific proteins. Ribosomal RNA is manufactured in the nucleolus (see page 15).

Fig. 2.7 Ribosomes.
Electron micrograph showing free ribosomes in the cytosol; they are small electron-dense particles 20–30 nm in diameter present either singly or in chains called **polyribosomes.**

Fig. 2.8 Nucleus.
Electronmicrograph showing typical cell nucleus. It is bounded by a double nuclear membrane (NM). The nucleolus (N) is clearly visible as an electron-dense circular area. Nucleus chromatin is divided into two types: heterochromatin (H) is dense-staining, while euchromatin (E) is light-staining.

THE NUCLEUS

The nucleus contains the cellular DNA and the nucleolus.

The nucleus is the largest single membrane-bound compartment in the cell and contains the cellular DNA (Fig. 2.8).

In light microscopic preparations, nuclei are spherical or ovoid in shape, generally measuring 5–10 μm in diameter, they stain with basic dyes such as hematoxylin (i.e. basophilic) and they contain a smaller spherical structure, the nucleolus, which synthesizes ribosomal subunits.

Nuclei are bound by two concentric membranes with different functional roles. The inner nuclear membrane contains specific membrane proteins that act as attachment points for filamentous proteins, termed **lamins**, which form a scaffolding to maintain the spherical shape. The outer nuclear membrane binds the perinuclear space, which is continuous with the lumen of the ER; it may be associated with ribosomes in a similar manner to rough ER.

The nuclear membrane is perforated by numerous pores which establish continuity between the cytosol and the nuclear lumen containing the chromatin (Fig. 2.9).

Nuclear DNA is tightly packed by association with special proteins and forms the chromatin.

The nucleus contains DNA wound around proteins called histones to form nucleosomes, which are regular repeating globular structures similar to beads on a string. The nucleosome string is then wound into filaments 30 nm in diameter, which make up the structure of chromatin. Further condensation into distinct chromosomes is possible during cell replication when chromatin forms large looped domains by attachment to DNA binding proteins. This relationship is shown in Figure 2.10.

The distribution of chromatin is not uniform, and this reflects varying degrees of unfolding according to whether genes are being transcribed. **Euchromatin** is seen as light-staining electron-lucent areas and represents actively transcribed cellular DNA. **Heterochromatin** is seen as a dense-staining area, often adjacent to the nuclear membrane, and is the highly condensed, transcriptionally inactive form.

The nucleolus is the site of formation of ribosomal RNA in the nucleus.

The nucleolus is a spherical area within the nucleus. It measures 1–3 μm in diameter, increasing in size with active gene transcription. Inactive cells have indistinct nucleoli, while metabolically active cells have large or multiple nucleoli. In H&E preparations nucleoli stain blue-pink because of their affinity for both acidophilic and basophilic dyes.

The nucleolus produces ribosomal RNAs, which are packaged with proteins to form ribosomal subunits and exported to the cytosol via the nuclear pore complexes.

Fig. 2.9 Nuclear pore.

ⓐ The double nuclear membrane (NM) bounding the perinuclear space (PNS) is perforated by nuclear pores (P) which appear as gaps in transmission electronmicrographs.

ⓑ Structurally the pores are rimmed by eight protein complexes to form the nuclear pore complex shown in this diagram. The pores form channels which allow transport of small molecules, but restrict movement of large molecules, between the cytosol and the nucleus. Movement of some proteins into the nucleus is desirable, however, and it is currently thought that the nuclear pore complex recognizes and actively transports specific peptide sequences in proteins destined for the nucleus. In a similar fashion, large ribosomal subunits produced in the nucleus are actively transported into the cytosol. The central granules of the pore complex are believed to be large proteins or components of ribosomes in transit between different cell areas.

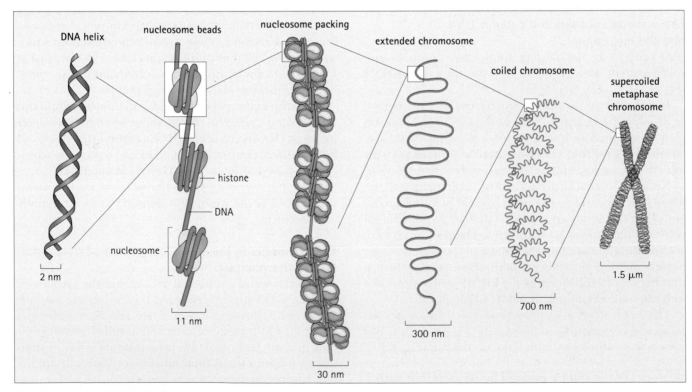

Fig. 2.10 Chromatin structure

DNA is organized around histones into nucleosomes. The nucleosomes are wound into a helix to form chromatin. In chromosomes this is then wound again into a supercoiled structure.

Three regions of the nucleolus can be distinguished by electron microscopy (Fig. 2.11):

- **pars amorpha** (pale areas), so-called nuclear organizer regions with specific RNA binding proteins, correspond to large loops of transcribing DNA containing the ribosomal RNA genes;
- **pars fibrosa** (dense-staining regions), correspond to transcripts of ribosomal RNA genes beginning to form ribosomes;
- **pars granulosa** (granular regions), correspond to RNA containing maturing ribosomal subunit particles.

The nuclear lamina is a scaffolding which maintains the shape of the nucleus.

The nuclear lamina is a network of protein filaments 20 nm thick that lines the internal nuclear membrane. It is composed of three proteins termed nuclear lamins A, B and C, which are organized into filaments and form a regular square lattice as a scaffold beneath the nuclear membrane.

It is thought that this nuclear lamina network interacts with nuclear membrane proteins and acts as a nuclear cytoskeleton, possibly interacting with chromatin in the spatial organization of the nucleus.

MITOCHONDRIA

The mitochondria are the most important sites of ATP production in cells.

Mitochondria are membrane-bound cylindrical organelles (Fig. 2.12) typically measuring 0.5–2 μm in length, which provide energy to cells through oxidative phosphorylation.

Mitochondria are believed to have evolved in human cells as symbiotic prokaryotic organisms similar to bacteria. In support of this hypothesis, each mitochondrion has its own DNA and systems for protein synthesis independent of the cell nucleus.

Each mitochondrion is constructed with two membranes, an outer membrane and an inner membrane, which define two inner mitochondrial spaces, the intermembranous space and the matrix space.

The outer membrane contains specialized transport proteins such as porin, which allow free permeability to molecules up to about 10 kDa molecular weight, from the cytosol into the intermembranous space.

The inner membrane is highly impermeable to small ions due to a high content of the phospholipid cardiolipin. This feature is essential to mitochondrial function as it permits the development of electrochemical gradients during the production of high-energy cell metabolites.

The inner membrane is folded into pleats (cristae), thereby increasing its surface area, and is the location of respiratory chain enzymes, as well as ATP synthetase, which is responsible for energy generation.

The intermembranous space contains:

- metabolic substrates which diffuse through the outer membrane;
- ATP generated by the mitochondrion;
- ions pumped out of the matrix space during oxidative phosphorylation. The matrix space contains enzymes to oxidize fatty acids and pyruvate as well as for the citric acid (TCA) cycle. It also contains mitochondrial DNA and specific mitochondrial enzymes for mitochondrial DNA transcription.

The morphology of mitochondria varies with cell type. In cells with a high oxidative metabolism, mitochondria are commonly large and serpiginous. In steroid hormone-secreting cells such as those of the adrenal cortex, the cristae are tubular structures rather than flat plates.

CELL NUCLEUS

- bounded by a double nuclear membrane
- contains the cellular DNA as chromatin
- contains the nucleolus which is responsible for making ribosomes
- moves substances in and out through nuclear pores

Fig. 2.11 Nucleolus.
Electronmicrograph showing the nucleolus from a cell actively producing protein. The pars amorpha (A), pars fibrosa (F) and pars granulosa (G) are clearly visible.

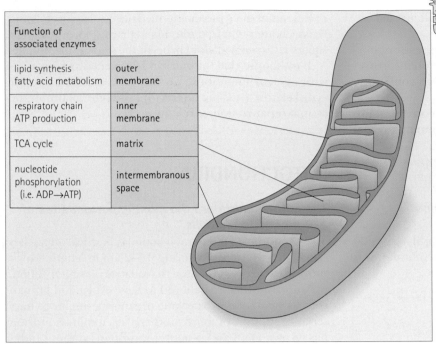

Function of associated enzymes		
lipid synthesis fatty acid metabolism	outer membrane	
respiratory chain ATP production	inner membrane	
TCA cycle	matrix	
nucleotide phosphorylation (i.e. ADP→ATP)	intermembranous space	

Fig. 2.12 Mitochondrion.
ⓐ Diagram of the structural organization of a mitochondrion accompanied by a table detailing the locations and functions of mitochondrial enzymes.
ⓑ Electronmicrograph of a mitochondrion. Note the outer membrane (OM), inner membrane (IM) and cristae (C).

MITOCHONDRIAL CYTOPATHY SYNDROMES

Mitochondrial DNA is not inherited in the same way as cellular DNA, and in man the whole mitochondrial complement of a developing embryo is derived from mitochondria present in the ovum (i.e. are maternally derived); there is no paternal contribution.

Abnormal mitochondrial DNA can impair mitochondrial function and lead to defective cell functioning, which mainly results in structural abnormalities of muscle and the nervous system, and metabolic abnormalities derived from failure of oxidative metabolism. Affected individuals can be considered to have mosaics of genetically different mitochondria, a concept termed heteroplasmy. If a large number of abnormal mitochondria are inherited then it is likely that severe disease will develop. If only a proportion are abnormal then the resulting disease may be less severe. The most common patterns of clinical disease are as follows:

- muscle weakness, particularly affecting the extraocular muscles;

- degenerative disease of the central nervous system; (e.g. loss of the optic nerve fibers, loss of cerebellar tissue or degeneration of brain white matter)

- metabolic disturbances, marked particularly by the

development of abnormally high levels of lactic acid. Such diseases may become manifest at any age from childhood into adult life and diagnosis can be assisted by muscle biopsy (Fig. 2.13), in which abnormal mitochondria can be seen in a large proportion of cases.

Fig. 2.13 Mitochondrial cytopathy.
Electronmicrograph of abnormal mitochondria in the muscle cell of a person with muscle weakness. Characteristic paracrystalline inclusions (PCI) are present, and are thought to be composed of excess mitochondrial protein which accumulates as a result of the genetic abnormality (compare with Fig. 2.12).

ENDOPLASMIC RETICULUM (ER) AND GOLGI

The endoplasmic reticulum and Golgi are involved in protein and lipid biosynthesis.

The ER and Golgi are two distinct regions of an inter-communicating membrane-bound compartment involved in the biosynthesis and transport of cellular proteins and lipids (Fig. 2.14).

They are arranged as deeply folded flattened membrane sheets or as elongated tubular profiles, their quantity depending on cellular metabolic requirements. Little ER is present in the majority of metabolically inactive cells, but cells which synthesize and secrete protein-containing molecules contain vast amounts. Most cells have only a relatively small quantity of smooth ER with the exception of cells secreting or processing lipids.

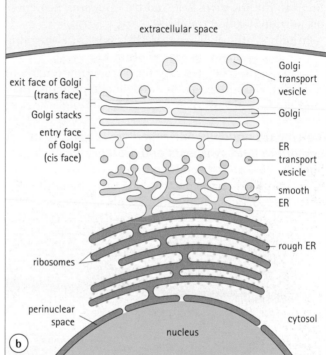

Fig. 2.14 Endoplasmic reticulum.
(a) Electron micrograph of rough ER composed of sheets of membrane with ribosomes on the cytosolic surfaces.
(b) Diagram of the relationship between ER and Golgi. The lumen of rough ER is continuous with the perinuclear space and with the lumen of smooth ER, while the Golgi forms a separate membrane system. Communication between ER and Golgi is mediated by small vesicles of ER, which break off, move through the cytosol and fuse with Golgi membrane.
(c) Diagram to show the spatial relationship between rough ER and smooth ER. Smooth ER cisternae are tubular.

Protein synthesis occurs through interaction of ribosomes, RNA and rough endoplasmic reticulum.

Protein synthesis begins in the cytosol where messenger RNA attaches to free ribosomes and translation produces the new peptide. The first portion of the RNA forms a signal sequence. Proteins destined to remain in the cytosol have a different signal sequence to those destined for entry into membranes or for secretion.

Ribosomes producing peptides with the signal sequence for a membrane or secreted protein become attached to the surface of ER where the rest of the peptide is translated (Fig. 2.15). The attachment of ribosomes to the ER gives it a studded appearance, hence this portion is called rough ER.

Protein synthesis by rough ER results in either the attachment of membrane proteins to ER membrane or retention of proteins destined for secretion or retention within the ER lumen. These newly made proteins then enter the smooth ER for transport to the Golgi.

The smooth endoplasmic reticulum is the site of membrane lipid synthesis and protein processing.

Smooth ER is a vital cell membrane system. As well as processing synthesized proteins it is the site of cell lipid synthesis, particularly membrane phospholipids. The lipid synthetic enzymes are located on its outer (cytosolic) face with ready access to lipid precursors.

Once synthesized and incorporated into the outer part of the smooth ER membrane lipid bilayer, phospholipids are flipped over into the inner part by specific transport proteins colloquially termed 'flipases'.

The Golgi is a membrane system involved in the sorting, packaging and transporting of cell products.

From the smooth ER, further processing of synthesized macromolecules takes place in the Golgi. To reach the Golgi, vesicles bud from the smooth ER and travel in cytosol to fuse with its inner face. Membrane proteins are incorporated into the Golgi membrane while luminal proteins enter the Golgi space (Fig. 2.16a).

The Golgi membrane system has three important roles:

- **modification** of macromolecules by the addition of sugars to form oligosaccharides;
- **proteolysis** of peptides into active forms;
- **sorting** of different macromolecules into specific membrane-bound vesicles for subsequent incorporation into a membrane, transport into the lumen of a specific membrane-bound organelle, or extracellular secretion.

To facilitate the roles of modification, proteolysis and sorting, the Golgi is divided into three functional components (Fig. 2.16): the cis face, the medial Golgi and the trans Golgi network.

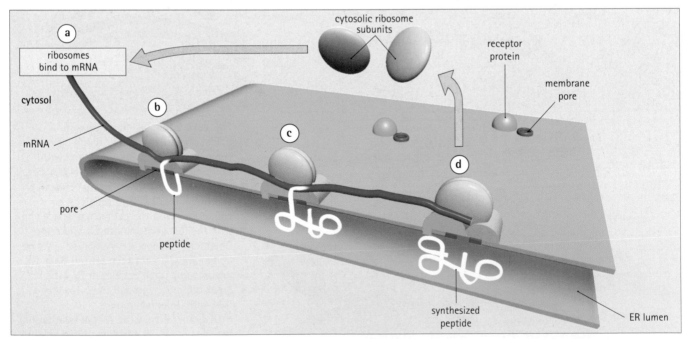

Fig. 2.15 Protein synthesis on rough endoplasmic reticulum.
(a) Free cytosolic ribosomes attach to messenger RNA and begin to produce a peptide.
(b) The ribosome attaches to a receptor on the ER membrane and the peptide is threaded into the ER lumen via a small protein-lined pore. At any one time several ribosomes may be transcribing the same messenger RNA strand.
(c) The original signal sequence that threads the peptide into the ER lumen is cleaved, and as the peptide is made it forms in the lumen. Some proteins (i.e. those destined to be integral membrane proteins) can also form directly within the ER membrane.
(d) After completion of peptide synthesis the ribosome detaches from the receptor protein and returns to the cytosolic free pool.

VESICLES

Very small membrane-bound bodies are called vesicles and are derived from several compartments.

Vesicles are small spherical membrane-bound organelles. They are formed by the budding off of existing areas of membrane and have two main functions. They:

- transport or store material within their lumina;
- allow the exchange of cell membrane between different cell compartments.

The main types of vesicle are:

- cell surface-derived endocytotic (i.e. pino- or phagocytotic) vesicle;
- Golgi-derived transport and secretory vesicles;
- ER-derived transport vesicles;
- lysosomes (see below);
- peroxisomes (page 22).

The cellular distribution of these vesicles can be determined by immunohistochemical staining for specific vesicle-associated proteins or specific vesicle contents.

Lysosomes are part of the acid vesicle system which is involved in degradation of proteins.

A lysosome is a membrane-bound organelle with a high content of hydrolytic enzymes operating in an acid pH. It thus functions as an intracellular digestion system, processing either material ingested by the cell or effete cellular components. This definition encompasses a variety of membrane-bound organelles derived from slightly different sources and with different functional roles.

Lysosomes are now considered to be only one part of the acid vesicle system, a group of vesicles so named because of their common membrane H^+-ATPase, which can decrease their luminal pH to 5. This low pH activates powerful acid hydrolase enzymes, which are derived from vesicles that bud from the Golgi.

The membrane proteins required for lysosomal function (particularly the membrane pump, which increases H^+ concentration to maintain the acid pH), are not present in the initial Golgi hydrolase vesicles (formerly called primary lysosomes), which appear as membrane-bound

Fig. 2.16 Golgi.

(a) Ultrastructurally Golgi is seen as parallel stacks of membrane (M) delineating Golgi lumen (L) from the cytosol (C). Transport vesicles (V) can be seen *en route* from ER.

(b) Golgi has three functional parts: the nuclear-facing **cis face** receives transport vesicles from smooth ER and phosphorylates certain proteins; the central **medial Golgi** adds sugar residues to both lipids and peptides to form complex oligosaccharides; the **trans Golgi network** performs proteolytic steps, adds sugar residues and sorts different macromolecules into specific vesicles which bud off the trans face.

Sorting is performed by specific membrane receptor proteins, which recognize signal groups on macromolecules and direct them into correct vesicles.

New membrane lipid synthesized in the smooth ER makes its way into the cell membrane via the Golgi.

vesicles with a dense core measuring 200–400 nm in diameter (Fig. 2.17a).

A functional lysosome, fulfilling the definition of acid environment plus hydrolases, results from the fusion of hydrolase vesicles with endosomes which contain the correct membrane proteins to form an endolysosome (formerly termed a secondary lysosome). Endolysosomes are larger than Golgi hydrolase vesicles, 600–800 nm in diameter, and also have an electron-dense core (Fig. 2.17b). They can fuse with other endosomes derived from phagocytosis to form phagolysosomes. In this way particulate matter brought into the cell is digested. Cells with a specific phagocytic function, such as certain white blood cells, have a well-developed acid vesicle system.

The relationships between members of the acid vesicle system are shown in Figure 2.18.

It is possible to demonstrate the presence of lysosomes by histochemical staining for acid hydrolases, the most reliable being the demonstration of acid phosphatases. Immunohistochemical reagents can also be used to detect specific hydrolases, for example cathepsin-B and β-glucuronidase.

Peroxisomes are membrane-bound vesicles important in metabolism of long fatty acids.

Peroxisomes are small membrane-bound organelles containing enzymes involved in the oxidation of several substrates, particularly β-oxidation of very long chain fatty acids (C18 and above).

Fig. 2.17 Lysosomes.
(a) Electronmicrograph of Golgi hydrolase vesicles, which are bounded by membrane (M) and have electron-dense core (C) composed of acid hydrolase enzymes. The membrane of this type of vesicle does not contain H^+-ATPase.
(b) Electronmicrograph showing several endolysosomes, which are produced by fusion of Golgi hydrolase vesicles with endosomes. Endolysosomes have a membrane containing H^+-ATPase, which can reduce pH to activate the hydrolases.

Effete organelles are eliminated from cells by first becoming wrapped in membrane derived from the ER. These bodies subsequently fuse with an endolysosome to form an autophagolysosome; this enables old or damaged organelles to be recycled in a process termed **autophagy**.

Following digestion of material by acid hydrolases, indigestible amorphous and membranous debris may be seen in large membrane-bound vesicles called residual bodies.

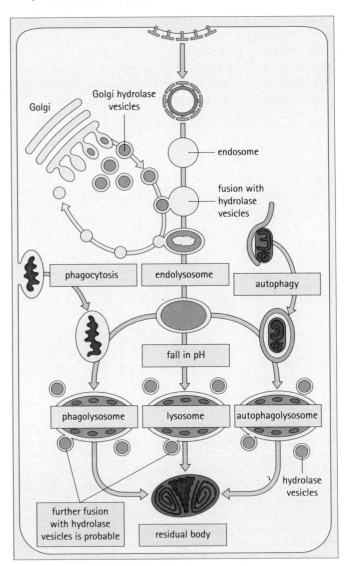

Fig. 2.18 Acid vesicle system.
Diagram of the relationships between the 'digestive' organelles of the acid vesicle system. Endosome forms from cell membrane and fuses with hydrolase-containing vesicles derived from the Golgi to form endolysosomes. The special Golgi membrane which forms the hydrolase vesicles is recycled back to the Golgi.

LYSOSOMAL STORAGE DISORDERS

In the acid vesicle system there are more than 30 defined and specific acid hydrolases which not only degrade abnormal large molecules but also recycle or process normal cell constituents.

Genetic defects in the production of specific acid hydrolases lead to an inability to degrade specific classes of molecule, which then accumulate in the acid vesicle system. Most of these defects are inherited as single gene autosomal recessive traits.

Lysosomal glycogen storage disease (acid maltase deficiency) leads to the accumulation of glycogen, which cannot be broken down (Fig. 2.19). Tay-Sachs disease results from a deficiency in an enzyme degrading one of the sphingolipids (hexosaminidase-A deficiency). Huge amounts of lipid accumulate in lysosomes and lead to severe neuronal degeneration.

Fig. 2.19 Acid maltase deficiency.
Electronmicrograph showing glycogen accumulation (G) in muscle cell cytoplasm and also within lysosomal bodies (L).

Ultrastructurally peroxisomes are small spherical bodies 0.5–1 μm in diameter with an electron-dense core. In some animals, but not in man, there is a central paracrystalline core termed a nucleoid.

Several enzymes in peroxisomes oxidize their substrate and reduce their O_2 to H_2O_2, while catalase, which is also present, decomposes H_2O_2 to O_2 and H_2O.

PEROXISOMAL DISORDERS

Several diseases are due to defects in the peroxisomal enzymes responsible for processing very long chain fatty acids, and are manifest by metabolic disturbances associated with acidosis, or with the storage of abnormal lipids in susceptible cells.

The most common example is adrenoleukodystrophy, in which impaired β-oxidation of fatty acids results in abnormal lipid storage in the brain, spinal cord and adrenal glands, leading to intellectual deterioration (dementia) and adrenal failure.

CYTOSKELETON

The cytoskeletal proteins form filaments which brace the internal structure of the cell.

Several functions of the cell are maintained by a set of filamentous cytosolic proteins, the cytoskeletal proteins, of which there are three main classes (depending on the size of their filaments):

- **microfilaments** (5 nm in diameter), composed of the protein **actin;**
- **intermediate filaments** (10 nm in diameter), composed of six main proteins, which vary in different cell types;
- **microtubules** (25 nm in diameter), composed of two **tubulin** proteins.

These filamentous proteins become attached to cell membranes and to each other by anchoring and joining proteins to form a dynamic three-dimensional internal scaffolding in the cell. This scaffolding is in a continual state of assembly and disassembly, but periods of stability subserve specific functional roles such as maintaining cellular architecture, facilitating cell motility, anchoring cells together, facilitating transport of material around the cytosol and dividing the cytosol into functionally separate areas.

Microfilaments are based on assemblies of the protein actin.

Actin accounts for about 5% of the total protein in most cell types. It is a globular protein (G-actin), which polymerizes to form filaments (F-actin) with all the actin subunits facing in one direction (polar filaments).

Actin

In association with other proteins, actin filaments, form a layer (the cell cortex, Fig. 2.20) beneath the cell membrane. The actin is arranged into a stiff cross-linked meshwork by linking proteins, the most abundant being filamin. This meshwork resists sudden deformational forces, but allows changes in cell shape by reforming, which is facilitated by actin-severing proteins.

Actin filament networks can provide mechanical support to the cell membrane by attachment to it via membrane-anchoring proteins; the best characterized of these are spectrin and ankyrin in red blood cells (see Fig. 7.2c), but similar proteins are present in most other cells. In addition, actin can become linked to transmembrane proteins in specialized areas of the plasma membrane, termed adherent junctions or focal contacts (see Figs 3.9 and 3.10), which are externally attached to other cells or extracellular structures; thus the actin filament network of one cell can become linked to other cells or structures.

Actin filaments can form rigid bundles to stabilize protrusions of cell membrane termed microvilli (see Fig. 3.15). In these bundles, actin is associated with small linking proteins, the most abundant being fimbrin and fascin.

In all cells, actin filaments interact with a protein called myosin to generate motile forces. Myosin is an actin-activated ATPase composed of two heavy chains and four light chains arranged into a long tail and a globular head. These myosin heads can bind to actin and hydrolyze ATP to ADP. The interaction between actin and myosin to produce contractile forces is shown in Fig. 5.3.

Polymerization of actin filaments is probably responsible for the forces that drive local outgrowths of cell cytoplasm, such as spikes and ruffles, which are particularly evident in motile cells and cells undergoing migration in embryogenesis.

There are several molecular variants (isoforms) of actin, which have specific distributions in different cell types, for example, isoforms restricted to smooth muscle or skeletal muscle.

Fig. 2.20 Cell cortex.
The cell cortex is composed of a stiff cross-linked meshwork of actin and actin-linking proteins, the most abundant being filamin. It forms a layer that lines the cytosolic face of the cell membrane.

Microtubules brace internal organelles and guide movement in intracellular transport.

Microtubules are present in all cells except red blood cells. They are formed from two protein subunits, α and β **tubulin**, which polymerize in a head-to-tail pattern to form protofilaments. These are arranged into groups of 13 to form hollow tubes 25 nm in diameter (Fig. 2.21).

Other cellular elements, such as centrioles and cilia, are also made up of tubulin in the form of doublet or triplet tubules (see below).

Microtubules are constantly polymerizing and depolymerizing in the cell and grow out from the microtubule organizing center. They are stabilized by associating with other proteins (microtubule-associated proteins or MAPs e.g. Tau protein), which convert the unstable microtubular network into a relatively permanent framework. Microtubules are also stabilized by proteins that cap the growing end and prevent depolymerization.

The centriole acts as a region which organizes the distribution of microtubules.

Microtubules originate in the microtubule-organizing center. This special region of the cell, known as the centrosome is an organelle which contains a pair of centrioles (the centriole, Fig. 2.22).

Each centrosome with its pair of centrioles surrounded by an amorphous electron-dense area of cytoplasm acts as the nucleation center for the polymerization of microtubules; these radiate from the centrosome in a star-like pattern called an aster. The protein forming the amorphous area is highly conserved in evolution and is present in both animal and plant cells. Each centrosome can act as the center for about 250 microtubules.

The centriole has two roles in the cell:
- it organizes the cytoplasmic microtubular network in both normal and dividing cells;
- it organizes the development of specialized microtubules in motile cilia (see Fig. 3.17).

Intermediate filament proteins vary between different functional classes of cells.

Intermediate filaments are a group of filamentous cytoskeletal proteins comprising six main types, which have a specific distribution in different cell types (Fig. 2.23). Ultrastructurally they form relatively ill-defined bundles or masses in the cytosol of cells.

Microtubule function

Microtubules form a network allowing transport around the cell, via the attachment proteins dynein, which moves down a microtubule toward the cell center, and kinesin, which moves up a microtubule toward the cell periphery. These attachment proteins are associated with the membranes of vesicles and organelles, and facilitate their movement around the cell. This process is particularly important in the transport of organelles down the long cell processes of nerve cells (see Chapter 6).

Microtubules also form a network (cytoskeleton) for membrane-bound cell compartments (e.g. they maintain the extended tubular arrangement of the ER).

Chromosomes are organized in cell division along the microtubular cell spindle (see Fig. 2.27).

Specialized motile components of the cell, cilia (see Fig. 3.17), are composed of microtubules bound together with other proteins.

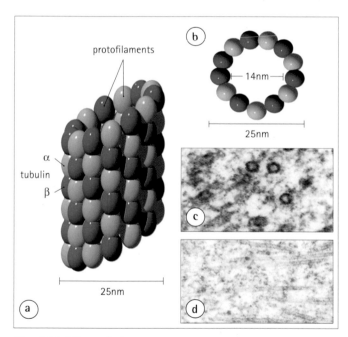

Fig. 2.21 Microtubules.
(a) Each microtubule is composed of 13 protofilaments of alternating α and β tubulin subunits. Microtubules are polar, with polymerization occurring at one end and depolymerization at the other.
(b) In cross-section each microtubule is 25 nm in diameter.
(c) Electronmicrograph showing the circular profiles of microtubules in cross-section.
(d) Electronmicrograph showing the faint parallel lines of microtubules in longitudinal section.

Fig. 2.22 Centriole.
(a) A centriole is composed of a cylindrical bundle measuring 200 x 400 nm composed of 9 microtubule triplets arranged together by linking proteins.
(b) In most cells, centrioles exist in pairs arranged at right angles to each other.
(c) In electron microscopic preparations, one centriole is usually visible in cross-section, revealing the circular (C) arrangement of tubules, while its partner is cut either longitudinally or slightly obliquely (O).

Intermediate filaments.

Intermediate filaments are anchored to transmembrane proteins at special sites on the cell membrane (desmosomes and hemidesmosomes, see Figs. 3.11 and 3.12) and spread tensile forces evenly throughout a tissue so that single cells are not disrupted.

Although intermediate filaments have several defined roles in cells as outlined below, detailed mechanisms of their function have not been elucidated, unlike those of the other cytoskeletal proteins.

In **epithelial cells of the skin**, keratin intermediate filaments become compacted with other link proteins to form a tough outer layer (see Fig. 3.27) and hence have an important structural role as an impermeable barrier, as well as being the main constituent protein of hair and nail.

In **neurons**, neurofilaments have long side arms, which probably help maintain the cylindrical architecture of nerve cell processes when subjected to lateral tensile forces in bending. They also anchor membrane ion channel proteins via a link protein ankyrin, to facilitate nerve conduction.

When cells are damaged, the intermediate filament network collapses to form a perinuclear spherical ball associated with abnormal or damaged cellular

proteins. It is possible that in this situation the intermediate filaments act to cocoon damaged cellular components in one spot for subsequent elimination by proteolysis. Following cell recovery, the intermediate filament network re-expands.

This phenomenon occurs in liver cells in response to persistent alcohol excess, when collapsed bundles of cytokeratin intermediate filaments (Mallory's hyaline) accumulate.

In the **nucleus**, the nuclear lamins form a square lattice on the inner side of the nuclear membrane, which probably acts with other link proteins in the organization of the nucleus.

The cell-specific restriction of distribution of intermediate filament proteins may be used for the histologic assessment of cell types, using immunohistochemical staining for the various filaments. This is particularly useful when small samples of malignant tumor are being assessed to determine their likely site of origin.

The detection of cytokeratin argues strongly for an epithelial origin, while the presence of desmin would suggest a muscle derivation, and glial fibrillary acidic protein (GFAP) is only seen in specialized central nervous system tumors.

- microfilaments are made of actin and have roles in movement and membrane stabilization

- microtubules are made of tubulin and have roles in intracellular transport as well as in scaffolding of internal membranes

- intermediate filaments are made of proteins which vary between different cell types and function to link separate cells into structural units

Intermediate filament	Localization
cytokeratins	epithelial cells
desmin	muscle (smooth and striated)
glial fibrillary acidic protein (GFAP)	astrocytic glial cells
neurofilament protein	neurons
nuclear lamin	nucleus of all cells
vimentin	many mesodermal tissues

Fig. 2.23 Intermediate filaments.
Table showing the location of different types of intermediate filament.

CELL INCLUSIONS AND STORAGE PRODUCTS

Accumulations of products within certain cells may occur in the form of cytoplasmic inclusions.

Lipofuscin pigment is mainly composed of phospholipid and is the result of 'wear and tear'.

Lipofuscin appears as membrane-bound orange-brown granular material within the cytoplasm. Derived from residual bodies containing a mixture of phospholipids from cell degradation, lipofuscin is commonly referred to as 'wear and tear' pigment, as it becomes more prominent in old cells. It is particularly common in tissues from elderly persons, and is most evident in nerve, heart muscle and liver cells.

Lipid is stored in cells as non-membrane-bound vacuoles.

Lipids may accumulate as non-membrane-bound vacuoles which appear as large clear spaces in the cytoplasm because paraffin wax processing dissolves out the fat. If the tissues are frozen and cut in a freezing microtome, the fat can be stained with certain dyes. Large fat vacuoles are a special feature of fat storage cells called adipocytes (see Fig. 4.19). Fat also accumulates in certain cells such as heptocytes in the liver in response to sub-lethal metabolic damage. The most common cause is chronic high alcohol ingestion.

Glycogen may impart a pale vacuolated appearance to cells.

Glycogen, a polymer and storage product of glucose, forms as granules in the cell cytoplasm and is only visible by electron microscopy. Demands for energy are met by conversion of glycogen to glucose.

In certain cells, the presence of large amounts of glycogen causes pale staining or apparent vacuolation of cell cytoplasm. Glycogen can be stained by the PAS method.

CELL DIVISION

Cell division for growth and renewal is achieved by the process of mitosis.

An essential feature of development is the ability of cells to divide and reproduce. In addition, death of mature cells in the adult needs to be compensated for by production of new cells.

Cells reproduce by duplicating their contents and dividing into two daughter cells. The phases involved in cell replication can be regarded as a cell cycle (Fig. 2.24). The phases of cell division are visible histologically and involve duplication of cellular cytoplasmic contents, duplication of DNA, separation of cellular DNA into two separate areas of the cell (mitosis, Figs 2.25 and 2.26) and finally cell division (cytokinesis).

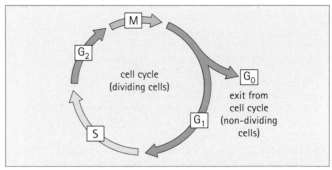

Fig. 2.24 Cells can enter a phase of proliferation in which they divide. Cells which leave the cycle are said to be in the G_0 phase.

Fig. 2.25 The cell cycle.
The DNA of cells is only replicated during certain phases of a cell's growth pattern, which takes place in several stages. The cell cycle is divided into two main periods: mitosis and interphase, which includes G_1, S and G_2 phases.

Cells which are not dividing are non-cycling or G_0 cells, while G_1 cells have just entered a phase of cellular growth. S phase cells actively synthesize DNA, G_2 cells have a double complement of cellular DNA and are resting prior to cell division, and M phase cells are in mitosis, which comprises 5 stages. In most tissues only a small proportion of cells will be in the cell cycle, the majority being differentiated cells in a G_0 phase. Stem cells may be in a G_0 phase and only come to re-enter the cell cycle if there is a demand, for example following cell death.

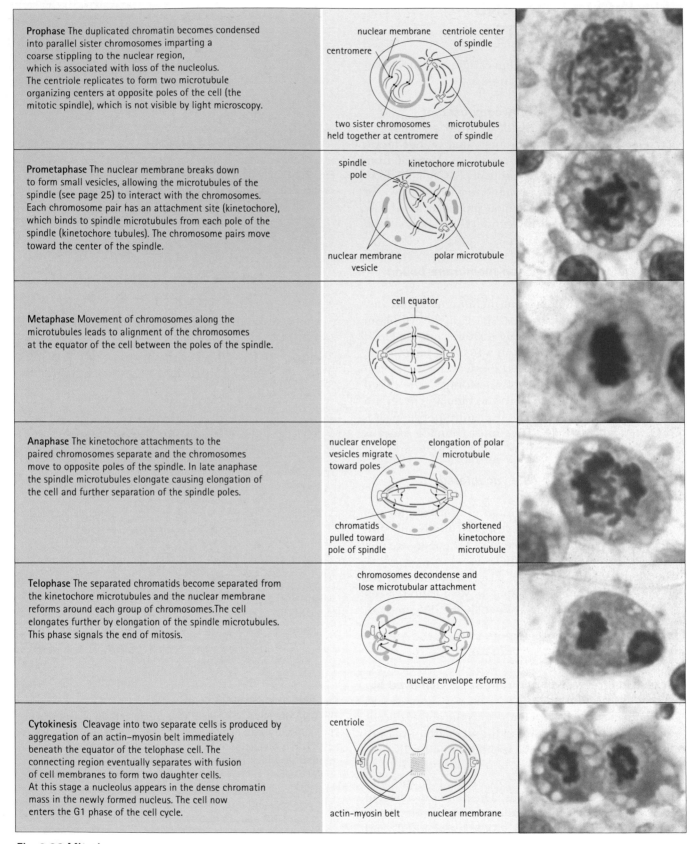

Prophase The duplicated chromatin becomes condensed into parallel sister chromosomes imparting a coarse stippling to the nuclear region, which is associated with loss of the nucleolus. The centriole replicates to form two microtubule organizing centers at opposite poles of the cell (the mitotic spindle), which is not visible by light microscopy.

nuclear membrane   centriole center of spindle
centromere
two sister chromosomes   microtubules
held together at centromere   of spindle

Prometaphase The nuclear membrane breaks down to form small vesicles, allowing the microtubules of the spindle (see page 25) to interact with the chromosomes. Each chromosome pair has an attachment site (kinetochore), which binds to spindle microtubules from each pole of the spindle (kinetochore tubules). The chromosome pairs move toward the center of the spindle.

spindle pole   kinetochore microtubule
nuclear membrane   polar microtubule
vesicle

Metaphase Movement of chromosomes along the microtubules leads to alignment of the chromosomes at the equator of the cell between the poles of the spindle.

cell equator

Anaphase The kinetochore attachments to the paired chromosomes separate and the chromosomes move to opposite poles of the spindle. In late anaphase the spindle microtubules elongate causing elongation of the cell and further separation of the spindle poles.

nuclear envelope   elongation of polar
vesicles migrate   microtubule
toward poles
chromatids   shortened
pulled toward   kinetochore
pole of spindle   microtubule

Telophase The separated chromatids become separated from the kinetochore microtubules and the nuclear membrane reforms around each group of chromosomes. The cell elongates further by elongation of the spindle microtubules. This phase signals the end of mitosis.

chromosomes decondense and
lose microtubular attachment
nuclear envelope reforms

Cytokinesis Cleavage into two separate cells is produced by aggregation of an actin–myosin belt immediately beneath the equator of the telophase cell. The connecting region eventually separates with fusion of cell membranes to form two daughter cells. At this stage a nucleolus appears in the dense chromatin mass in the newly formed nucleus. The cell now enters the G1 phase of the cell cycle.

centriole
actin-myosin belt   nuclear membrane

Fig. 2.26 Mitosis.

Different cell populations can be defined according to their pattern of growth.

In adults, not all cells are capable of division. Several different populations of cells can be defined based on their capacity to replicate:

- **static cell populations** are cells which do not divide in the developed tissue;
- **stable cell populations** do not normally divide;
- **renewing cell populations** normally divide constantly.

Nerve cells and cardiac muscle cells, for example, divide and form tissues during embryogenesis. Once tissues are formed the cells do not divide again. Stable cell population, for example liver cells, divide in order to replace cells lost through disease. Skin and gut lining cells are renewing cell populations which divide continually to replace shed cells. Blood cell populations have a short life span and are constantly renewed.

Stem cells are partly committed cells which function as a dividing population to produce a range of specialized cells.

Some cells become only partly committed down a line of differentiation. They then act as a pool of dividing cells to replenish more specialized cell populations. These partly committed cells are called stem cells, and it is now known that such cells are the basis for continued renewal of many constantly dividing cell types.

Several types of renewing cell populations are thought to originate from common stem cells, for example the different cells of the blood originate from a common hemopoietic stem cell, and enterocyte stem cells probably give rise to the different cell types lining the gut.

Following stem cell division, two types of cell may result: new stem cells to maintain the stem cell population, and committed cells, which differentiate along one cell line, but may still divide in what are termed amplification divisions.

A stem cell must reproduce itself each time it divides to maintain the stem cell population.

Cell division to produce gametes for reproduction is achieved through the process of meiosis.

Normal cells have two sets of complementary (homologous) chromosomes derived from the maternal and paternal germ cells at fertilization and are therefore called **diploid**, or 2n cells.

The germ cells (ova and spermatozoa), which are destined to fuse in fertilization to produce an embryo, have half the normal complement of chromosomes (i.e. are haploid, n, cells). They are the product of a modified form of cell division, **meiosis**.

In meiosis (Fig. 2.27), complementary chromosomes become paired on the mitotic spindle following S phase of the cell cycle (see Fig. 2.25) with the maternal set attached to one pole and the paternal set attached to the opposite pole; the pole to which maternal- and paternal-

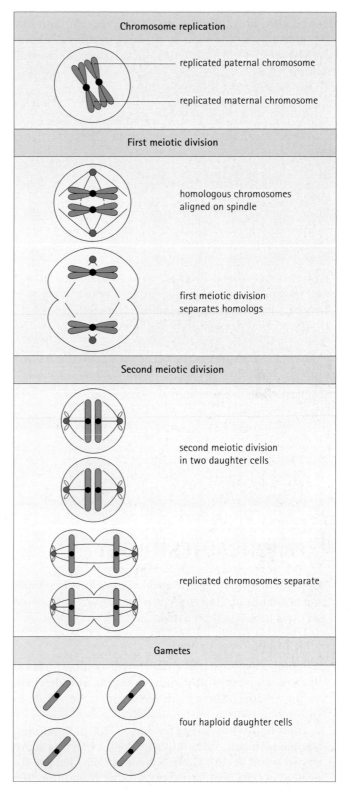

Fig. 2.27 Meiosis.
Meiosis results in the formation of four daughter cells, each with half the normal chromosomal complement (i.e. n, haploid).

derived chromosomes become attached is random for each chromosome. This is in contrast to mitosis where complementary chromosomes do not align across the spindle.

Thus, in meiosis, maternal and paternal complementary chromosomes are separated, migrating to opposite ends of the spindle by a first meiotic division. Once segregated in this way a second division (virtually identical to a mitotic division, see Fig. 2.26) separates replicated chromosomes. The result of meiosis is four daughter nuclei, each containing one set of chromosomes.

ANTI-CANCER DRUGS

Many drugs used to treat cancer act specifically on cells in the cell cycle (see Fig. 2.24), the aim being to remove abnormally growing cells.

Unfortunately these drugs act on normal body cells as well as cancer cells and have adverse effects particularly on renewing cell populations, which depend on a high proportion of cells being in cycle.

Thus, blood cell production, hair production and gut-lining cell production are all impaired by the administration of such anti-cancer drugs.

CELL DEATH

Programmed cell death is a normal means of controlling dividing cell populations.

In many replicating tissues, and particularly during embryogenesis, control of the cell population is achieved by controlling the rate of cell death. Normal cells require a balance of signals which maintain their viability. In the absence of a correct pattern of signals, certain genes are switched on which bring about carefully controlled dissolution of the cell. Because of the genetic control of this process it is referred to as programmed cell death, and contrasts with cell death that occurs in many diseases or is brought about by deleterious stimuli.

The most important form of programmed cell death is **apoptosis**. In this process the cell becomes fragmented and is ingested by adjacent cells (Fig. 2.28).

PRACTICAL HISTOLOGY

General principles can be applied usefully when looking at cells either in cytologic preparations or in tissue sections to assess their activity, as outlined below.

NUCLEUS

A metabolically inactive cell has a compact round nucleus which typically stains intensely as little chromatin is being transcribed. No nucleoli are visible as ribosome production is minimal.

A protein-synthesizing cell has a large pale-staining nucleus with large or multiple nucleoli, reflecting active transcription of chromatin. Similar nuclear changes are evident in cells in an active phase of multiplication (see Fig. 2.25).

A dead cell has a shrunken nucleus, which appears as an amorphous compact mass of intensely staining material. This later fragments into separate particles, and is completely lysed, leaving the cell devoid of any discernible nucleus.

CYTOPLASM

Examination of cell cytoplasm should concentrate on the intensity and distribution of acidophilic (pink) and basophilic (purple) elements.

A granular intensely pink-staining cytoplasm contains accumulations of organelles that take up acidic dye, which are usually mitochondria or secretory granules, (e.g. neurosecretory granules, or specialized granules, such as those seen in white blood cells).

A diffuse purple tint to the cytoplasm indicates the presence of cytoplasmic RNA in the form of ribosomes, and thus active protein production.

Large non-staining areas are generally large secretory vacuoles, such as those seen in those mucin-secreting cells. In some cell types they may represent fat.

Normal cells are arranged in close contact with each other and are united by cell junctions. Early in the process of apoptosis there is synthesis of enzymes needed to cause cell dissolution, but this is not associated with structural changes. This is termed **priming**. In development many cells are primed for apoptosis and survive only if rescued by a specific trophic factor.

The apoptotic cells lose surface specializations and junctions, shrinking in size. The nuclear chromatin condenses beneath the nuclear membrane. In contrast to necrosis, cell organelles remain normal. Endonuclease enzymes cleave chromosomes into individual nucleosome fragments.

There is splitting of the cell into several fragments known as **apoptotic bodies**. Nuclear fragmentation also occurs. Each fragment contains viable mitochondria and intact organelles. The process takes a few minutes only.

Apoptotic fragments are recognized by adjacent cells, which ingest them by phagocytosis for destruction. Some fragments degenerate extracellularly, while others are ingested by local phagocytic cells, not shown on this diagram.

Although apoptosis is a physiological process, it can also be induced by pathological conditions.

Fig. 2.28 Apoptosis.
Apoptosis of cells is a programmed and energy-dependent process designed specifically to switch cells off and eliminate them. This controlled pattern of cell death, termed programmed cell death, is very different from that which occurs as a direct result of a severe damaging stimulus to cells (termed necrosis).

NUCLEAR CHANGES IN CANCER

A cell containing a very large nucleus relative to the amount of cytoplasm is generally in a phase of cell division. Cells with inappropriately large nuclei raise the suspicion of cancerous change. For example cells on the surface of the uterine cervix should have small nuclei unless there is abnormal cell growth such as that associated with the development of a malignancy.

In any specialized cell type, all the nuclei in adjacent cells should be roughly the same size and have the same staining characteristics. In cancer, however, nuclei vary in size and shape (nuclear pleomorphism) and commonly show dense-staining chromatin in a coarse clumped pattern (nuclear hyperchromatism).

DIAGNOSTIC CYTOLOGY

Cytology is the study of cellular form and refers to an important specialty in laboratory medicine, which concentrates on establishing the diagnosis of disease by examination of small numbers of cells.

Cells for examination are obtained from patients either by scraping the surface of epithelia (e.g. the uterine cervix or gastric lining),by aspirating solid tissues with a needle or by collecting cells from body fluids such as sputum or urine.

The ultimate aim is to detect abnormalities in cell structure that point to the presence of disease. In clinical medicine the most important aspect is the recognition of changes which herald the development of cancer (neoplastic changes).

---

1. CELL MEMBRANE

(a) is structurally based on a lipid bilayer
(b) contains proteins which only act as enzymes
(c) surrounds the nucleus in a single layer
(d) surrounds individual ribosomeswithin the cell
(e) is maintained by vesicles derived from the Golgi

2. MITOCHONDRIA

(a) replicate independently from the cell
(b) are the main site for oxidative phosphorylation
(c) have a highly impermeable outer cell membrane
(d) vary in morphology between different cell types
(e) contain their own genetic material

3. LYSOSOMES

(a) lysosomes have a membrane H^+-ATPase capable of maintaining an acid environment
(b) the enzymes contained in lysosomes are also present in peroxisomes

(c) vesicles from the Golgi take acid hydrolases to lysosomes
(d) fusion of an endosome with a vesicle containing acid hydrolases forms an endolysosome
(e) lysosomal storage diseases are caused by lack of specific lysosomal enzymes leading to accumulation of a metabolic product

4. IN DIVIDING CELLS

(a) the nuclear membrane is fragmented during separation of chromosomes
(b) the nucleolus is involved in ribosomal biogenesis and is a prominent structure in dividing cells
(c) prophase and metaphase both occur in the S phase of the cell cycle
(d) the final daughter cells which derive from meiosis are haploid
(e) control of the overall population may be regulated by apoptosis

3. Epithelial Cells

INTRODUCTION

Epithelial cells are a specialized component of many organs. They are characterized by common structural features, especially their arrangement into cohesive sheets, but have diverse functions made possible by many specialized adaptations. Many of the physical properties of epithelial cells rely on their attachment to each other which is mediated by several types of cell junction. The specialized functions of epithelial cells are mediated through both structural modifications of their surface as well as by internal modifications which adapt cells to manufacture and secrete a product.

Epithelial cells are specialized for absorption, secretion or to act as a barrier.

Epithelial cells form very cohesive sheets of cells called epithelia, which function mainly as:
- a covering or lining for body surfaces, for example skin, gut and ducts;
- the functional units of secretory glands such as salivary tissue and liver.

Epithelial cells are firmly joined together by adhesion specializations. These special structures serve to anchor the cytoskeleton of each epithelial cell to its neighbors and to anchor the epithelium to underlying or surrounding extracellular matrix materials.

Epithelial cells are further specialized by modifications of their surfaces to fulfill their specific role, which may be absorption or secretion, or to act as a barrier (see pages 39-47).

The classification of epithelial cells is based on their shape and how they are stacked together.

The traditional nomenclature and classification of different types of epithelium are based on the two-dimensional shape of cells as observed by early light microscopy, and ignore any specialized functional attributes. Thus, the nomenclature now appears rather simplistic given the present detailed knowledge of the biology of these cells.

Traditionally cells are classified into three main cell groups according to their shape. These groups are: **squamous** (flat plate-like, Fig. 3.1), **cuboidal** (height and width similar, Fig. 3.2), and **columnar** (height 2–5 times greater than width, Fig. 3.3).

Epithelial cells form either a single layer in which all of the cells contact underlying extracellular matrix (simple epithelium), or several layers where only the bottom layer of cells is in contact with the extracellular matrix (stratified epithelium, Fig. 3.4).

Pseudostratified epithelium (Fig. 3.5) contains epithelial cells that appear to be arranged in layers, but are all in contact with the extracellular matrix. A transitional epithelium is a further special type of stratified epithelium which is mainly restricted to the lining of the urinary tract (see Chapter 15), and varies between cuboidal and squamous depending on the degree of stretching.

Epithelia are also grouped according to whether they occur as a surface or glandular component.

The traditional morphologic classification has limitations. In the past, great emphasis was placed on the distribution of the different morphologic types of epithelium

simple squamous epithelium

extracellular support matrix (basement membrane)

(a)

(b)

Fig. 3.1 Simple squamous epithelium.
(a) A simple squamous epithelium is composed of a single layer of cells, which are flat and plate-like.
(b) In histologic sections, the nuclei (N) appear flattened and the cytoplasm is indistinct.

Although squamous refers to any flat epithelium, its use is restricted as many flat epithelia are given more specific names, the flat epithelium lining blood vessels being called endothelium, and that lining the abdominal and pleural cavities, mesothelium.

and whether they were stratified or simple, surface or glandular; such classification is now outmoded. Although two epithelia may be described as cuboidal, their function and biology may be so different that it is misleading to equate them.

However, provided this limitation of nomenclature is realized, the use of a morphologic classification of epithelia is still descriptively valuable.

The traditional terms used to describe epithelia are found throughout this book, but are always qualified to give insight into their function.

Fig. 3.2 Simple cuboidal epithelium.
(a) A simple cuboidal epithelium is composed of a single layer of cells whose height, width and depth are the same. Note they are not strictly cuboidal.
(b) In histologic section, such cells usually have a centrally placed nucleus (N).

Fig. 3.3 Simple columnar epithelium.
(a) A simple columnar epithelium is composed of cells whose height is 2–3 times greater than their width.
(b) The nuclei (N) of columnar cells are basal and arranged in an ordered layer.

Fig. 3.4 Stratified squamous epithelium.
(a) A stratified epithelium is composed of several layers such that cells high up in the epithelium are not in contact with the underlying extracellular matrix.
(b) Stratified squamous epithelium derives its name from the flattened (squamous) appearance of cells in the superficial part of the epithelium (S). Cells in the basal (B) and middle (M) layers of this type of epithelium are in fact pyramidal or polygonal and are not flattened.

Fig. 3.5 Pseudostratified columnar epithelium.
(a) In a pseudostratified epithelium, several layers of nuclei suggest several layers of cells, but in fact all cells are in contact with the underlying extracellular matrix.
(b) Routine histologic preparations show several layers of nuclei.

EPITHELIAL CELL JUNCTIONS

Specialized structures are present in epithelia which link the individual cells together into a functional unit.

The structural integrity of epithelium is maintained by adhesion of the constituent cells both to each other and to structural extracellular matrix. These adhesions are mediated by two main systems:

- cell membrane proteins acting as specialized cell adhesion molecules;
- specialized areas of cell membrane incorporated into cell junctions.

There are three types of cell junctions: **occluding junctions** link cells to form an impermeable barrier; **anchoring junctions** link cells to provide mechanical strength; and **communicating junctions** allow movement of molecules between cells.

Occluding junctions bind cells together and maintain the integrity of epithelial cells as a barrier.

Occluding junctions have two main functions:

- prevention of diffusion of molecules between adjacent cells, thereby contributing to the barrier function of the epithelial cells in which they are present.
- prevention of lateral migration of specialized cell membrane proteins, thereby delineating and maintaining specialized cell membrane domains.

The occluding function is performed by intramembranous proteins (Fig. 3.6), which mediate the adhesion of adjacent cells;

Ultrastructurally an occluding junction is seen as a focal area of close apposition of adjacent cell membrane. This has lead to its alternative name of **tight junction**.

Occluding junctions are particularly well developed in the epithelial cells lining the small bowel, where they:

- prevent digested macromolecules from passing between the cells:
- confine specialized areas of the cell membrane involved in absorption or secretion to the luminal side of the cell.

Occluding junctions are also important in cells that actively transport a substance, for example the active transport of an ion, against a concentration gradient. In this situation occluding junctions prevent back diffusion of the transported substance (Fig. 3.7).

Anchoring junctions link the cytoskeleton of cells both to each other and to underlying tissues.

Anchoring junctions (Fig. 3.8) provide mechanical stability to groups of epithelial cells so that they can function as a cohesive unit.

The actin network interacts with two separate types of junction:

- adherent junctions link the actin filament network between adjacent cells (Fig. 3.9);
- focal contacts link the actin filament network of a cell to the extracellular matrix (Fig. 3.10).

Fig. 3.6 Occluding junction.

(a) Occluding junctions are particularly evident between epithelial cells that have secretory or absorptive roles. A collar of occluding junction is present between each cell, sealing individual cells into a tight barrier. The intramembranous proteins that form these junctions are arranged as serpiginous intertwining lines (**sealing strands**), which stitch the membrane of adjacent cells together.

(b) An occluding junction is seen ultrastructurally as an area of close apposition of adjacent areas of cell membrane (CM) corresponding to the site of membrane attachment proteins.

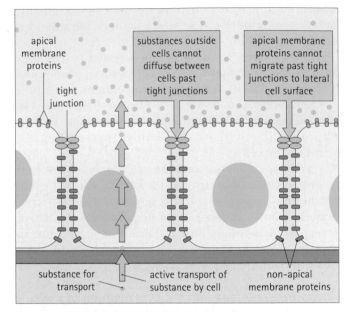

Fig. 3.7 Occluding junction (tight junction).
Cells that transport molecules against a concentration gradient have occluding junctions to prevent back diffusion of the transported substance.

In addition, it is desirable to concentrate specialized cell membrane components into certain areas of the cell, for example a transport protein in the apical cell membrane. Cells use occluding junctions to prevent lateral migration of specialized membrane proteins, thus establishing specialized membrane domains.

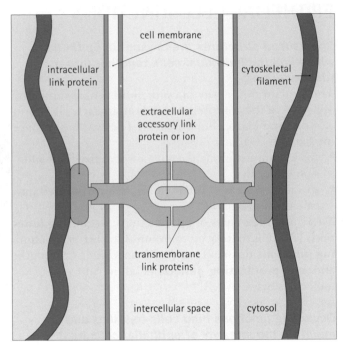

Fig. 3.8 Anchoring junction (general structure).
Cytoskeletal filaments of adjacent cells are joined through intracellular link proteins, which attach the filaments to transmembrane link proteins. These can then interact with similar proteins on adjacent cells. The extracellular interaction may be mediated by additional extracellular proteins or ions, such as Ca^{++}. Different (or multiple) link proteins and transmembrane proteins operate for the different classes of junction.

Fig. 3.9 Adherent junction.
Actin fibers in adjacent cells are linked by actin-binding proteins (α-actinin and vinculin) to a transmembrane protein, which is one of a group of cell surface glycoproteins mediating cell adhesion (**cadherins**). The type in adherent junctions is E-cadherin, which links cells in the presence of Ca^{++}.

Ultrastructurally, an adherent junction is a fuzzy plaque (P) of electron-dense material adjacent to the cell membrane (CM), corresponding to the location of α actinin and vinculin, into which actin filaments (A) are inserted. The intercellular junctional component (i.e. extracellular component of adjacent E-cadherin molecules and Ca^{++}) is not visible, but is evident as a lucent area between the adjacent membranes.

Fig. 3.10 Focal contact.
Bundles of actin filaments interact with actin-binding proteins (α-actinin, vinculin and talin) to link with a transmembrane link protein, which is one of a class of cell adhesion molecules termed an **integrin** (see Fig. 4.9).

The intermediate filament network interacts with two separate types of junction:

- desmosomes connect the intermediate filament networks of adjacent cells (Fig. 3.11);
- hemidesmosomes connect the intermediate filament network of cells to extracellular matrix (Fig. 3.12).

Adherent junctions are most common toward the apex of adjacent columnar and cuboidal epithelial cells, where they link submembranous actin bundles into a so-called **adhesion belt**. They are prominent in the cells lining the small intestine where they form a zone visible by light microscopy as an eosinophilic band (the **terminal bar**).

In embryogenesis, adherent-type junctions transmit motile forces generated by the actin filaments across whole sheets of cells. They are thus essential in mediating the folding of epithelial sheets to form early organs in the embryo.

Desmosomes provide mechanical stability in epithelial cells subject to tensile and shearing stresses, and are particularly well developed in stratified squamous epithelium covering the skin.

Desmosomes are so characteristic of epithelial cells that their detection in malignant tumors of uncertain nature is indicative of an epithelial as opposed to a lymphoid or support cell origin.

A **junctional complex** describes the close association of several types of junction between adjacent epithelial cells and is a manifestation of the requirement for several types of epithelial cell attachment in order to maintain structural and functional integrity (Fig. 3.13).

DISEASE OF CELL JUNCTIONS — PEMPHIGUS

In pemphigus, the body produces abnormal antibodies to the proteins forming desmosome junctions in the skin; this prevents normal adhesion between the desmosomes. Affected people develop widespread skin and mucous membrane blistering as the desmosomal junctions between adjacent squamous cells of the skin fall apart. Immunohistochemical staining can be used to demonstrate the abnormal antibodies adhering to the intercellular space between the diseased epidermal cells.

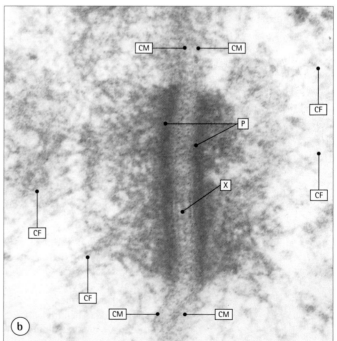

Fig. 3.11 Desmosome.

ⓐ Each desmosome consists of an intracellular plaque composed of several link proteins (the main types being desmoplakins), into which cytokeratin intermediate filaments (**tonofilaments**) are inserted. The cell adhesion is mediated by transmembrane proteins called desmogleins.

ⓑ The disc-shaped adhesion plaques (P) in adjacent cells are seen as electron-dense areas into which cytokeratin filaments (CF) are inserted. The cell membranes (CM) between adhesion plaques are about 30 nm apart and there may be an electron-dense band between cells in some desmosomes (X).

Fig. 3.12 Hemidesmosome.

(a) A hemidesmosome is similar to a desmosome except that it interacts with extracellular matrix rather than with an adjacent desmosome on another cell. In contrast to a desmosome, the cytokeratin filaments (tonofilaments) commonly terminate end-on rather than looping through. The proteins in the hemidesmosome differ from those in desmosomes.

(b) Ultrastructurally, a hemidesmosome consists of a dense plaque (P) composed of intracellular link proteins including desmoplakins, into which cytokeratin intermediate filaments (CF) are inserted. Linkage is to the extracellular matrix (M) and by a series of fine anchoring fibrils (F) composed of type VII collagen.

Fig. 3.13 Junctional complex.

A junctional complex is commonly seen toward the apex of cuboidal and columnar cells. Immediately below the cell apex an occluding junction (O) is followed by an adherent junction (A), and below this by desmosomes (D). This example is obtained from cells lining the small bowel where such complexes are well developed. In other epithelia, particularly those in which occluding junctions are not required, such fully developed complexes are uncommon.

Communication junctions allow direct cell–cell communication.

Communication junctions (gap junctions) allow selective diffusion of molecules between adjacent cells and facilitate direct cell to cell communication (Fig. 3.14).

Gap junctions are usually present at relatively low density in most adult epithelia, but are found in large numbers during embryogenesis, when they probably have a role in the spatial organization of developing cells. Gap junctions are also important in cardiac and smooth muscle cells where they pass signals involved in contraction from one cell to another.

The basement membrane anchors of epithelial cells to underlying tissues.

The attachment of epithelial cells to underlying support tissues at hemidesmosome and focal contacts is mediated by a specialized layer of extracellular matrix materials, the basement membrane (see Fig. 4.11). Basement membrane contains a special form of matrix protein called Type IV collagen, which is synthesized by the epithelial cells.

By light microscopy, basement membrane is just visible as a linear structure at the base of epithelia. It can be stained with the PAS technique.

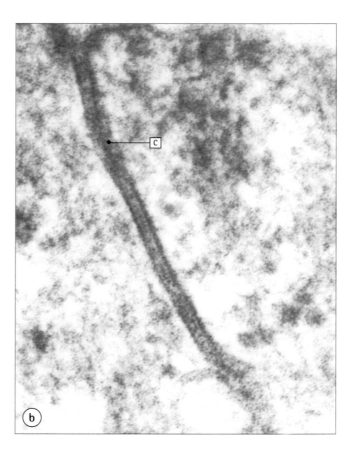

Fig. 3.14 Gap (communication) junction.

(a) Diagram showing a small part of a gap junction. Each junction is a circular patch studded with several hundred pores, each formed by six protein subunits traversing the cell membranes and termed a **connexon**. Pores on adjacent cells are aligned, allowing small molecules to move between cells.

(b) Ultrastructurally, a cross-section of a gap junction is seen as a flat area of closely apposing cell membranes, between which the connexons (C) can just be seen as dot-like granules.

EPITHELIAL CELL SURFACE SPECIALIZATIONS

The surface of epithelial cells can be adapted to allow a specialized function.

The surface of epithelial cells is highly developed to fulfill specialized functions:

- the main adaptation requirement is for increased surface area, which in different cell types is subserved by microvilli, basolateral folds and membrane plaques;
- the need to move substances over their surface is met by motile cell projections termed cilia.

Microvilli are surface specializations to increase the surface area of cells.

Microvilli are finger-like projections of the apical cell surface (Fig. 3.15). Small microvilli are found on the surface of most epithelial cells but are most developed in absorp-

tive cells, such as kidney tubule cells and small bowel epithelium. The shape of microvilli is maintained by a bundle of actin filaments, which form a core running through each villus; it is anchored to the actin cortex of the cell. In epithelial cells of the small bowel, the actin core is also linked to the actin network of adherent junctions between adjacent cells.

The cell membrane which covers microvilli bears specific cell surface glycoproteins and enzymes involved in the absorptive process. This cell surface specialization is just about visible ultrastructurally as a fuzzy coating, but is much more evident when enzyme histochemistry or immunohistochemistry is used to detect specific proteins, such as lactase and alkaline phosphatase (see Fig. 3.19).

Stereocilia are extremely long forms of microvilli and, despite their name, have nothing to do with true cilia (see page 41). They are found on epithelial cells lining the epididymis and are the sensors of cochlear hair cells (see Chapter 19).

Fig. 3.15 Microvilli.

(a) Each microvillus is a finger-like extension of cell membrane, which is stabilized by a bundle of actin filaments held rigidly 10 nm apart by actin-binding proteins. The actin bundle is bound to the lateral surface of the microvillus by a helical arrangement of myosin molecules, which bind on one side to the actin and on the other to the inner surface of the cell membrane. The bundle is also adherent to the apex of the microvillus in an amorphous area of anchoring proteins which may represent capping proteins for the actin filaments to prevent their depolymerization.

At the base of the microvillus the entering actin bundle is stabilized by the actin/spectrin cell cortex, under which are cytokeratin intermediate filaments.

(b) Electronmicrograph showing the surface of a cell lining the small bowel. Microvilli (M) form finger-like projections, each having an actin filament (AF) core that enters the cell and merges with the actin cortex (AC), which is also known as the terminal web.

Basolateral folds increase cell surface area.

Basolateral folds are deep invaginations of the basal or lateral surface of cells (Fig. 3.16).

Basal folds are particularly evident in cells involved in fluid or ion transport, and are commonly associated with high concentrations of mitochondria, which provide the energy for ion and fluid transport. The presence of basal folds and mitochondria imparts a striped appearance to the basal cytoplasm of such cells, giving rise to the descriptive term 'striated epithelial cells'.

Basal folds are seen in renal tubular cells (see Fig. 15.18) and in the ducts of many secretory glands.

Cell surface area can be similarly increased by folding of lateral cell membrane, which can be seen in some epithelial cells, particularly absorptive cells lining the gut.

Membrane plaques are a specialized structure seen in urothelium.

Membrane plaques are rigid areas of the apical cell membrane found only in epithelium lining the urinary tract. They can fold down into the cell when the bladder is empty and unfold to increase the luminal area of the cell when the bladder is full (see Fig. 15.39).

Fig. 3.16 Basal folds.

Electronmicrograph showing deep infolding of basal cell membrane (BF) of a distal tubule kidney cell. This facilitates cell membrane transport of ion by greatly increasing cell surface area.

Cilia are motile surface projections of cells involved in transport.

Cilia are hair-like projections, 0.25 μm in diameter, which arise from the surface of certain specialized cells and have a role in moving fluid over the surface of the cell or to confer cell motility.

Each cilium is a highly specialized extension of the cytoskeleton and is composed of an organized core of parallel microtubules (the axoneme). These microtubules are bound together with other proteins to produce energy-dependent movement of the filaments, which results in beating from side to side (Fig. 3.17).

Cilia are particularly evident in:
- epithelium lining the respiratory tract, where they move mucus over the cell surfaces (see Fig. 10.2);
- epithelium lining the fallopian tube, where they convey released ova to the uterine cavity (see Fig. 17.12).

A similar axonemal structure to that of cilia is found in the flagellum of spermatozoa (see Fig. 16.8).

Fig. 3.17 Cilia.

(a) Diagram of a cross-section of a cilium. The nine outer doublet tubules are made of tubulin, while arms composed of the protein dynein occur every 24 nm down the length of the cilium and interact with adjacent doublets as a 'molecular motor' to produce bending. Links composed of another protein, nexin, are more widely spaced (every 86 nm) and hold the microtubules in position. Radial spokes extend from each of the nine outer doublets toward a central pair of tubules at 29 nm intervals, while the central sheath projections are present every 14 nm.

(b) Ultrastructural appearance of a cilium in cross- section. Because the different constituent proteins are periodically spaced at different intervals along the length of the axoneme, not all are visible in any one plane of section.

(c) In longitudinal section, the base of each cilium (C) is seen to arise as a specialized derivative of the centriole (the basal body, BB). Here, the outer doublets of the cilium arise directly from the outer triplet of the centriole. (CM, cell membrane; Cy, cytoplasm.

(d) Micrograph of a ciliated epithelium. Cilia (C) form a hair-like layer at the apical cell surface. As they are very fragile they may not be well preserved in poorly fixed or processed tissue.

CILIAL DEFECTS AND DISEASE

Genetic defects in genes coding for ciliary proteins give rise to uncoordinated or absent ciliary beating in ciliated epithelia. This causes the **immotile cilia syndrome**.

Ultrastructurally, elements of the cilia may be absent or abnormal (Fig. 3.18).

There are several possible consequences of such abnormality:

- in embryogenesis the defective cilia are unable to move cell layers correctly and the major organs do not assume their normal anatomic positions, e.g. right-sided heart;
- development of air sinuses in the skull, which is dependent on normal cilial action, is impaired;
- failure of mucus removal from the lung results in recurrent and severe chest infections. Eventually, prolonged stagnation of secretions and recurrent bacterial infections lead to permanent dilation of the large air passages, which fill with stagnant infected secretions and lead to premature death;
- infertility is common because ovum transport along the fallopian tube depends on normal ciliary function, and ciliary proteins make up the motile tail of spermatozoa.

Fig. 3.18 Immotile cilia syndrome.
Electronmicrograph of cilia from a person with recurrent chest infections since childhood. The outer dynein arms are absent and there are abnormal single microtubules (M), which prevent normal motility. Compare with Fig. 3.17b.

Cell surface proteins can act as enzymes or adhesion molecules or be used for cell recognition.
The surface of epithelia is invested with a layer of protein, glycoprotein and sugar residues, which, in many cells, can be resolved ultrastructurally as an amorphous fuzzy coating to the cell membrane. By virtue of the sugar content it is stainable by techniques such as the PAS method (see page 6). This coat is the **glycocalyx**.

Enzyme histochemical and immunohistochemical methods can be used to detect specific enzymes in this surface coat (Fig. 3.19), and it is apparent that epithelial cells at different sites have different functional attributes in terms of enzyme activity despite similarities in their morphology.

Surface proteins are also used in a variety of cell recognition and adherence mechanisms, often of great importance to the function of the immune system.

SECRETORY ADAPTATIONS

Some organelles develop to adapt a cell for secretion of macromolecules.
Certain epithelial cells have structural specializations related to their role in the production and secretion of macromolecules, such as enzymes, mucins and steroids. In addition, epithelial cells can be adapted for the secretion and transport of ions. Such cells are characterized by an expansion of the specific organelle systems which are involved in the elaboration and secretion of the respective macromolecules (see pages 42-44).

Protein-secreting epithelial cells have large nuclei and abundant rough ER.
Although all cells contain the apparatus to produce structural proteins, certain cells are specialized to secrete a protein product and have the following characteristics:

Fig. 3.19 Small bowel alkaline phosphatase activity.
The localization of cell membrane-associated alkaline phosphatase on the surface of epithelial cells lining the small bowel is shown. Note that the enzyme activity (demonstrated as a red stain deposit) is confined to the apical surface of the cells.

- a well-developed rough ER, which often results in purple coloration of the cytoplasm in H&E stained sections (see plasma cell, Chapter 8);
- distinct polarity with basal rough ER, a supranuclear Golgi just visible as an ill-defined lucent area of the cytoplasm, and an apical zone containing granules filled with packaged protein ready for secretion by exocytosis.

The staining characteristics of the apical portion of the cells depend on the nature of this protein (Fig. 3.20).

Fig. 3.20 Protein–secreting epithelial cells.
The cells shown in this micrograph are from the pituitary gland and are producing different peptide hormones, which impart different staining characteristics to the cells (eosinophilic, E; pale staining, P).

Mucin-secreting epithelial cells have a greatly expanded Golgi system.

Mucins (mixtures of glycoproteins and proteoglycans) have important functions in body cavities, for example as a lubricant in the mouth and as a barrier in the stomach.

Cells which produce and secrete mucin (Fig. 3.21) are characterized by the following features:
- a well-developed basal rough ER makes the protein core of mucins and imparts a faint blue color to the basal cytoplasm;
- a well-developed supranuclear Golgi is the main site of protein glycosylation, but is not clearly visible by light microscopy;
- large secretory vesicles of mucin at the cell apex impart an unstained vacuolated appearance to the apical cell cytoplasm.

Mucin-secreting cells may be part of a surface epithelium, when they are termed goblet cells, for example in epithelia lining the gut (see Fig. 11.44) and respiratory tract. In addition, mucin-secreting cells can be aggregated into specialized glands, for example in the genital tract, respiratory tract and intestinal tract.

Steroid-secreting epithelial cells have an extensive smooth endoplasmic reticulum system.

Cells producing steroid hormones (Fig. 3.22) are mainly found in the adrenal gland, ovary and testis, and have the following characteristics:
- a well-developed smooth ER which gives the cytoplasm a granular pink appearance;
- free lipid (lipids are the precursors of the steroid hormones) in vacuoles in the cell cytoplasm, which

Fig. 3.21 Mucin–secreting epithelial cells.
(a) Micrograph of mucin-secreting surface epithelium showing the purple basal cytoplasm due to well-developed basal ER, and the unstained vacuolated appearance of the apical cytoplasm due to large secretory vesicles of mucin (MV).
(b) Micrograph of mucin-secreting epithelial cells aggregated into a gland.

imparts a fine vacuolated appearance to the cells;

- prominent mitochondria with tubular rather than flattened cristae. Mitochondria are involved in the biosynthesis of steroids from lipid, but the functional significance of the tubular shape of their cristae is not clear.

Ion-pumping epithelial cells have many mitochondria and a large surface area.

Cells in the kidney tubules and in the ducts of some secretory glands transport ions and water, while acid-producing

Fig. 3.22 Steroid-secreting epithelial cells.
According to their cytoplasmic composition, steroid-secreting cells vary in appearance in H&E stained sections from granular pink-staining cells, which contain many mitochondria and little lipid, to pale pink-staining and vacuolated cells, which contain abundant lipid and dilated smooth ER. The cells shown here are from the adrenal gland and have a pale and finely vacuolated appearance.

Fig. 3.23 Ion-pumping epithelial cells.
Micrograph of striated duct epithelial cells from salivary gland. Folding of the cell membrane (F) containing the active membrane protein produces a fine striped appearance, while the large numbers of mitochondria impart a granular pink-staining appearance to the basal part of the cell. Tight junctions are only visible ultrastructurally.

cells of the stomach transport H$^+$ ions (see Fig. 11.29). Ion transport is mediated by membrane ion pumps; these use ATP as a source of energy for the exchange of ions between cytosol and extracellular space.

The structural specializations of ion-pumping epithelial cells (Fig. 3.23) are as follows:

- the cell membrane is folded to increase the active surface area of membrane containing the membrane protein that acts as the ion pump;
- large numbers of mitochondria are closely apposed to the membrane folds to supply ATP;
- tight junctions between the cells prevent back diffusion of pumped ions.

In cells of the intestine, gall bladder and kidney, the ion pumps move sodium and water from the apical surface to be absorbed, while in secretory glands, the cells move ions and fluid out of the apex of the cell, resulting in secretion of watery fluid (e.g. sweat).

Epithelial secretion is divided into four types.

There are four mechanisms of secretion of cell product by epithelial cells: **merocrine**, **apocrine**, **holocrine** and **endocrine** (Fig. 3.24).

Secretions from the apex of the cell onto a surface or into a lumen are termed exocrine, while secretions from the side or base of the cell, which enter the bloodstream directly, are termed endocrine.

Epithelial cells are grouped into glands to allow focused production of a secreted product.

A gland is an organized collection of secretory epithelial cells. In many epithelia, secretion is performed only by occasional specialized cells (e.g. mucin-secreting goblet cells) scattered among other non-secretory cells (Fig. 3.25).

Fig. 3.24 Types of cell secretion.
Secretion of cell produce may occur by exocytosis from the cell apex into a lumen (**merocrine** secretion); pinching off of apical cell cytoplasm containing cell product (**apocrine** secretion); shedding of the whole cell containing the cell product (**holocrine** secretion); or endocytosis from the cell base into the blood stream (**endocrine** secretion, see Fig. 14.1).

Fig. 3.25 Secretory cells and glands.

(a) Diagram of secretory cells and glands.

(b) Single cells in a surface epithelium secreting mucin. These are called goblet cells (G).

(c) H&E stained section showing a straight tubular colonic gland, which is typical of glands in the gut. Secretory cells (S) line straight tubules and discharge their mucin secretions onto the surface.

(d) H&E stained section of a sweat gland from the skin showing the arrangement of a coiled tubular gland. Secretory cells are present in the distal part and there is zoning of secretory function, with an area of protein-secreting cells (P) being followed by an area of ion-pumping cells (I), which add fluid to the secretion in the lumen. The distal part of the gland, (D) has no secretory function, but is specialized for transporting secretions, having tight junctions to prevent back diffusion of ions; such tubules are termed ducts.

(e) H&E section of a branched gland showing the arrangement of secretory epithelial cells into acini (A), and main excretory duct (MD). The myoepithelial cells (see Fig. 5.12) are not readily visible at this low magnification.

When more secretions are required, the surface area of secretory epithelium can be increased by invagination of the surface to form straight tubular glands or by the formation of more complex coiled or branched glands, which may be divided into specialized zones for the secretion of different products .

The most structurally refined glands are those which have a branched architecture with secretory cells arranged in islands termed acini. Transport of secretion from this type of exocrine gland is via a series of ducts lined by columnar epithelium with apical junctional complexes to prevent escape of the secretions (Fig. 3.26).

While most glands form part of other tissues (e.g. mucous glands in the respiratory tract), many are anatomically distinct (e.g. salivary glands, pancreas, liver).

Gland secretions are under hormonal and innervatory control, and all glands have a rich vascular supply to provide the necessary metabolites.

Fig. 3.26 Gland duct.
Ducts carry exocrine secretion from a gland and discharge it onto an epithelial surface or into a body cavity. Ducts are lined by a tall columnar epithelium (E) and contain no specialized secretory cell. Note pink-stained secretion (S) in the lumen.

BARRIER FUNCTION OF EPITHELIUM

Many epithelia function as a barrier and this role is associated with certain specializations.

- occluding junctions prevent diffusion of molecules between cells and therefore prevent diffusion of substances from one side of an epithelium to the other;
- the apical cell membrane of epithelial cells lining the urinary tract (i.e. urothelial transitional epithelium) contains a high proportion of sphingolipids. These not only form membrane plaques (see page 40), but are also believed to resist fluid and electrolyte movements out of the cells in response to the osmotic effect of concentrated urine.
- desmosomal and hemidesmosomal junctions provide a tight mechanical linkage between cells and extracellular matrix to resist shearing forces, and allow an epithelium to function as a mechanical barrier.
- stratified squamous epithelial cells may undergo keratinization, a process in which the cytoskeleton of superficial cells of the epithelium becomes tightly condensed with other specialized proteins into a resilient mass. This results in cell death and the formation of a tough impervious and protective layer (keratin) from the remaining cell membranes and cytoplasmic contents (Fig. 3.27).

Keratinization ultimately transforms the cells into nonliving proteinaceous material which remains attached to underlying cells by existing anchoring junctions. The surface keratin layer is mechanically strong, but flexible; it is relatively inert and acts as a physical barrier, particularly preventing ingress of microorganisms. The intercellular phospholipid renders the epithelium impermeable to water.

Immunohistochemical techniques can identify epithelial cells and are useful in biopsy diagnosis of cancer.

Epithelial cells have the following characteristics detectable by immunohistochemical techniques (see page 8).

- expression of the cytokeratin class of intermediate filament proteins. This is not a feature of other classes of cells, for example support cells or lymphoid cells;

- expression of a class of cell surface glycoprotein (epithelial membrane antigen, EMA);

- possession of a specialized stainable epithelial product by some epithelia, for example prostate-specific antigen and prostate-specific acid phosphatase in the ducts and acini of the prostate gland, thyroglobulin in cells of the thyroid gland, and γγ-enolase in cells of neuroendocrine lineage.

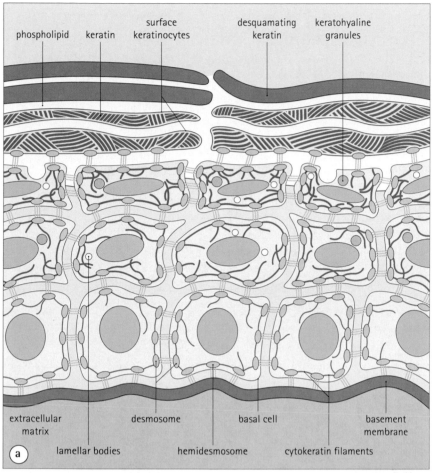

phospholipid · keratin · surface keratinocytes · desquamating keratin · keratohyaline granules

extracellular matrix · lamellar bodies · desmosome · hemidesmosome · basal cell · cytokeratin filaments · basement membrane

a

Fig. 3.27 Keratinization.

(a) Basal cells of keratinizing squamous epithelium are anchored by hemidesmosomes and desmosomes to basement membrane and adjacent cells, and contain abundant cytokeratin intermediate filaments (tonofibrils). As the cells differentiate and move up the stratified epithelium they remain tightly bound by desmosomal junctions, but the cytokeratin proteins change to higher molecular weight forms and the cells develop lamellar bodies. Lamellar bodies are membrane-bound granules containing phospholipids which are secreted by exocytosis into the extracellular space and form a lamellar sheet between cells in the upper epithelium. Cells in the upper part of the epithelium express genes coding for a variety of specialized proteins which interact with the cytokeratin filaments and the cell membrane to produce a resilient and mechanically robust compact mass (**keratin**). Small granules (**keratohyaline granules**) contain some of these specialized proteins. A prominent protein (**involucrin**) associates with and thickens the cell membrane.

b

(b) H&E section of keratinized squamous epithelium. Note the purplish keratohyaline granules (KHG) and the absence of nuclei in the surface keratin layer (K).

c

(c) Keratinizing squamous epithelium stained to show involucrin (brown), which is only present in the upper keratinizing part of the epithelium.

TUMORS OF EPITHELIAL CELLS

Cells may lose their normal growth control mechanisms and give rise to a tumor (neoplasm). Many such abnormal growths remain localized (benign neoplasms), but some invade adjacent tissues and metastasize to other parts of the body (malignant neoplasms).

A malignant neoplasm arising from squamous epithelial cells is termed a squamous carcinoma, while carcinoma derived from glandular epithelium is called an adenocarcinoma (Fig. 3.28).

In most cases, cells of a carcinoma resemble those of their tissue of origin. The diagnosis of malignancy is based on the presence of abnormal cytology (see page 32), and by locating cells that have invaded other tissues. In some cases, a carcinoma bears little resemblance to its cell of origin (undifferentiated carcinoma); such tumors commonly present with metastases and their site of origin may not be clear. In this situation it is essential to use immunohistochemistry and electron microscopy to confirm the diagnosis.

Fig. 3.28 Adenocarcinoma.
H&E section of colonic epithelium showing normal glandular epithelium (G) and carcinoma (C) forming gland-like structures (i.e. adenocarcinoma).

1. **THERE ARE SEVERAL DISTINCT FEATURES OF EPITHELIAL CELLS:**

   (a) squamous epithelial cells are flat and plate-like
   (b) a pseudostratified epithelium has all its cells in contact with the underlying extracellular matrix
   (c) a simple columnar cell is typically 2–3 times higher than its width
   (d) cell division occurs at all layers in a stratified squamous epithelium
   (e) transitional epithelium is a characteristic cell lining the urinary tract

2. **EPITHELIAL CELLS HAVE JUNCTIONS OF VARYING TYPES:**

   (a) occluding junctions prevent lateral diffusion of membrane proteins
   (b) adherent junctions interact with the actin filaments in cells
   (c) desmosomal junctions interact with the actin filaments in cells
   (d) hemidesmosomes anchor cells to basement membrane
   (e) gap junctions have a role in intercellular communication

3. **IN EPITHELIAL CELLS:**

   (a) microvilli are braced by the actin cytoskeleton
   (b) membrane plaques are a feature of transitional epithelium
   (c) cilia are based on the intermediate filaments
   (d) the glycocalyx is seen within the rough ER and stores lipids
   (e) the characteristic type of intermediate filament is cytokeratin

4. **EPITHELIAL CELLS HAVE A SECRETORY ROLE:**

   (a) endocrine secretion occurs when a cell enters the bloodstream
   (b) mucin-secreting cells have a well developed Golgi, this being the main site of protein glycosylation
   (c) ion-pumping cells have many lysosomes to export transported solutes
   (d) merocrine secretion occurs when a secreted product is exocytosed from the cell onto a surface or into a lumen
   (e) apocrine secretion occurs when the whole cell is shed as the secreted product

4. Support Cells and the Extracellular Matrix

INTRODUCTION

The cells which form tissues can be divided into two types: **parenchymal cells** which subserve the main function of a tissue; **support cells**, which provide the structural scaffolding of a tissue . Support cells comprise a set of highly developed cell types with complex metabolic functions and produce an extracellular matrix which largely defines the physical characteristics of a tissue.

Support cells and their associated extracellular matrix are commonly termed **connective tissue**. However we believe that this term does not emphasize the highly specialized nature of this class of tissues.

This chapter covers general characteristics and types of support cell, and describes the main components of the extracellular matrix materials which form the essential support scaffolding to tissues.

Support cells produce extracellular matrix materials, which are important for spatial organization and mechanical stability.

Support cells are vital in providing mechanical stability to tissues. These are included within the class of connective tissue cells. They have the following common characteristics:

- embryological derivation from mesenchyme (Fig. 4.1);
- production of a variety of extracellular matrix materials;
- when mature, formation of sparsely cellular tissues in which matrix is the main component;
- cell adhesion mechanisms that interact with extracellular matrix materials rather than other cells.

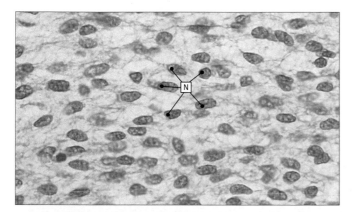

Fig. 4.1 Embryonic mesenchyme.
Mesenchyme is an embryonic tissue and may develop from any of the three germ layers. It is characterized by spindle-shaped cells with large nuclei (N), which develop into a variety of cell types in embryonic life, thus forming the family of support cells.

The support cells (see pages 57–63) are fibroblasts, chondrocytes, osteoblasts, myofibroblasts and adipocytes. Fibroblasts secrete extracellular matrix components in most tissues; chondrocytes secrete the extracellular matrix components of cartilage; and osteocytes secrete the extracellular matrix components of bone. Myofibroblasts secrete extracellular matrix components and also have a contractile function, and adipocytes store lipid.

In addition, support cells produce the specially organized extracellular matrix material that forms tissues such as the transparent cornea of the eye and tendons to anchor muscles to bone.

Adipocytes, the specially adapted lipid-storing support cells not only act as an energy store, but also have a cushioning and padding function.

EXTRACELLULAR MATRIX

The extracellular matrix is mainly composed of fibrillar proteins surrounded by glycosaminoglycans.

The extracellular matrix produced in most support cells is composed of two major materials: glycosaminoglycans (GAGs) and fibrillar proteins. In addition, there are small amounts of structural glycoprotein present in the extracellular matrix, with important roles in cell adhesion.

The general structure of support tissue is a scattered network of support cells producing an organized, abundant extracellular network of fibrillar proteins arranged in a hydrated gel of GAGs. Other cells (e.g. epithelial cells, contractile cells) are anchored to this tissue by cell matrix-anchoring junctions (see page 38).

Glycosaminoglycans are large polysaccharides which help give turgor and determine the diffusion of substances through extracellular matrix.

GAGs are large, unbranched polysaccharide chains composed of repeating disaccharide units (70–200 residues). They can be divided into four groups according to their structure: hyaluronic acid; chondroitin sulfate and dermatan sulfate; heparan sulfate and heparin; and keratan sulfate (Fig. 4.2). They form the hydrated gel matrix of support tissues, the properties of which are determined by their charge and spatial arrangement. There is great variability in GAG distribution in different tissues reflecting local requirements for specific pore sizes and charges in the extracellular matrix.

Many of the proteins which form the backbone of proteoglycans have been isolated and characterized.

Glycosaminoglycan	Sulfation	Protein-linked	Distribution
Hyaluronic acid	no	no	cartilage synovial fluid, skin, support tissue
Chondroitin sulfate	yes	yes	cartilage, bone, skin, support tissue
Dermatan sulfate	yes	yes	skin, blood vessels, heart
Heparan sulfate	yes	yes	basement membrane, lung arteries
Heparin	yes	yes	lung, liver, skin, mast cell granules
Keratan sulfate	yes	yes	cartilage, cornea, vertebral disk

Fig. 4.2 Glycosaminoglycans.
There are four main groups of glycosaminoglycans, which have different tissue distributions. Sulfation causes the molecules to be highly negatively charged and contributes to their ability to retain Na^+ ions and water. With the exception of hyaluronic acid, the glycosaminoglycans become linked to proteins to form proteoglycans. The presence of specific types of glycosaminoglycan in different tissues confers special attributes to the extracellular matrix, particularly with regard to diffusion or binding of other extracellular substances.

GAGs have the following properties:

A high negative charge because in all GAGs one of the repeating units is an amino sugar (N-acetylglucosamine or N-acetylgalactosamine), which is commonly sulfated (SO_3^-), and in most GAGs the second sugar is uronic acid with a carboxyl group (COO^-).

Strongly hydrophilic behavior because they cannot fold into compact structures and therefore have a large, permanently open coil conformation.

Retention of positive ions (e.g. Na^+) together with water, thereby maintaining tissue architecture by virtue of an inherent turgor which tends to prevent deformation by compressive forces.

With the exception of hyaluronic acid, covalent attachment to proteins to form proteoglycans, which are huge molecules capable of maintaining a large hydration space in the extracellular matrix. The spatial organization and charge of proteoglycans facilitate selective diffusion of different molecules probably by allowing variation in pore size of the matrix gel. This is particularly important in the basement membranes of the kidney glomerulus (see Fig. 15.7).

Fibrillar proteins determine the tensile properties of support tissues.

There are four major proteins that form fibrils in extracellular matrix:
- collagen;
- fibrillin;
- elastin;
- fibronectin.

The role of these fibrillar proteins is to provide different tensile properties to support tissues and provide anchorage for other cellular elements in tissues.

The collagens are a large family of proteins and comprise the most important fibrillar extracellular matrix components.

The collagens are a family of closely related proteins which can aggregate to produce either filaments, fibrils, or meshworks which then interact with other proteins to provide support in the extracellular matrix. There are at least 20 types of collagen polypeptide chains (α chains) produced from different genes which combine to produce different morphologic forms (Fig. 4.3). The collagens can be divided into several families according to the types of structure they form:
- **fibrillar collagens**: types I, II, III, V, XI;
- **facit collagens** (fibril-associated collagen with interrupted triple helix): types IX, XII, XIV;
- **short chain collagens**: types VIII, X;
- **basement membrane collagens**: type IV;
- **other collagens**: types VI, VII, XIII.

Collagen types I, II and III are arranged as rope-like fibrils and are the main forms of fibrillar collagen.

Collagen fibers (type I collagen) resist tensile stresses in tissues, thus their orientation and cross-linking vary according to the local environment. In histologic preparations, collagen fibers appear as pink-staining material and have a dominant role in providing tensile strength to tissues (Fig. 4.4).

Reticular fibers (also called reticulin) are thin fibrils (about 20 nm in diameter) of type III collagen (Fig. 4.5). They form a loose mesh in many support tissues and are particularly evident in a zone beneath basement membranes, where they are thought to have a support function as part of the fibroreticular lamina (see Fig. 4.11c).

Reticular fibers can be considered as a fine scaffolding supporting specialized extracellular matrix components. In lymph nodes, spleen and bone marrow, reticular fibers form the main extracellular matrix fibers supporting the hemopoietic and lymphoid tissues. In parenchymal organs, such as the liver and kidney, reticular fibers form a network supporting specialized epithelial cells.

Type IV collagen assembles into a meshwork rather than fibrils and is restricted to basement membrane formation (see page 55).

Type VII collagen forms the anchoring fibrils of some basement membranes.

Type VIII collagen forms a hexagonal lattice in Descemet's membrane in the cornea of the eye.

Although collagen is mainly produced by fibroblasts (see page 57), it can be produced by other mesenchyme-derived cells of the support cell family, as well as by a variety of epithelial and endothelial cells which produce the type IV collagen of basement membranes. Collagen fibers are constructed of precursor proteins (α chains)

Fig. 4.4 Collagen fibers.
In H&E stained preparations collagen fibers appear as pink-stained material, which is often difficult to delineate from other structures that stain equally pink (e.g. support cells, walls of blood vessels). Special stains can be used to stain collagen (see Fig. 4.13). Immunohistochemical staining can also be performed for different molecular types of collagen, but is seldom used in the routine examination of tissues.

Fig. 4.5 Reticular fibers.
Reticular fibers cannot be seen in H&E sections, but can be stained by silver impregnation methods. In this micrograph, reticular fibers in a lymph node are seen as fine black lines, with lymphoid cells stained red in the background (V, vessel).

Type	I	II	III	IV	V	VI	VII	VIII	IX	X	XI
Morphology	large banded collagen fiber	small banded collagen fiber	small banded collagen fiber	sheet-like layers	thin fibrils	thin fibrils	short striated fibrils	chains and lattices	fibril	short chain	fibril
Distribution	skin dermis, tendon, bone, ligaments, fascia, fibrous cartilage, cornea, loose fibrous tissue	hyaline and elastic cartilage, vertebral disks, vitreous of eye	blood vessels parenchymal organs, bone marrow, lymphoid tissues, smooth muscle, nerves, lung, fetal skin	basement membranes, external laminae, lens capsule	basement membrane of placenta, smooth and skeletal muscle	ubiquitous	anchoring fibrils in basement membrane of skin and amnion	endothelium	cartilage	mineralizing cartilage	cartilage

Fig. 4.3 Molecular forms of collagen.

Fig. 4.6 Fibrillar collagen.

(a) Fibrillar collagen is formed from three polypeptide (α) chains, which are initially secreted with both amino and carboxyl terminal extensions to prevent collagen forming inside cells. Initial assembly of these chains is into a triple helix (**procollagen**).

(b) Cleavage of the amino and carboxyl extensions to leave the functional mid domains (**tropocollagen**) allows the molecules to align themselves into linear arrays to form long filaments. The individual collagen molecules are 300 nm long, and are arranged with a 67 nm overlap between adjacent molecules. This gives rise to a periodicity of 67 nm.

(c) Electronmicrograph of collagen showing the periodicity of 67 nm.

(d) Electronmicrograph of collagen in transverse section.

(e) The initial filaments (collagen **microfibrils**) become arranged into **fibers**, and the fibers into larger **bundles** by tight cross-linking between adjacent molecules via lysine residues; this contributes to the mechanical strength of collagen fibers in tissues.

wound together to form rigid linear triple helix structures which are then secreted by fibroblasts. After proteolytic cleavage, the triple helical portions are assembled into long filaments and incorporated into cross-linked fibers and bundles (Fig. 4.6)

DISEASES DUE TO DISORDERS OF COLLAGEN

There are many inherited diseases caused by mutations in genes coding for collagen. The main effect is reduced tensile strength in support tissues, leading to abnormal tissue laxity or susceptibility to injury.

Important types of disease:

OSTEOGENESIS IMPERFECTA is a syndrome in which defective collagen formation is caused by genetic abnormalities and leads to abnormally fragile bones. Individuals affected by this disease suffer repeated fractures after relatively minor trauma. There are several genetic subtypes of disease, although most cases are due to point mutations in genes coding for type I collagen.

EHLERS–DANLOS SYNDROMES are characterized by abnormally extensible skin and joint laxity leading to recurrent dislocations. There are several genetic subtypes of disease. However, in some individuals this phenotype is due to mutations in genes for type I collagen.

Elastin is a protein which assembles into stretchable and resilient fibers and sheets.

Elastin is a hydrophobic protein which assembles into filaments and sheets by cross-linking (Fig. 4.7) and is the main component of elastic fibers. Like collagen, elastin is produced by fibroblasts.

Elastic fibers are formed by the interaction of elastin and fibrillin. The fibrillin microfibrils appear to organize secreted elastin so that it is deposited between the microfibrils to form distinct elastic fibers (Fig. 4.8). As their name implies, they confer elasticity to tissues and allow them to recoil after stretching. Elastic fibers are important constituents of many support tissues.

Fig. 4.7 Elastin.
(a) Elastin has a random coil structure in the relaxed state that can stretch, but reforms as a different random coil on relaxation.
(b) Elastin molecules are covalently linked into arrays which can reversibly stretch and recoil, and may be arranged as fibers or sheets.

Fig. 4.8 Elastic fiber.
(a) Elastic fibers are composed of glycoprotein microfilaments (fibrillin) surrounding and organizing a core region of cross-linked elastin.
(b) Ultrastructurally, the elastin core appears as an electron-dense area (E) with microfilaments (M) arranged peripherally. The microfilaments are prominent in early formed elastic tissue, and decrease in number with aging.

(c) In H&E stained tissues, elastic fibers (E) stand out as glassy bright pink-stained structures, taking up acidic dyes such as eosin with much greater avidity than collagen fibers. (F, fibroblast).
(d) Elastic fibers can be stained by special techniques. In this example, elastic fibers (E) in the dermis of the skin are stained blue by toluidine blue and contrast with the pale-staining collagen (C).

Microfibrils contain fibrillin and are important components of elastic fibers.

Fibrillin, a recently characterized fibril-forming glycoprotein, is the main component of extracellular microfibrils. Microfibrils, 8–12 nm in diameter, are one constituent of elastic fibers (see Fig. 4.8). They are also found in the extracellular matrix of renal glomeruli (mesangium) and the suspensory fibers of the lens.

Microfibrils are prominent in elastic-containing extracellular matrix, particularly in lung, skin and blood vessel walls. The microfibrils are believed to mediate adhesion between different components of the extracellular matrix.

MUTATIONS IN GENES FOR FIBRILLIN CAUSE MARFAN'S SYNDROME

People who have Marfan's syndrome are unusually tall, have a very wide arm span, are prone to develop subluxation of the lens and are also prone to develop rupture of the aorta.

The abnormality in this condition has been associated with absence of fibrillin which interacts with elastin in tissues. It is easy to understand why the lens dislocates, as its suspensory fibers normally contain fibrillin. It is also easy to understand how a lack of elastic recoil in the aorta would weaken the wall and predispose to rupture. It is assumed that the growth of long bones is somehow constrained by the presence of fibrillin, and hence bones grow longer in its absence.

Fibronectin mediates adhesion between a wide range of cells and extracellular matrix components.

Fibronectin is a multifunctional glycoprotein and exists in three main forms. These are:

- a circulating plasma protein;
- a protein that transiently attaches to the surface of many cells;
- insoluble fibrils forming part of the extracellular matrix, when fibronectin dimers cross-link to each other by disulfide bonds.

The functional importance of fibronectin stems from its ability to adhere to several different tissue components because it possesses sites which bind collagen and heparin, as well as cell adhesion molecules.

Fibronectin is recognized by fibronectin receptor proteins in cell membranes, allowing cell adhesion to extracellular matrix. Such a fibronectin receptor is one of the class of cell surface receptors called integrins (Fig. 4.9). When tissues grow, fibronectin binds to cell surfaces via integrins and is thought to have an important role in organizing the subsequent deposition and orientation of early collagen fibrils through its collagen attachment sites.

Because fibronectin receptors are linked to intracellular actin, the orientation of the internal cytoskeleton of a cell influences the orientation of the extracellular matrix.

Extracellular structural glycoproteins.

Several non-filamentous proteins mediate interaction between cells and extracellular matrix and interact with specific receptors on the cell surface. The distribution of such proteins varies between different tissues. The best characterized of these proteins are laminin, tenascin and entactin.

Laminin, a sulfated glycoprotein, is a major component of basement membranes. It is produced by most epithelial and endothelial cells, and is a cross-shaped molecule with binding sites for specific cell receptors (integrins) (Fig. 4.9), heparan sulfate, type IV collagen, and entactin (see below). The multiple binding ligands for laminin make it a major extracellular link molecule between cells and extracellular matrix. There are several forms specific to different tissues.

Entactin is a sulfated glycoprotein that is a component of all basement membranes and binds with laminin. It is thought to function as a link protein binding laminin to type IV collagen.

Tenascin, an extracellular glycoprotein involved in cell adhesion, is particularly expressed in embryonic tissue and thought to be important to cell migration in the developing nervous system.

BASEMENT MEMBRANE

Basement membranes are specialized sheets of extracellular matrix which lie between parenchymal cells and support tissues

Basement membranes are specialized sheet-like arrangements of extracellular matrix proteins and GAGs, and act as an interface between parenchymal cells and support tissues.

They are associated with epithelial cells, muscle cells and Schwann cells, and also form a limiting membrane around the central nervous system.

Basement membranes have five major components: type IV collagen (Fig. 4.10), laminin, heparan sulfate, entactin, and fibronectin. With the exception of fibronectin, these are synthesized by the parenchymal cells. In addition, there are numerous minor and poorly characterized protein and GAG components.

The general structure of basement membrane has been well characterized (Fig. 4.11). Superimposed on this, minor protein and carbohydrate components are specific to certain tissues. Thus, for example, the renal basement membrane differs from that of the skin.

Fig. 4.9 Integrins.

Integrins are a class of cell adhesion molecule, 16 have been functionally characterized. They comprise two protein subunits.

The **fibronectin receptor** shown in the diagram is the best characterized of the integrin family, possessing a cytosolic domain binding to actin (via talin, and a recently described protein termed fibulin), a transmembrane domain, and extracellular domains binding to fibronectin. Thus, this molecule links the intracellular actin network with extracellular matrix at focal contacts (see Fig. 3.10). The laminin receptor also belongs to the integrin family.

Integrins may bind to other cell surface proteins, thus acting as intercellular adhesion molecules. In addition, some integrins bind to extracellular matrix components and allow cell–matrix adhesion, the main extracellular matrix ligands being fibronectin, laminin, collagens, tenascin and thrombospondin.

Fig. 4.10 Basement membrane.

The basement membrane can be demonstrated by immunostaining for constituent proteins such as laminin (4.10a) and type IV collagen (4.10b).

Fig. 4.11 Basement membrane.

(a) H&E preparations fail to show distinct basement membrane because it is only 0.05μm thick and stains poorly; however, a high content of glycoprotein renders it stainable with PAS, when it appears as a faint magenta-stained line (BM).

Specific components of basement membrane can be detected with immunohistochemical staining, for example laminin and type IV collagen.

(b) By electron microscopy, basement membrane resolves into several layers (**laminae**). The **lamina densa** (D) is a dark-staining band 30–100 nm thick. Between this and the attached cell (C) is a lucent zone, the **lamina lucida** (L), which is usually 60 nm wide. On the other side of the lamina densa is a rarefied layer of variable thickness, **the fibroreticular lamina FR**, which merges

with fibrous proteins of the extracellular matrix. The structure seen by light microscopy with PAS and silver stains and referred to as basement membrane, is a combination of all these laminae, but particularly the fibroreticular lamina. The term **basal lamina** strictly should refer to the lamina densa as an ultrastructural feature. However, with the detection of specific basal lamina components by light microscopy using immunohistochemistry the terms basement membrane and basal lamina are commonly used interchangeably.

(c) The fibroreticular lamina anchors basement membrane to adjacent extracellular matrix by three main mechanisms, which vary according to site and are illustrated in this diagram.

The main functions of basement membrane are cell adhesion, diffusion barrier and regulation of cell growth.

Basement membrane has three main functions.

First, it forms an adhesion interface between parenchymal cells and underlying extracellular matrix, the cells having adhesion mechanisms to anchor them to basement membrane, while basement membrane is tightly anchored to the extracellular matrix of support tissues, particularly collagen. Where such an interface occurs in non-epithelial tissues, for example around muscle cells, it is referred to as an **external lamina**.

Second, the basement membrane acts as a molecular sieve (permeability barrier) with pore size depending on the charge and spatial arrangement of its component GAGs. Thus basement membrane of blood vessels prevents large proteins leaking into the tissues, that of the kidney prevents protein loss from filtered blood during urine production, and that of the lung permits gaseous diffusion.

Third, basement membrane probably controls cell organization and differentiation by the mutual interaction of cell surface receptors and molecules in the extracellular matrix. These interactions are the subject of intense research, particularly in the investigation of mechanisms that might prevent the spread and proliferation of cancer cells throughout the body.

CELL ADHESION TO EXTRACELLULAR MATRIX

Adhesion of cells to the extracellular matrix is mediated by four main types of junction.

The organization of cells into functional tissues and organs depends on the support functions of the extracellular matrix and the cells that produce it. While various types of intercellular junction tie cells together (see pages 36-37), the junctions between cells and the extracellular matrix are equally important in maintaining structural integrity.

Junctions between cells and extracellular matrix include the following:

- hemidesmosomes (see Fig. 3.12) – anchor the intermediate filament cytoskeleton of cells to basement membrane;
- focal contacts (see Fig. 3.10) – anchor the actin cytoskeleton to basement membrane. The interaction is mediated through the fibronectin receptor (see Fig. 4.9).
- laminin receptors (see Fig. 4.9) – anchor cells to basement membrane where laminin is a major component;

- non-integrin glycoproteins (possessed by many cells) – bind to collagen and other cell matrix components.

SUPPORT CELL FAMILY

Support cells derive from embryonic mesenchyme.

During embryogenesis, a proportion of developing mesenchymal spindle-shaped cells differentiate into the following types of support cells: fibroblasts, myofibroblasts, lipoblasts, osteoblasts and chondroblasts.

The addition of 'blast' to the root name of a support cell indicates that the cell is actively growing or secreting extracellular matrix material. Support cells in a quiescent phase in tissues are indicated by the use of the suffix 'cyte' (e.g. fibrocyte, osteocyte, chondrocyte).

Fibroblasts and fibrocytes populate fibrocollagenous tissue, which is the most important of the support tissues.

Fibroblasts (Fig. 4.12) produce fibrocollagenous (fibrous) tissue, which is composed mainly of collagen fibers associated with GAGs, elastic fibers and reticular fibers (Fig. 4.13). Fibrocollagenous tissue is described as loose when collagen fibers are thin, haphazardly arranged and widely spaced, or dense when collagen fibers are broad and virtually confluent. The degree of organization and collagen orientation varies from site to site according to local tissue stresses. Highly organized dense fibrocollagenous tissue forms tendons and ligaments.

Fibrocollagenous tissue is the major support tissue in most organs, and has the following specific functions:

- support of nerves, blood vessels and lymphatics; vessels and nerves are a conspicuous feature, particularly in loose fibrocollagenous support tissue;
- separation of functional layers in organs and tissues (e.g. separation of mucosa from underlying tissues). its loose arrangement and variable elastic content allow mobility and stretching;
- support for transient and resident immune cell populations (i.e. macrophages, lymphocytes, plasma cells, mast cells);
- formation of fibrous capsule, which surrounds most parenchymal organs, such as the liver, spleen and kidneys;
- formation of fibroadipose tissue, which is a component of most tissues, by enclosing and blending with adipocytes.

Fibroblasts are extremely robust cells, and resist damaging stimuli that kill most other cell types, such as nerves, epithelial cells or muscle. They are important in tissue repair (see page 64).

Myofibroblasts have features which overlap between fibroblasts and smooth muscle cells.

Myofibroblasts resemble fibroblasts by light microscopy, but ultrastructurally contain aggregates of actin fibers associated with myosin to subserve a contractile function (see page 75). In this respect they resemble smooth muscle cells, discussed later on page 72. They are not prominent in support tissues, being found only in small numbers, and identifiable by immunohistochemical or ultrastructural methods.

Myofibroblasts develop during repair after tissue damage, and may originate either by proliferation of the normally inconspicuous tissue myofibroblasts, or possibly by differentiation of fibrocytes. They produce collagen and their contractile properties contribute to retraction and shrinkage of early fibrocollagenous scar tissue.

Fig. 4.12 Fibroblasts and fibrocytes.

(a) In the embryo, collagen-secreting cells develop from mesenchyme and appear as plump spindle shaped cells separated by early secreted collagen (C), which stains pink in H&E preparations.

(b) In the adult, active collagen-secreting cells are called fibroblasts and are characterized by a large oval nucleus and large nucleolus, a tapering bipolar spindle-shaped morphology with small additional cell processes and basophilic cytoplasm reflecting active protein synthesis.

(c) Once collagen secretion has stopped the fibroblasts lose their voluminous basophilic cytoplasm and the nucleus shrinks, reflecting non-transcription of DNA. The cells are now called fibrocytes to indicate this inactivity.

(d) Ultrastructurally, fibroblasts have a well-developed rough endoplasmic reticulum (RER), Golgi and secretory vesicles, reflecting active collagen secretion. Mitochondria (M) are numerous. Collagen fibers (C) are visible adjacent to the cells. Fibroblasts also secrete elastic and reticular fibers, and when they form reticular fibers in lymphoid tissue and bone marrow, they have a highly branched stellate shape and are often called reticulum cells.

Fig. 4.13 Fibrocollagenous (fibrous) tissue.

(a) Fibrocollagenous tissue contains many extracellular matrix components, with collagen fibers being predominant. Only collagen (C) is evident in H&E sections, staining light pink. Fibroblasts (F) are widely scattered and inconspicuous. Immune cells (i.e. lymphocytes [L], plasma cells, macrophages, mast cells) are occasionally found.

(b) The collagen fibers (C) in loose fibrocollagenous tissue can be stained by dyes with affinity for collagen (e.g. Van Gieson, shown here). The bundles are haphazardly arranged and of varying thickness.

(c) In most loose fibrocollagenous tissues elastic fibers are present, but are usually inconspicuous in H&E preparations. They are revealed by special stains (elastic stain) as wavy black-staining fibers (E), which contrast with the orange-stained collagen (C). Elastic fibers form a minor and variable component of most fibrocollagenous tissues.

(d) Stains for the GAG component of fibrocollagenous tissue reveal that the unstained areas of the H&E preparations are rich in this extracellular material (seen here stained blue with Alcian blue stain). (C, collagen). In contrast with loose fibrocollagenous tissue, dense irregular fibrocollagenous tissue has little space for GAGs and appears uniformly pink with few architectural features. Collagen-secreting fibroblasts are widely spaced and inconspicuous.

Chondroblasts and chondrocytes form cartilage which is closely associated with bone.

Chondroblasts elaborate a special support tissue called cartilage which is composed mainly of GAGs associated with collagen fibers. Developing from embryonic mesenchyme, chondroblasts first appear as clusters of vacuolated cells with a rounded morphology. These contrast with the spindle-shaped cells of surrounding undifferentiated mesenchyme, which develop into fibroblasts and form a confining sheet of cells termed the **perichondrium**.

Chondroblasts contain abundant glycogen and lipid and their active synthesis of extracellular matrix proteins is indicated by their basophilic cytoplasm, which is due to a high content of rough endoplasmic reticulum (Fig. 4.14a).

Growth of cartilage results from proliferation of chondroblasts within established matrix (interstitial growth) and also by development of new chondroblasts from the perichondrium (appositional growth). After depositing cartilage matrix, chondroblasts become less metabolically active and have small nuclei with pale, indistinct cytoplasm (i.e. they become chondrocytes, Fig. 4.14b).

Fig. 4.14 Chondroblasts and chondrocytes.
(a) Chondroblasts are metabolically active and have large vesicular nuclei with prominent nucleoli. Their cytoplasm is pale and vacuolated because of a high lipid and glycogen content, and tends to draw away from the extracellular matrix when fixed and embedded in paraffin, forming a space called a lacuna (L).
(b) Chondrocytes are smaller than chondroblasts, with densely staining nuclei and less cytoplasm, reflecting their low level of metabolic activity.

Cartilage has two main extracellular components:

• fibrous proteins (predominantly type II collagen), which confer mechanical stability;

• abundant GAGs, which resist deformation by compressive forces.

The collagen fibers are thin and arranged in an interwoven lattice, which merges into the extracellular matrix of adjacent support tissues. The major GAGs are hyaluronic acid, chondroitin sulfate and keratan sulfate which are bound to a core protein called aggrecan to form a large proteoglycan. These are attached to the collagen lattice by so-called link protein.

Because of its high content of sulfated GAGs cartilage stains with basic dyes such as hematoxylin, which gives it a slightly blue color in H&E preparations; this is particularly evident around the chondrocytes.

The arrangement of extracellular matrix in cartilage confers important properties:

• the tightly bound proteoglycans form a hydrated matrix with an inherent turgor that resists deformation by compressive forces;

• small molecules can diffuse freely through the extracellular matrix.

Classification of cartilage on the content of specific fibrous proteins.

The three types of cartilage – hyaline cartilage, fibrocartilage and elastic cartilage – are distinguished by their fibrous protein content. Hyaline cartilage contains type II collagen only (Fig. 4.15). It forms the temporary skeleton in fetal development until it is replaced by bone, the growing point in long bones in childhood, the articular surface in joints (see Chapter 13), and acts as a support tissue in the respiratory passages (see Fig. 10.8).

Fibrocartilage contains both type II and type I collagen (Fig. 4.16), and is a component of intervertebral discs, tendon attachments to bones, and the junctions between the flat bones of the pelvis. Elastic cartilage contains elastic fibers in addition to type II collagen (Fig. 4.17). It is located in the auricle of the ear, the walls of the external auditory canal and Eustachian tubes (see Chapter 13), and in the epiglottis of the larynx (See Fig. 10.6).

Osteoblasts and osteocytes form bone which contains an extracellular matrix material termed osteoid.

Osteoblasts elaborate the support matrix of bone, osteoid, which subsequently calcifies to form bone.

Osteoid is composed mainly of type I collagen, which is associated with the extracellular GAGs, chondroitin sulfate and keratan sulfate. Two glycoproteins, sialoprotein and osteocalcin, are mainly found in the bone matrix and bind calcium, hence they may have a role in bone mineralization. The cytology and structure of bone and its matrix are discussed in Chapter 13.

Fig. 4.15 Hyaline cartilage.

This hyaline cartilage is from a child and therefore in a state of growth. The perichondrium (P) is a layer of spindle-shaped fibroblasts with associated type I collagen, which merges with the outer layer of the pink-staining extracellular matrix of the hyaline cartilage. New chondroblasts develop from the perichondrium and allow appositional growth.

The chondroblasts show artifactual vacuolation, forming the characteristic lacunae around the cell bodies. Many in this sample are in small clusters (C), which will eventually move apart as the cells secrete extracellular matrix material during interstitial growth.

Hyaline cartilage is associated with perichondrium in most sites except where it lines joints.

Fig. 4.16 Fibrocartilage.

(a) In this H&E section of fibrocartilage, small inactive chondrocytes are dispersed in a pink-stained extracellular matrix in which coarse collagen fibers (C) are visible. These are type I collagen fibers, and merge with the type I collagen fibers in surrounding fibrocollagenous support tissue.

(b) The presence of type I collagen is highlighted in this Van Gieson stained section of fibrocartilage in which it stains red.

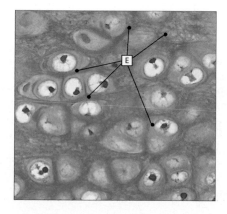

Fig. 4.17 Elastic cartilage.

The structural arrangement of elastic cartilage is similar to that of hyaline cartilage, with a perichondrial layer and chondrocytes set in an extracellular matrix, but differs because it contains elastic fibers.

These appear as bright pink-staining linear bundles running between cells (E), and confer great resilience and elastic recoil in the cartilage. The elastic fibers can be highlighted with special staining methods.

Adipose tissue stores fat and has a role in heat regulation in the young.

Adipocytes are characterized by their intracellular storage of fat. There are two types of fat-storing tissue, unilocular and multilocular adipose tissue.

Unilocular adipose tissue ('white fat') develops from embryonic mesenchyme with the formation of spindle-shaped cells (lipoblasts) containing small fat vacuoles (Fig. 4.18). These mature into adipocytes, storing fat which is used as a source of energy by other body tissues (Fig. 4.19).

Ultrastructurally, adipocytes have prominent smooth endoplasmic reticulum and numerous pinocytotic vesicles, these being involved in lipid biosynthesis and transport. Each cell is surrounded by an external lamina and there is an extracellular matrix composed of reticular fibers (type III collagen).

Multilocular adipose tissue 'brown fat' is most prominent in the newborn, its development in the fetus being separate from that of unilocular adipose tissue. Its function is to metabolize fat to produce heat in the neonatal period (Fig. 4.20).

Ultrastructurally, multilocular adipose cells contain huge numbers of mitochondria in addition to lipid vacuoles; this correlates with their function of heat generation through mitochondrial metabolism of fatty acids.

The high mitochondrial density is responsible for both the eosinophilia seen histologically and the brown color seen macroscopically, which gives this tissue its alternative name of 'brown fat'. Multilocular adipose tissue does not usually persist in adult life: it becomes lost during childhood, although small amounts may remain in certain sites (Fig. 4.21).

Fig. 4.18 Lipoblasts.

(a) In the fetus, the first indication of differentiation into a fat-storing cell is when the spindle-shaped mesenchymal cells (M) accumulate fat in their cytoplasm in multiple small vacuoles (V).

(b) The vacuoles fuse to form a larger perinuclear vacuole and the cell is recognized as a maturing lipoblast (L), losing its spindle shape. With increased fat storage the cytoplasm becomes attenuated around a single huge lipid vacuole and the nucleus is displaced to one side.

Each developing lipoblast produces extracellular matrix material and a basement membrane forms around each cell.

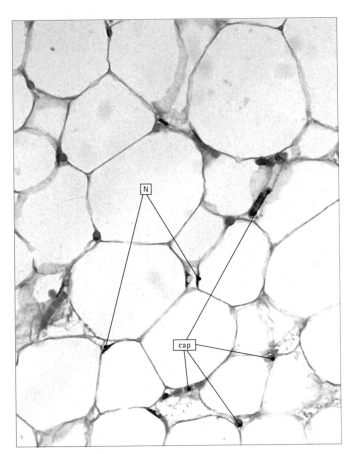

Fig. 4.19 Unilocular adipose tissue.

Unilocular (white) adipose tissue cells (adipocytes) are 50—150 μm in size and polyhedral in shape.

In H&E-stained preparations, as here, they appear as stringy wisps of cytoplasm surrounding an empty vacuole because embedding in wax involves immersion in lipid solvents which remove all of the fat. Close examination reveals inconspicuous flattened nuclei (N) to one side of the cells.

Numerous fine arborizing capillary vessels (cap) transfer metabolites to and from the cells.

Unilocular adipose tissue is the main form of fat-storing cell in the adult, and is adapted as a support tissue and as an energy store by means of:

- receptors for growth hormone, insulin, glucocorticoids, thyroid hormones and norepinephrine (noradrenalin) that modulate the uptake and release of fat;

- a rich capillary blood supply and innervation by the autonomic nervous system. Local release of norepinephrine stimulates the release of stored fat into the blood;

- organization into pads by sheets of fibrocollagenous tissue at certain sites to act as deformable shock-absorbing support tissues, particularly in the soles of the feet, the buttocks, around the kidneys and in the orbit around the eye.

Fig. 4.20 Multilocular adipose tissue.
Multilocular adipose tissue is so-termed because cells contain multiple small lipid droplets. It develops as a cluster of plump eosinophilic cells differentiating from fetal mesenchyme, and has a restricted distribution, being concentrated in support tissues in the neck, shoulders, back, perirenal and para-aortic regions.

As shown in this micrograph, two populations of cells can be seen: lipid-rich cells (L) with a central nucleus and multiple small unstained vacuoles, and polyhedral-shaped cells (P) with a granular, pink-stained cytoplasm, a central nucleus and only occasional lipid vacuoles.

A capillary vascular supply together with thin fibrocollagenous septa divide the tissue into small lobules.

Fig. 4.21 Mixture of unilocular and multilocular adipose tissue.
Certain adipose tissue, particularly in the subcutaneous tissue over the back and shoulders, contains a mixture of both unilocular (U) and multilocular (M) adipose tissue.

TISSUE DAMAGE IS REPAIRED BY PROLIFERATION OF SUPPORT CELLS AND SECRETION OF MATRIX TO FORM SCAR TISSUE

Following tissue damage (e.g. by infection), the loss of specialized cells can be rectified by regrowth only if the architecture of the support tissues (particularly basement membrane) is preserved; for example, epithelial cells lining the lung can regrow following some types of pneumonia.

If damage has been severe and the specialized support tissue architecture is destroyed, such regrowth is usually not possible, and the area of dead tissue is repaired by means of the growth of non-specialized support tissue which forms a fibrous scar.

Chemical mediators produced by damaged tissue attract phagocytic cells, such as neutrophils and monocytes (see Chapter 7) from the blood into the tissue. These cells ingest the dead cells, while inactive support cells, particularly fibroblasts, are stimulated to proliferate by the secretion of growth factors (e.g. platelet-derived growth factors and fibroblast growth factor).

The stimulated support cells are multipotential, and can differentiate into endothelial cells, myofibroblasts and fibroblasts, the damaged area being replaced by a mixture of these cell types which form new blood vessels and lay down collagen. The resulting fibrocollagenous tissue is termed a **fibrous scar**.

During this process of healing by fibrous repair, which is one of the basic responses to cell death in most body tissues, active fibroblasts assume a multipotential role and behave in a similar manner to the primitive mesenchyme from which they were derived, by differentiating into a variety of cell types.

This ability to transform into a variety of cell types in adult life to facilitate healing and repair is an important attribute of the support cell family.

1. COLLAGEN

(a) type I is the main collagen in skin
(b) type IV is the main type in bone
(c) type III is the main type in reticulin
(d) is secreted by fibroblasts as procollagen molecules.
(e) is one of the matrix components of osteoid.

2. GLYCOSAMINOGLYCANS

(a) are composed of repeating sugar residues.
(b) are weakly hydrophilic
(c) may be attached to proteins to form proteoglycans
(d) include hyaluronic acid, dermatan sulfate, heparin and fibronectin
(e) have a very dense folded structure which gives turgor to the tissue extracellular matrix

3. BASEMENT MEMBRANE

(a) contains type I collagen
(b) contains laminin
(c) contains glycosaminoglycans
(d) links to epithelial cells via integrin receptors
(e) acts as a permeability barrier.

4. THERE ARE SEVERAL TYPES OF SUPPORT TISSUE

(a) fibrocollagenous tissue is the major support tissue in most organs.
(b) chondroblasts elaborate the specialized extracellular matrix of cartilage.
(c) hyaline cartilage contains type II collagen and forms the main component of the auricle of the ear.
(d) unilocular adipose tissue produces heat in the neonatal period.
(e) following severe tissue damage, fibrocollagenous tissue is formed in healing to produce a fibrous scar.

5. Contractile Cells

INTRODUCTION

Several cell types are specialized to generate motile forces through contraction. This chapter presents an overview of the main types of contractile cell. The general structure of each type of cell is described together with details of their fine structure and how this relates to the molecular basis of contraction.

There are four main groups of contractile cells.

Contractile cells are specially adapted to generate motile forces by the interaction of the proteins actin and myosin (contractile proteins).

There are four groups of contractile cell: muscle cells, myoepithelial cells, myofibroblasts and pericytes. Muscle cells are the main type and comprise striated (voluntary) muscle, cardiac muscle, and smooth (involuntary) muscle. Myofibroblasts have a contractile role in addition to being able to secrete collagen. Pericytes are smooth, muscle-like cells that surround blood vessels. Myoepithelial cells are an important component of certain secretory glands.

Different arrangements of actin and myosin in each type of contractile cell, together with important structural adaptations, modulate and control contraction.

Fig. 5.1 Skeletal muscle.
In cross-section skeletal muscle cells have a roughly hexagonal profile with individual cells moulded together. Nuclei (N) are arranged beneath the cell membrane. Fibrocollagenous septa (S) contain blood vessels.

SKELETAL MUSCLE

Skeletal muscle cells form the structural basis of muscles (see Chapter 13), which are responsible for voluntary movement under the influence of the nervous system, and for maintenance of posture. The attachment of muscle to the skeletal system is discussed in Chapter 13.

Each skeletal muscle fiber is a multinucleate syncytium formed by fusion of individual cells in development.

In embryogenesis, each skeletal muscle cell forms from the fusion of many hundreds of precursor cells (myoblasts), so in the adult each is a syncytium containing hundreds of nuclei which are located just beneath the cell membrane. Each skeletal muscle cell is a long thin cylindrical structure, typically 50–60 μm in diameter in an adult and up to 10 cm long depending on its location (Fig. 5.1).

In adult muscle there is a resident population of muscle precursor cells (satellite cells) which can divide to form new muscle cells after tissue damage.

In addition to contractile proteins, skeletal muscle cell cytoplasm contains numerous mitochondria, as well as abundant glycogen to provide energy. Each muscle cell is surrounded by an external lamina (see page 55).

Because of long usage, special terms are often used to describe skeletal muscle cell components. These are: sarcolemma (cell membrane), sarcoplasm (cell cytoplasm), and sarcoplasmic reticulum (endoplasmic reticulum).

Skeletal muscle contracts as a result of organized assemblies of actin and myosin.

The contractile elements of skeletal muscle cells (myofibrils) are thin cylindrical structures 1–2 μm in diameter. They are composed of overlapping, repeating assemblies of thick (mainly myosin) and thin (mainly actin) filaments.

Any one muscle fiber has hundreds of myofibrils running parallel along its length, the alternating zones of thick and thin filaments giving rise to the descriptive term striated muscle (Fig. 5.2a).

Ultrastructurally, the thick and thin filaments are held in place by plates of accessory proteins, visible as lines, which divide the myofibrils into functional units called sarcomeres (Fig. 5.2b). Sarcoplasm, mitochondria, and other cellular elements are packed between the myofibrils.

There is a regular arrangement of contractile proteins within each sarcomere, with each thick filament being surrounded by six thin filaments (Figs 5.2c, d). Contraction of muscle occurs as thick and thin filaments slide past each other (Fig. 5.3) and is therefore accompanied by a decrease in the width of the light bands. The width of the dark bands remains unchanged.

Accessory proteins maintain the alignment of actin and myosin filaments.

Skeletal muscle function depends on a precise alignment of actin and myosin filaments within each myofibril. This is achieved by accessory proteins which link the different components and hold them in register with each other. These proteins can only be visualized using immuno-histochemical techniques.

Fig. 5.2 Myofibrils.

ⓐ Individual skeletal muscle cells appear to have cross-striations in longitudinal section due to the presence of stacks of myofibrils composed of alternating, overlapping zones of thick (dark-stained) and thin (light-stained) filaments.

ⓑ Ultrastructurally, several zones of staining can be discerned along myofibrils. The A (dark) band refers to the thick filament band and includes a zone where the thin filaments overlap the thick filaments. The H zone is a pale-staining area in the centre of the A band and indicates where no thin filaments overlap the thick filaments. The I (light) band is the zone of thin filaments that does not overlap the thick filaments, while the Z line is a

dark band in the centre of the I band and the M line runs down the centre of the H band. The unit delineated between two Z disks is termed a sarcomere.

ⓒ Diagram to show the arrangement of filaments in a sarcomere. The thin filaments are composed mainly of actin, the thick filaments mainly of myosin.

ⓓ When viewed in cross-section at the level of overlap between the A and I bands as in ⓑ, each myofibril is seen to have a regular spaced arrangement of thick and thin filaments, such that each thick filament is surrounded by six thin filaments arranged in an approximately hexagonal lattice.

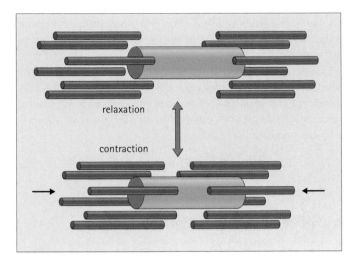

Fig. 5.3 Muscle contraction.
During muscle contraction the thin filaments of the myofibrils slide over the thick filaments. This is reversed on muscle relaxation.

Fig. 5.4 Myosin molecule.
Each myosin molecule is composed of two tadpole-shaped heavy chains, the tails of which coil around each other, with four small light chains attached to the head portions. The coiled, rod-like tail portions of many myosin molecules aggregate and pack together in a regular staggered array to form the filament, while the head portions project out in a regular helical pattern.

MYOFIBRILS

Thin filaments are mainly formed from actin

Thin filaments are 8 nm in diameter and composed mainly of the protein actin. Each thin filament (F-actin) is formed by the polymerization of many single molecules of globular actin (G-actin). These actin filaments are polar, all G-actin molecules pointing in the same direction.

To form a complete thin filament, two actin filaments become attached by their tail ends to α-actinin in the Z line so that they face in opposite directions (i.e. away from the Z line).

Thick filaments are mainly formed from myosin

Thick filaments are composed mainly of the protein myosin. Like the actin filament, the myosin filament is polar. To form a complete heavy filament, two myosin filaments become attached by their tail ends so that they face in opposite directions (i.e. away from the M line) (Fig. 5.4). Different molecular types (isoforms) of myosin are present in different types of skeletal muscle fiber.

ACCESSORY PROTEINS OF MUSCLE

Actinin holds actin filaments in a lattice arrangement in the Z disk. Other Z disk proteins include filamin, amorphin, and Z protein.

Myomesin holds myosin filaments in a lattice arrangement in the region of the M line. Current models of the M line lattice suggest that additional, as yet uncharacterized, proteins are also involved.

Titin (connectin) is an extremely long elastic protein, which runs parallel to the filament array and links the ends of the thick filaments to the Z disk, maintaining their ends in register with the lattice of thin filaments.

Desmin filaments (one of the class of intermediate filament proteins) link adjacent myofibrils to each other and maintain their register. In addition, they link myofibrils to the cell membrane.

C protein is a myosin-binding protein localized in seven stripes running parallel to the M band in the first half of the A band.

Contraction of skeletal muscle is mediated by a cycle of binding and release between actin and myosin.

In muscle contraction the actin filaments slide along the myosin filaments. This is driven by the heads of the myosin molecules, which bind to actin and, in a sequence of binding and release movements, 'walk' along the actin filament. This repetitive binding and release is powered by the hydrolysis of ATP (Fig. 5.5) and myosin can be regarded as an ATPase that is activated by the binding of actin.

Control of muscle contraction is achieved by proteins that bind to actin and prevent muscle contraction by blocking the myosin–actin interaction (Fig. 5.6). This is reversed by high concentrations of Ca++ ions in the cell cytoplasm (Fig. 5.7).

Fig. 5.5 Use of ATP by myosin binding to actin.
A myosin molecule uses the energy of ATP to move along an actin filament.
(a) ATP bound to myosin is hydrolyzed to ADP and phosphate (Pi).
(b) This causes myosin to bind loosely to actin.
(c) Pi is released and myosin binds tightly to actin.
(d) This binding initiates molecular folding of the myosin molecule to cause the movement of the molecule relative to the actin filament. ADP is released, fresh ATP binds, and the myosin returns to its non-attached state.

The cycle repeats and the myosin head 'walks' along the actin filament.

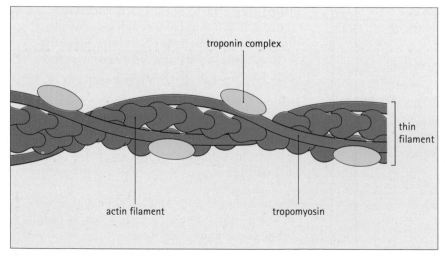

Fig. 5.6 Control of muscle contraction.
Tropomyosin is a long rod-like protein that winds around an actin filament to stabilize and stiffen it.

The troponin complex, which regulates the binding of actin to myosin, is attached to tropomyosin and composed of three separate polypeptides termed troponin T, I and C. Troponin T binds the complex to tropomyosin and positions the complex on the actin filament at the site where actin would bind to myosin. Troponin I physically prevents myosin binding to actin. Troponin C binds Ca++ ions, which cause a confrontational change in the troponin complex, allowing myosin access to the actin filament.

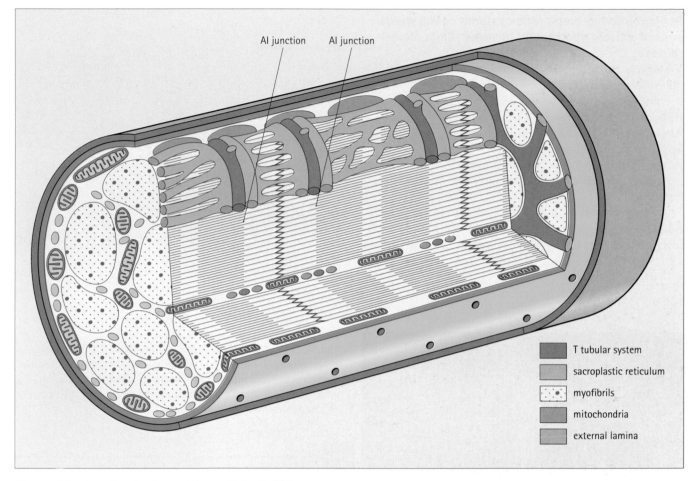

Al junction   Al junction

T tubular system

sacroplastic reticulum

myofibrils

mitochondria

external lamina

Fig. 5.7 Muscle cell excitation and intracellular Ca^{++} ions.
Following a nerve signal, excitation of the muscle cell membrane is conveyed to the interior of the cell via a series of membranous channels (the transverse tubular system of T tubules) which extend from the muscle surface to surround each myofibril.

Running alongside each T tubule are two portions of sarcoplasmic reticulum, called terminal cisternae, which contain a high concentration of Ca^{++} ions and have electrically sensitive Ca^{++} ion channels in their wall. Membrane excitation of the T tubule system causes these Ca^{++} ion channels to open, thus allowing Ca^{++} ions to flood into the sarcoplasm.

In the resting state, muscle cells have little intracellular free Ca^{++} ions, and a sudden increase in free cytosolic Ca^{++} ions initiates muscle contraction.

Membrane pumps (Ca^{++} -ATPase) in the sarcoplasmic reticulum pump the Ca^{++} ions back into the sarcoplasmic reticulum rapidly (within about 30 ms) and stop contraction.

The close association of T tubules and sarcoplasmic reticulum form three tubules in cross-section (a membrane triad). In human muscle there is a membrane triad surrounding every myofibril in the Al junction region; thus there are two triads to each sarcomere.

The force of muscle contraction is transmitted to the extracellular matrix by a series of link proteins

The cytoskeleton of each skeletal muscle fiber is linked to the external lamina by a series of link molecules. Actin filaments inside the cell are linked to the protein dystrophin. Dystrophin then links with a complex composed of several glycoproteins that bridge through the muscle cell membrane to the cell surface. On the outer surface of the muscle cell the glycoprotein complex links to the protein merosin, which is a laminin component of the basement membrane. In this way, forces generated inside the muscle are transferred to the extracellular matrix in the external lamina.

If there is a genetic absence of one of the linking proteins then muscle fibers are prone to undergo tearing on contraction and the affected person develops one of the many forms of muscular dystrophy.

It is being increasingly recognised that the different forms of muscular dystrophy can be related to defects in structural proteins in the muscle fibers. Duchenne muscular dystrophy is described on page 230.

Special internal membrane systems called triads control muscle contraction by regulating calcium release.

There is a specialized internal membrane system in skeletal muscle called the T-tubular system. This extends from the surface membrane as thin tubules which extend deep through the muscle fiber running along the region of the AI junction (Fig. 5.8). Running alongside, and in close apposition to each T tubule are two extensions of the sarcoplasmic reticulum containing a very high calcium concentration. In cross-section these three tubes form a triad (Fig. 5.9).

In response to membrane depolarization in the T-tubular system calcium channels in the membrane of the sarcoplasmic reticulum release calcium into the cytosol of the muscle fiber, causing contraction.

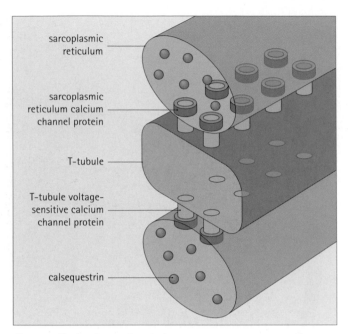

Fig. 5.9 Skeletal muscle triad.
The SR Ca^{++} channel protein lines up with the Ca^{++} channel protein in the T-tubular system. Depolarization of the T-tubular system causes opening of the SR calcium channels. Calcium, which is held in the SR lumen by calsequestrin, can then be released into the muscle cytoplasm.

Fig. 5.8 This is an electron micrograph of a skeletal muscle triad. The T-tubule is seen as a small open tube (T) and on each side are extensions of the sarcoplasmic reticulum. In humans the sarcoplasmic reticulum contains electron-dense material making these relatively indistinct structures in comparison to illustrations taken from animal material. A single triad is shown at higher magnification in the inset.

SKELETAL MUSCLE

Each muscle fiber is surrounded by an external lamina

Striated muscle is based on close alignment of actin and myosin filaments

Actin is arranged as thin filaments anchored to the Z line

Myosin is arranged as thick filaments anchored to the M line

Membrane triads couple membrane excitation to calcium release into the cytoplasm

Cytosolic calcium regulates contraction

CARDIAC MUSCLE

Cardiac muscle is a form of striated muscle but differs significantly from skeletal muscle.

Like skeletal muscle, cardiac muscle is a type of striated muscle and is characterized by a similar arrangement of actin and myosin filaments to mediate contraction. The important differences between cardiac muscle and skeletal

Fig. 5.10 Cardiac muscle.

(a) Cardiac muscle cells appear as elliptical or lobulated structures in transverse section. Their nuclei are centrally placed and have irregular shapes, and fibrocollagenous septa containing small blood vessels run between fibers. Between individual cardiac muscle cells there is a rich capillary blood supply.

(b) In longitudinal section, cardiac muscle appears as a series of anastomosing cords of cells which branch and join with adjacent fibers at cell junctions (intercalated disks, ID), seen as dark lines by the immunocytochemical method for alpha-B crystallin.

(c) Ultrastructurally, cardiac muscle cells contain myofibrils with thick and thin filament systems virtually identical to those in skeletal muscle, but composed of different structural isoforms.

Mitochondria are prominent and make up a much larger proportion of cell volume than in skeletal muscle. Several regions of the intercalated disk structure can be resolved showing desmosome-like junctions (D), adherent-type junctions (A), and, in the lateral portions of the intercalated disk, prominent communicating gap junctions (G).

(d) Diagram of the structural arrangement of adjacent cardiac muscle cells. Cells are bound together by desmosomal junctions at interdigitating areas at the ends of adjacent cells to form the intercalated disk. Gap junctions facilitate transmission of the contractile stimulus between cells.

muscle are as follows:
- cardiac muscle cells are mononuclear and much shorter than those of skeletal muscle;
- long cardiac muscle fibers are produced by linking numerous cardiac muscle cells end to end via anchoring-type cell junctions;
- a population of stem cells, analogous to satellite cells of skeletal muscle (see page 230), is not present in cardiac muscle, and so regeneration following damage cannot occur.

Individual cardiac muscle cells are linked into long chains by specialized cell junctional systems.

Instead of fusing to form syncytia as for skeletal muscle, (see page 227), cardiac muscle cells align into long chains and develop cell junctions, which anchor each cell to its neighbor (Fig. 5.10).

In the adult, a cardiac muscle cell is about 15 μm in diameter and about 100 μm long with a centrally positioned nucleus. Intercellular junctions, which can be seen in light microscopic preparations as faint lines running transversely across fibers, are termed **intercalated disks**. These contain three types of cell junction:
- desmosomal junctions tightly link adjacent cells via anchors involving the intermediate filaments (see Fig. 3.11).;
- adherent-type junctions anchor the actin fibers of the sarcomeres to each end of the cell (see Fig. 3.9);
- communicating gap junctions (see Fig. 3.14) facilitate the passage of membrane excitation (communication) and thereby synchronization of muscle contraction.

The molecular basis of contraction of cardiac muscle is very similar to that of skeletal muscle.

Contraction of cardiac muscle cells is regulated by cytosolic Ca^{++} ion concentration in a manner virtually identical to that for skeletal muscle (see Figs 5.5 and 5.6) but:
- the cardiac muscle transverse (T) tubular system consists of much wider invaginations of the cell surface;
- sarcoplasmic reticulum associated with the T tubules is neither as regular nor as well organized as in skeletal muscle;
- the association of cardiac sarcoplasmic reticulum with T tubules takes the form of dyads rather than triads, and is located in the region of the Z lines rather than the AI junction.

SMOOTH MUSCLE

Smooth muscle is the main contractile cell in the walls of viscera and in blood vessels.

Smooth muscle cells have a much less organized system of contractile proteins than striated skeletal and cardiac muscle cells. Forming the contractile portions of the wall of most hollow viscera (e.g. gut, urinary bladder and uterus), as well as the contractile elements in blood vessel walls and secretory gland ducts, smooth muscle cells are found in situations requiring sustained slow or rhythmic contractions not under voluntary control.

Individual smooth muscle cells are anchored together into functional units by basement membrane material.

Smooth muscle cells are typically spindle-shaped and, depending on site, vary in size from 20 μm (small blood vessels) to 400–500 μm (uterus). Each cell has a single, centrally located nucleus which is elongated or elliptical in shape (Fig. 5.11).

In cross-section, smooth muscle cells have polygonal profiles, but in longitudinal section appear as linear bundles.

Each smooth muscle cell is surrounded by an external lamina (see page 55) to which cell membranes adhere; small groups of cells are organized into bundles by fine collagenous tissue containing blood vessels and nerves.

Contraction of smooth muscle cells is mediated by a dispersed arrangement of actin and myosin which is very different to striated muscle.

Ultrastructurally, smooth muscle does not show the highly organized system of contractile proteins (i.e. myofilaments) seen in striated muscle, but has an arrangement where bundles of contractile proteins crisscross the cell and are inserted into anchoring points (focal densities). Focal densities are similar to adherent junctions and are studded around the cell membrane.

Tension generated by contraction is transmitted through the focal densities to the surrounding network of external laminae, thus allowing a mass of smooth muscle cells to function as one unit. The abundant intermediate filaments of smooth muscle, desmin, are also inserted into the focal densities.

Energy is supplied by numerous mitochondria which tend to be located, along with endoplasmic reticulum and other organelles around the nucleus, in an area devoid of contractile filaments.

Although each smooth muscle cell is surrounded by an external lamina, this is deficient where the cells communicate with each other via gap junctions. These junctions, which are also termed nexus junctions in smooth muscle, are widespread and allow spread of membrane excitation between cells.

A characteristic feature of smooth muscle cells is the presence of numerous invaginations of cell membrane forming structures that resemble caveoli. It is thought that these invaginations function in a similar way to the specialized transverse (T) tubular system of striated muscle by controlling the entry of Ca^{++} ions into the cell following

Fig. 5.11 Smooth muscle.

ⓐ In longitudinal section smooth muscle cells have abundant pink cytoplasm and are characterized by elongated, centrally placed nuclei.

ⓑ In transverse section it is apparent that each cell has a polygonal profile and the centrally placed nuclei are evident.

ⓒ The external lamina surrounding each smooth muscle cell binds individual cells into a functional mass and is highlighted by silver staining which detects Type IV collagen and glycoproteins.

ⓓ Ultrastructurally, smooth muscle cells are surrounded by an external lamina (EL) and have centrally placed nuclei (N). The irregularly arranged contractile proteins (CP) give rise to dense staining at the periphery of each cell, while mitochondria and other organelles are located in a perinuclear lucent zone (PLZ).

ⓔ Gap junctions (G) connect adjacent cells at defects in the external lamina.

ⓕ A terminal sac of the endoplasmic reticulum (ER) lies closely apposed to endocytotic vesicles (V) at the surface of the smooth muscle cell. The external lamina (EL) is visible.

ⓖ Contractile proteins are inserted into focal densities around the cell membrane. With contraction each cell assumes a short, compact, rounded shape.

membrane excitation. Terminal sacs of Ca^{++} ion-containing endoplasmic reticulum terminate beneath the cell membrane close to these vesicles.

SMOOTH MUSCLE CONTRACTION

Thin filaments of actin (an isoform specific to smooth muscle) are associated with tropomyosin (see Fig. 5.6) but, in contrast to striated muscle, there is no troponin.

The thick filaments are composed of myosin, but of a different type to that in skeletal muscle and will only bind to actin if its light chain is phosphorylated; this phenomenon does not occur in skeletal muscle.

Although Ca^{++} ions in smooth muscle cells cause contraction as in striated muscle, the control of Ca^{++} ion movements is different. In relaxed smooth muscle free Ca^{++} ions are normally sequestered in sarcoplasmic reticulum throughout the cell. On membrane excitation, free Ca^{++} ions are released into the cytoplasm and bind to a protein called calmodulin (a calcium-binding protein). The calcium–calmodulin complex then activates an enzyme called myosin light-chain kinase, which phosphorylates the myosin light chain and permits it to bind to actin. Actin and myosin subsequently interact by filament sliding to produce contraction in a similar way to that for skeletal muscle.

In the cell membrane of smooth muscle cells are calcium channels which can open and let calcium into the cell. Some of these channels are activated by hormones (ligand-gated channels) while others are activated by membrane depolarization (voltage-gated channels). These channels provide another mechanism for initiation or modulation of contraction.

Contraction of smooth muscle can be modulated by surface receptors activating internal secondary messenger systems. Expression of different receptors allows smooth muscle in different sites to respond to several different hormones.

Compared with skeletal muscle, smooth muscle is able to maintain a high force of contraction for very little ATP usage.

The molecular basis of contraction in smooth muscle differs from that in skeletal muscle.

The contraction mechanism of smooth muscle differs from that for striated muscle. Because the contractile proteins are arranged in a crisscross lattice inserted circumferentially into the cell membrane, contraction results in shortening of the cell, which assumes a globular shape in contrast to its elongated shape in the relaxed state (Fig. 5.11g).

Smooth muscle can be arranged into two functional types termed unitary and multi-unit.

Most smooth muscle is present in the walls of hollow viscera (e.g. gut, ureter, fallopian tube) where it is arranged in sheets with cells aligned circumferentially or longitudinally, with contraction resulting in reduction of the lumen diameter.

In these so-called unitary smooth muscles, cells tend to generate their own low level of rhythmic contraction, which may also be stimulated by stretch, and is transmitted from cell to cell via the gap junctions. Such smooth muscle is richly innervated by the autonomic nervous system (see Chapter 6), which increases or decreases levels of spontaneous contraction rather than actually initiating it. Physiologically, this is termed tonic smooth muscle and is characterized by slow contraction, no action potentials, and a low content of fast myosin.

A second arrangement of smooth muscle is typified by that in the iris of the eye. Here, rather than simply modulating spontaneous activity, autonomic innervation precisely controls contraction, resulting in opening and closing of the pupil. Similar neurally controlled or multi-unit smooth muscle is found in the vas deferens and some large arteries. Physiologically, this is termed phasic smooth muscle and is characterized by rapid contraction associated with an action potential, and a high cell content of fast myosin.

SUPPORT CELL FUNCTION OF SMOOTH MUSCLE

Smooth muscle cells have to secrete elements of their extracellular matrix

Depending on the site, smooth muscle cells produce collagen, elastin, and other components of the extracellular matrix. Thus they have a support cell function as well as a contractile cell function. In most situations this support cell function is limited to manufacturing extracellular matrix to anchor the smooth muscle.

MYOFIBROBLASTS

Myofibroblasts are important in tissue responses to injury.

Myofibroblasts are spindle-shaped cells that secrete collagen (i.e. fibroblast-like), but also have well defined contractile properties similar to those of smooth muscle (i.e. myoid).

In conventional histologic sections myofibroblasts cannot be readily distinguished from fibroblasts, but immunohistochemical detection of their content of smooth muscle actin and desmin (not seen in fibroblasts) and ultrastructural demonstration of contractile proteins shows that they are distinct. Myofibroblasts lack an external lamina, in contrast to true smooth muscle cells.

In normal tissues, myofibroblasts are inconspicuous and commonly form an inactive population of cells, for example in the alveolar septa of the lung and around the crypts of glands in the gut. They also form a sparse population in loose collagenous support tissue.

Following tissue damage, however, myofibroblasts become active and proliferate, and their role appears to be to repair defects resulting from tissue death. They secrete collagen to provide a firm scaffold to consolidate a damaged area (fibrous scar). As healing proceeds, each myofibroblast contracts and pulls the extracellular matrix together to reduce the physical size of the damaged area.

PERICYTES

Pericytes are found around vessels and can act as mesenchymal stem cells.

Pericytes are spindle-shaped cells which are found circumferentially arranged around capillaries and venules (see Fig. 9.11). They are surrounded by external lamina and, in normal tissues, show little cytoplasmic differentiation ultrastructurally, but contain actin and myosin immunohistochemically, suggesting a contractile function.

Following tissue injury, pericytes proliferate and assume the role of primitive mesenchymal cells, being able to differentiate into myofibroblasts, as well as mesenchymal tissue which develops into collagenous support tissue and new blood vessels.

MYOEPITHELIAL CELLS

Secretions from glands are expelled by the contractile function of myoepithelial cells.

Myoepithelial cells are found in exocrine glands including highly developed glands such as the breast, where they form a major population surrounding glandular acini and ducts and squeeze secretions from the glandular lumina.

Myoepithelial cells are generally inconspicuous in routine H&E sections, appearing as a layer of flat cells running around acini and ducts. They have dark-staining rounded nuclei and clear or vacuolated cytoplasm.

Around acini, myoepithelial cells have a stellate, multiprocessed morphology in three dimensions and form a contractile meshwork which encloses secretory units of glands. Around ducts they are fusiform in shape and surround the periphery of ducts in a way analogous to barrel hoops.

Ultrastructurally, myoepithelial cells contain contractile proteins arranged in a similar manner to that in smooth muscle and have numerous desmosomal connections with adjacent cells.

Immunohistochemically they can be detected by their content of the muscle-specific intermediate filament desmin (Fig. 5.12).

Myoepithelial cells are controlled by the autonomic nervous system and on stimulation contract and expel glandular secretions.

Fig. 5.12 Myoepithelial cells.
Myoepithelial cells in this section from salivary gland can be shown by an immunoperoxidase technique that demonstrates desmin, which is the muscle-specific intermediate filament and stains brown.

1. **SKELETAL MUSCLE CELLS**

   (a) have thin filaments made of actin which are anchored to the Z band
   (b) have thick filaments made of desmin which are anchored to the M band
   (c) regulate contraction by control of calcium release from sarcoplasmic reticulum
   (d) are surrounded by an external lamina
   (e) contain multiple nuclei in each cell

2. **CARDIAC MUSCLE CELLS**

   (a) are mononuclear and linked by intercellular junctions to form a fiber
   (b) are striated in a similar way to skeletal muscle
   (c) can regenerate following cell damage
   (d) regulate contraction by release of calcium from sarcoplasmic reticulum
   (e) have communicating junctions linking fibers to facilitate contraction

3. **SMOOTH MUSCLE CELLS**

   (a) have single nuclei
   (b) use actin and myosin to develop contractile forces
   (c) are surrounded by an external lamina
   (d) have membrane receptors for hormones
   (e) may generate their own level of rhythmic contraction

4. **MYOFIBROBLASTS, PERICYTES AND MYOEPITHELIAL CELLS ARE ALL TYPES OF SPECIALIZED CONTRACTILE CELL**

   (a) myoepithelial cells are found in exocrine glandular tissue such as the breast
   (b) myoepithelial cells are stellate cells, with multiple processes, which surround secretory units of glands.
   (c) myoepithelial cells are controlled by autonomic innervation
   (d) pericytes may assume the role of primitive mesenchymal cells
   (e) myofibroblasts proliferate and are involved in repair following tissue damage

6. Nervous Tissue

The nervous system allows rapid and specific communication between widely spaced areas of the body by the action of specialized nerve cells (neurons) which gather and process information and generate appropriate response signals.

The nervous system is divided into two main parts:

- the **central nervous system** (CNS) comprising the brain and spinal cord;
- the **peripheral nervous system** (PNS) comprising the nerves which run between the CNS and other tissues, together with nerve 'relay stations' termed ganglia.

NERVE CELLS (NEURONS)

Nerve cells are responsible for direct communications between different groups of cells.

Neurons form a network of highly specific connections between different groups of cells in order to:

- gather information from sensory receptors;
- process information and provide a memory;
- generate appropriate signals to effector cells.

A neuron is divided into several regions, each with a different function.

Neurons (Fig. 6.1) are characterized by:

- a cell body containing the nucleus and most of the organelles responsible for maintaining the cell;
- a long cell process (**axon**) stretching from the cell, often over a long distance, which is responsible for transmitting signals from the neuron to other cells;

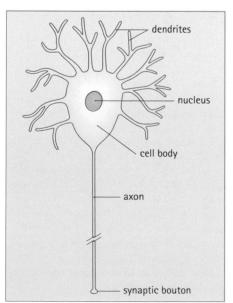

Fig 6.1 General structure of a neuron.
Neurons consist of a cell body, axon and dendrites, the axon carrying impulses to its terminal, the synaptic bouton, which makes contact with another cell. The dendrites connect with synaptic boutons from other neurons.

- numerous short cell processes (**dendrites**) which increase the surface area available for connecting with axons of other neurons;
- specialized cell junctions (**synapses**) between its axon and other cells to allow direct cell communication.

The functional attributes of the nervous system are determined mainly by the network of connections between neurons rather than on specific structural features of individual neurons.

Neurons have a characteristic cytology reflecting a high metabolic activity.

Neurons are highly metabolically active as they not only maintain a massive surface area of cell membrane, but also constantly require energy to develop electrochemical gradients. This activity is reflected in their histologic appearance (Fig. 6.2), in which the nucleus is typically large and

Fig. 6.2 Neuron.
ⓐ Electron micrograph of a neuron showing the axon (A) containing mitochondria and cytoskeletal filaments, and the cell body containing a nucleus, (N), dark staining lysosomal bodies, (L), and abundant rough endoplasmic reticulum (Nissl substance), (NS).
ⓑ Micrograph showing a neuron with a large nucleus, (N),containing a prominent nucleolus. Within the cell body purple-staining Nissl substance, (NS), composed of rough endoplasmic reticulum can be seen. The axon (A) stretches away from the cell body.

rounded, with a large central nucleolus, reflecting a high degree of transcriptional activity. There is abundant rough endoplasmic reticulum, which synthesizes the necessary proteins, and is visible in the cytoplasm in H&E sections as purple-stained granules, the so-called **Nissl substance**, which is present in the cell body (perikaryon) and dendrites but not the axon. There is also a well developed Golgi to produce secretory products, and large numbers of mitochondria to supply the high energy requirements. Lysosomes are numerous because of a high turnover of cell membrane and other cell components, and residual bodies containing lipofuscin are often prominent, particularly in the elderly.

The cytoskeleton of the neuron is vital for axonal transport

The cytoskeleton of neurons is highly organized to maintain the unique shape of these cells, and particularly axons, which may be up to 1 m long.

Neurofilament protein, the intermediate filament of nerve cells, is thought to act as an internal scaffold to maintain the shape of the axon and cell body. In the axon, certain membrane proteins are anchored in place in an organized pattern by attachment to cellular neurofilaments.

There is also a highly organized network of microtubules, which transport substances and organelles up and down the axon.

The metabolic maintenance of the long cell process of the axon requires a transport system for organelles, enzymes, and metabolites from the cell body which is largely directed by the microtubular cytoskeleton. Enzymes and elements of the cytoskeleton are transported down the axon at a speed of 1–5 mm/day by an unknown mechanism (**slow axonal transport**). Membrane-bound organelles, such as neurosecretory vesicles, are transported at speeds of 400 mm/day (anterograde fast axonal transport). This method is mediated by microtubular transport mechanisms using the molecule kinesin as a molecular motor.

The return of effete organelles as well as recycled membrane from the synaptic ending back to the neuronal cell body for processing occurs at a rate of 300 mm/day (retrograde fast transport). This is mediated by microtubular transport mechanisms using the molecule dynein as a molecular motor.

Neurons have different shapes reflecting differences in function.

Several types of neuron can be identified according to the pattern of axons and dendrites (Fig. 6.3). These appearances are only apparent when special staining methods are used to highlight cellular anatomy.

MOTOR NEURONS have a large cell body to provide metabolic support for the large axon. They also have many dendritic processes and are therefore classed as multipolar neurons.

SENSORY NEURONS are commonly unipolar cells, which are characterized by the possession of one major process. This divides into two branches, one running to the central nervous system and one to a sensory area of the body.

INTERNEURONS are generally small, simple cells with short processes that provide local connections within the central nervous system. Many such cells are bipolar in type, having two main processes of equivalent size: one dendritic and one axonal.

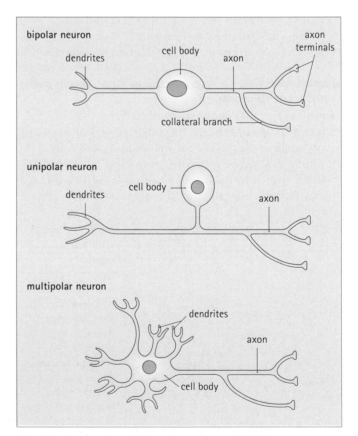

Fig. 6.3 Types of neuron.
There are many different types of neuron, which are shaped according to their function. Bipolar cells are commonly interneurons, while unipolar cells tend to be sensory neurons and multipolar cells are often motor neurons.

In addition to these general types of neuron, there are many types of neuron that are unique to a particular part of the brain, for example the Purkinje cells, which are large multi-processed cells in the cerebellum (Fig. 6.27b).

Neurons transmit signals by changes in the electrical polarity of the cell membrane.

Neuron signaling is controlled by an electrical (ionic) gradient across the cell membrane. Firing is associated with depolarization of the cell membrane which, in a resting axon, has a negative membrane potential of –70 mV. This depolarization is propagated along the axon of the cell at up to 100 m/sec.

The cell membrane of neurons is divided into several regions, each containing highly specialized membrane proteins. **Membrane ion pumps** maintain the baseline electrical gradient between the outside and inside of the cell and are widely distributed in the cell membrane. **Ion channel proteins** modify the electrochemical gradient across the neuron cell membrane by forming pores or gates which can switch their permeability to ions in response to specific signals (gated channels).

- **Ligand-gated channels** close or open in response to binding to chemical transmitter substances and are located mainly in synapses.
- **Voltage-gated channels** are involved mainly in the explosive and rapid depolarization that occurs as nerve cells fire, and are widely distributed in the cell membrane.

If an area of the axon membrane is locally depolarized and the current is small, then no gated channels will open. The current flows down the axon by passive local spread for a small distance before dissipating because of leakage from the membrane. In this situation, the axon behaves like an electrical cable, simply conducting a current along its surface with the speed of conduction related to the resistance and capacitance of the axon.

If an area of axon membrane is depolarized and the current is large, Na^+ and K^+ gated channels open and

THE NEURON

- divided into cell body, axon, dendrites, terminal bouton

- highly metabolically active cell with abundant lysosomes and rough endoplasmic reticulum (termed Nissl substance)

- cytoskeleton is vital for function, especially neurofilaments (architecture) and microtubules (axonal transport)

- the axon is specialized for conduction of electrical depolarization (action potential) mediated by ion channels in the cell membrane.

lead to an explosive change in the membrane potential, termed an **action potential**.

The opening of voltage-gated channels to produce an action potential can be considered as a local amplification system for membrane depolarization; the current does not now dissipate over a small length of the axon, but propagates to the end of the axon by causing a chain reaction triggering of gated ion channels along the way.

Action potentials propagate along an axon at the speed of passive local spread, which is determined by the resistance and capacitance of the axon; the larger the diameter of the axon, the greater is the speed of propagation.

Nerve cells signal to each other through structures called synapses.

A synapse is a special type of cell junction that allows direct communication between cells; a transmitter substance is secreted in a highly localized fashion by one cell and received uniquely by the other.

MOTOR NEURON DISEASE

Motor neuron disease is a progressive disease, mainly seen in old age, in which symptoms include weakness in voluntary muscles caused by death of motor neurones. The disease progresses to severe paralysis, leading to death in 2–3 years. The reason for the peculiar susceptibility of motor neurones to spontaneous death is not known. All motor neurons are vulnerable, and the particular symptoms in each case depend on which groups of motor neurons are most severely involved. Death of motor neurons in the brain stem produces the symptom complex called **progressive bulbar palsy**; of the lower motor neurons of the spinal cord produces **progressive muscular atrophy**. The most common pattern is called **amyotrophic lateral sclerosis** and is due to death of motor neurons in the cerebral cortex, brain stem and spinal cord.

Each synapse has vesicles containing neurotransmitter substances.

The terminal end of an axon is swollen to form a synaptic bouton, which is closely applied to the surface of a target cell, leaving a small gap 20 nm wide (the synaptic cleft). The cell membrane on each side of the synaptic cleft contains special membrane proteins and receptors involved in neurotransmission.

Ultrastructurally the cell membrane on each side of the synaptic cleft is slightly thickened and the synaptic bouton contains mitochondria, microtubules, and neurofilaments, as well as membrane-bound vesicles 40–65 nm in diameter (neurosecretory vesicles, Fig. 6.4). The appearance of these vesicles is variable; most are small and round with a clear center, others are elliptical. Certain neurosecretory granules (dense-core granules) have an electron-dense core with a pale 'halo' beneath the membrane.

In tissue sections it is possible to detect transmitter substances in neurons and their terminals by immunochemistry, using antibodies specific for the transmitter.

Neurosecretory granules also contain unique nontransmitter proteins which are vital to their function.

Again, these may by detected by immunochemistry, for example, synaptophysin, which is a glycoprotein in the membrane of neurosecretory granules, and chromogranins, proteins involved in the packaging of transmitter into dense-core vesicles.

Neurosecretory vesicles release transmitter by fusion with the presynaptic membrane.

When a wave of depolarization reaches the synaptic bouton, it triggers the release of a transmitter substance from the neurosecretory granules by exocytosis (Fig 6.5). The transmitter substance then diffuses across the synaptic cleft and is able to interact with receptors in the postsynaptic membrane of the target neuron. The membrane of the synaptic vesicle is recovered as a coated pit and recycles back to an endosome compartment in the nerve terminal. There is thus a constant recycling of membrane in the nerve terminal. Neurosecretory vesicles also arrive in the axon terminal by transport from the cell body but others are formed locally by budding off from the endosome compartment in the synapse. Neurotransmitter substances can be imported into vesicles formed from the endosome compartment from the nerve terminal by reuptake systems.

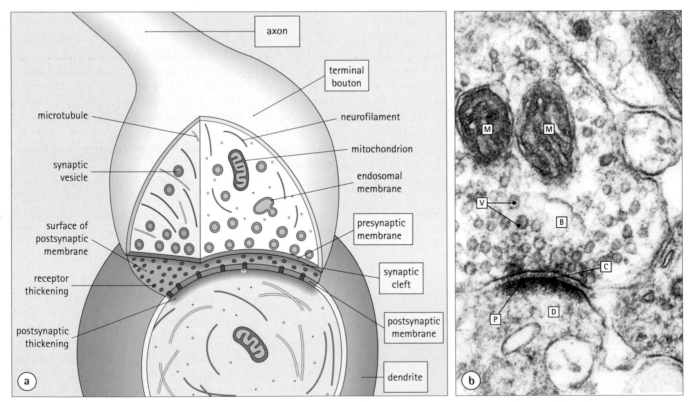

Fig. 6.4 Synapse.
(a) Diagram showing an axon terminating as a synaptic bouton on the surface of a neuron. The postsynaptic membrane bears arrays of receptors for the neurotransmitter contained in the synaptic vesicles. Vesicles are released into the synaptic cleft by exocytosis.

(b) Electronmicrograph showing the synaptic bouton, (B), making contact with dendrite, (D). The bouton contains small vesicles, (V), mitochondria, (M), and cytoskeletal filaments. The synaptic cleft, (C), contains faint granular material above the thickened postsynaptic membrane, (P).

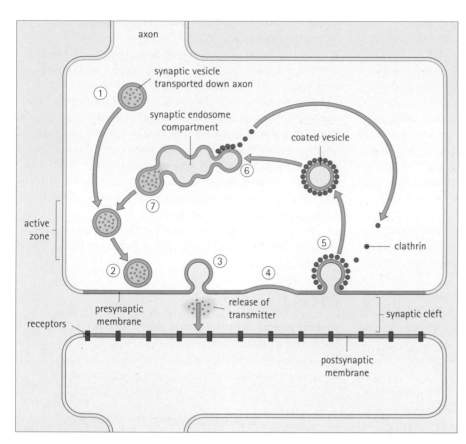

Fig. 6.5 Turnover of synaptic vesicles.
Synaptic vesicles (NSV) are formed in the neuronal cell body and are transported down the axon ①. Once in the terminal bouton, proteins in the NSV membrane direct vesicles to an area just above the presynaptic membrane termed the active zone. Vesicles from the active zone bind to special docking proteins in the presynaptic membrane and become primed for exocytosis ②. Exocytosis is associated with release of the transmitter substance into the synaptic cleft ③ and integration of the membrane of the vesicle with the presynaptic membrane ④. The protein clathrin associates with vesicle membrane and forms coated vesicles which recycle the vesicle membrane back into the nerve terminal ⑤. Recycled vesicle membrane fuses with an endosome membrane compartment in the nerve terminal ⑥ and clathrin is released. New synaptic vesicles can bud off from the endosome compartment ⑦. Transmitter substances which are free in the nerve terminal can be imported into these recycled vesicles via special membrane pumps.

NEUROSECRETION IS MEDIATED BY PROTEINS IN THE SYNAPTIC VESICLE AND PRESYNAPTIC MEMBRANE.

Many of the proteins involved in neurosecretion have now been characterized (Fig. 6.6).

The membrane of the synaptic vesicle contains an anchoring protein (synaptobrevin) which ties the vesicle to a docking protein in the presynaptic membrane (syntaxin) by a group of linking proteins (composed of proteins called αSNAP, βSNAP, SNAP25, and NSF).

The membrane of the synaptic vesicle and the adjacent presynaptic membrane contain proteins which can bring about membrane fusion and allow exocytosis. In the resting state a calcium-sensitive trigger protein (synaptotagmin) prevents the linking complex from allowing membrane fusion.

If an action potential reaches the terminal bouton, voltage-sensitive calcium channels open and increase the concentration of calcium in the nerve terminal. This releases the trigger protein and allows membrane fusion to take place, leading to exocytosis.

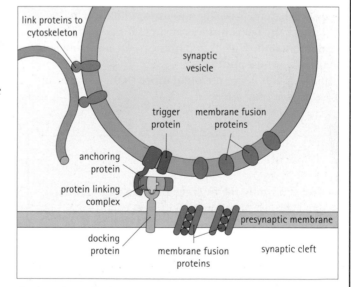

Fig 6.6 Synaptic docking and exocytosis.
Many of the proteins involved in the exocytosis of synaptic vesicles are characterized. Fusion of vesicle to presynaptic membrane only takes place when an increase in calcium causes an alteration in the configuration of proteins involved in docking.

Three possible effects of transmitter release are depolarization, hyperpolarization or altered cell sensitivity.

When a released transmitter binds to receptors on the postsynaptic cells there are three possible effects: depolarization, hyperpolarization or altered cell sensitivity.

The target cell **depolarizes** if the transmitter substance binds to a ligand-gated receptor (i.e. Na^+ ion channel protein) and causes it to open, allowing ions to diffuse into the neuron. If many receptors are activated at the same time, the alteration in membrane potential causes activation of voltage-gated ion channels, leading to an action potential.

Only a small group of transmitter substances act in this way, which generally results in rapid neural transmission. These include acetylcholine, which is the major transmitter in this group, and glutamate.

The target cell **hyperpolarizes** if the transmitter substance binds to a ligand-gated receptor that admits small negative ions into the cell. Hyperpolarization inhibits depolarization.

The main transmitter substances causing hyperpolarization are γ-aminobutyric acid and glycine.

The overall **sensitivity of a cell** to stimulation is altered if the transmitter substance binds to one of the class of non-channel linked receptors. These receptors generate secondary messengers (e.g. cAMP) within the target neuron, to modify the overall sensitivity of the cell to depolarization mediated by the ligand-gated receptors. Such behavior is called neuromodulation.

Many of the transmitters causing altered cell sensitivity are monoamines (e.g. dopamine, serotonin), but some are small neuropeptides.

In any given nerve terminal more than one transmitter substance may operate.

SYNAPSES

- are formed by the interaction of an axon terminal and the cell membrane of a target cell

- key components are terminal bouton, presynaptic membrane, synaptic cleft, postsynaptic membrane, neurosecretory vesicles

- neurotransmitter release is triggered by membrane depolarization which leads to increased calcium concentration inside the nerve terminal

- exocytosis of neurosecretory vesicles is mediated by a set of characterized proteins

- membrane of neurosecretory vesicles is recycled within the nerve terminal

Synapses form different patterns of connection between neurons.

Within the central nervous system, synapses form in a diversity of combinations between axons and dendrites, axons and cell bodies, axons and other axons (Fig. 6.7).

Because axons may be excitatory, inhibitory, or modulatory, certain synapses are formed from the coincidence of many axons from different neurons onto one part of a target neuron. The target neuron can then integrate the overall input into an appropriate output. Such functional clusters of synapses are commonly isolated from the adjacent nervous system by support cells of the brain such as astrocytes.

The neuromuscular junction (see Chapter 13) is a specialized form of synapse between a motor nerve axon and skeletal muscle.

MYELIN

Myelin wraps around axons and increases speed of conduction.

The speed of conduction along nerves is limited by the electrical capacitance and resistance of the axon.

Fig. 6.7 Patterns of synapse.
(a) Diagram to illustrate the combination of synapses. Synapses can form between axons and dendrites, axons and cell bodies, axons and other axons.
(b) Electron micrograph showing two axo-axonic synapses (S) onto the same axon (A). Firing of (A) will depend on the integration of these separate inputs.

Because wide axons have a lower capacitance than narrow ones, increasing the diameter of axons is a useful means of increasing the speed of nerve conduction. This is inefficient, however, as giant axons require high metabolic upkeep.

The speed of conduction along axons can also be increased if leakage of current from the membrane is minimized by insulation.

The two functions of insulation and reduction of electrical capacitance are performed by a substance called **myelin**, which is produced by specialized support cells. These cells, which wrap layers of membrane containing the lipid-rich insulating layer around axons, are called **oligodendrocytes** in the central nervous system and **Schwann cells** in the peripheral nervous system.

A Schwann cell myelinates only one axon, but an oligodendrocyte may myelinate several adjacent axons. Although largely identical in structure, there are minor differences in the composition of myelin formed by these two cell types.

Myelin can be stained by histologic methods with affinity for the lipid or protein components of the myelin sheath, and such methods highlight the structural difference in the central nervous system between neuron-rich areas low in myelin (gray matter) and tracts of axons with abundant myelin (white matter).

Myelin is a spiral layer of closely apposed cell membranes.

The myelin sheath is formed by the oligodendrocytes or Schwann cells wrapping spiral layers of cell membrane around the axon. Each layer of cell membrane is linked to its neighbor by specialized cell adhesion proteins.

Myelination begins with the invagination of a single axon into the support cell, which brings its outer cell membranes into close apposition and seals them together to form a sheet of internal membrane (the mesaxon, Fig. 6.8). The line of fusion is mediated by proteins in the outer surfaces of the cell membrane, and ultrastructurally forms a line (the intraperiod line). Myelination

Fig. 6.8 Myelin.

(a) Diagram to show myelin formation. First an axon invaginates a myelin-forming cell and the outer leaflets of the myelin-forming cell's membrane fuse to form the mesaxon.

The myelin-forming cell then wraps layers of the mesaxon around the axon; the inner cytoplasm is lost when the inner leaflet of the cell membrane fuses to form the major dense line. Myelin forms into numerous lamellae of fused membrane, the lamellae being separated by alternating major dense lines and mesaxon (intraperiod line).

(b) Low-power electronmicrograph showing an axon (A) surrounded by myelin (M) and the nucleus, (N), of a Schwann cell.
(c) Medium-power electron micrograph showing the fine structure of myelin. The axon (A) is surrounded by myelin lamellae, (M). Note the outer mesaxon, (OM). The areas of cytoplasm in the myelin represent Schmidt–Lantermann incisures, (S) (Fig. 6.9), and the inner collar of cytoplasm, (IC).
(d) High-power electronmicrograph showing the fine detail of myelin lamellae; the dark lines are the major dense lines while the intraperiod lines are barely visible in between.

then proceeds as the support cell wraps numerous layers of the mesaxon around the axon. A tight spiral composed of double-thickness cell membrane fused together forms because the cytoplasm of the support cell is excluded from most of the space between the membrane layers.

The inner surfaces of the cell membranes also fuse together and form a dense line, the **major dense line**.

The thickness of the myelin sheath depends on the number of layers (lamellae) wrapped around the axon.

In addition to the specialized cell adhesion proteins, the cell membrane of the support cells that forms myelin also contains special lipids – for example, the glycolipid galactocerebroside, which is abundant in myelin.

The myelin insulation is not continuous along axons, being limited by the size of the myelinating cell. The small bare areas of axon between myelin sheaths are termed the **nodes of Ranvier** and are physiologically important.

CELL MEMBRANES IN MYELIN ARE LINKED TOGETHER BY SPECIALIZED PROTEINS.

The layers of cell membrane which are wrapped to form myelin are tightly bound together by special proteins. The proteins involved are different for CNS myelin and PNS myelin.

In the myelin of the central nervous system, proteolipid protein (PLP) links the exoplasmic surfaces of myelin membranes together. The cytoplasmic surfaces are linked through interactions with another protein called myelin basic protein (MBP).

In the peripheral nervous system P0 protein associates with myelin basic protein to form the major dense line. P0 protein accounts for about 50% of protein in PNS myelin.

Myelin-associated glycoprotein (MAG) is expressed on the surface of oligodendrocytes and is one of the member of immunoglobulin-like proteins, acting as a cell surface ligand-binding protein.

Peripheral myelin protein-22 is involved in formation and maintenance of myelin in the peripheral nervous system.

ABNORMALITIES IN MYELIN PROTEINS CAUSE DISEASE OF NERVOUS SYSTEM

Several inherited diseases of the nervous system are now recognized to be caused by abnormalities in the genes coding for myelin-related proteins.

Dominantly inherited hereditary motor and sensory neuropathy type 1 (HMSN -1) is caused by mutations in peripheral myelin protein-22 (PMP-22) in 90% of affected families. Patients develop weakness and impaired sensation caused by degeneration of the myelin in peripheral nerves.

Deletion of the gene for peripheral myelin protein-22 (PMP-22) gives rise to hereditary neuropathy with liability to pressure palsies. Patients are unusually susceptible to nerve damage following relatively trivial pressure to nerves.

Mutations in the proteolipid protein (PLP) gene can cause two disorders. In Pelizaeus-Merzbacher disease, affected children develop degeneration of their CNS myelin and develop progressively severe mental disability. Other mutations can cause degeneration of myelin in the spinal cord leading to spastic paraparesis. The gene for PLP is on the X chromosome and so these diseases are manifest in males.

Myelin is maintained by extensions of cytoplasm from the parent myelin-forming cell.

The cell membranes forming myelin are a dynamic structure. The cytoplasm of the myelin-forming support cell remains in the myelin sheath at three sites to maintain the cell membrane. These sites are located:

- adjacent to the axon (**inner collar**);
- between the internodal myelin lamellae of peripheral nervous system myelin formed by Schwann cells (**Schmidt-Lantermann incisures**);
- at each end of the myelin segment adjacent to the nodes of Ranvier (**paranodal area**, see below);
- adjacent to the cell body on the outer aspect of the myelin (**outer collar**).

The cytoplasm in all these areas is in continuity with that of the cell body of the support cells so that the membrane forming the myelin can be maintained (Fig. 6.9).

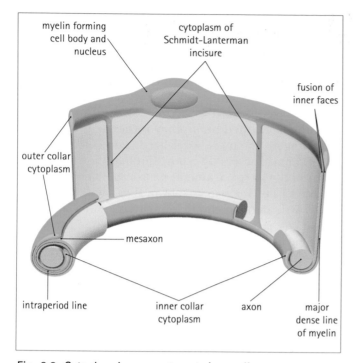

Fig. 6.9 **Cytoplasmic compartments in myelin.**
If the myelin around an axon is theoretically unwrapped, the relationships between the cytoplasmic compartments become evident.

The inner collar and outer collar run along and parallel to the axon, while the cytoplasm of the Schmidt-Lantermann incisures is wrapped around the axon in between myelin lamellae. These zones of cytoplasm are continuous with the cell body of the myelin-forming cell and serve to maintain the membrane forming the myelin.

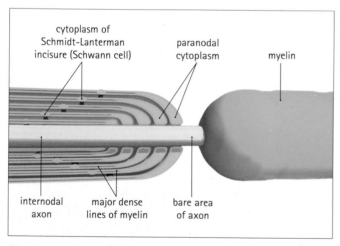

Fig. 6.10 **Node of Ranvier.**
Diagram of a node of Ranvier in longitudinal section. At the end of a myelin segment the myelin lamellae give way to a series of paranodal loops containing cytoplasm. The adjacent bare area of axon is generally slightly wider than the internodal axon and is the region containing the voltage-gated Na^+ channels, which are necessary for the formation of action potential. Compare the Schmidt-Lantermann incisures in this plane with those in Fig. 6.9.

The nodes of Ranvier contain bare areas of axon devoid of myelin.

Myelination of an axon is not continuous along its length, but occurs in small units 1–2 mm long, each unit being formed by an individual support cell. The small space between each unit of myelin is the node of Ranvier and has an important physiologic role in increasing the efficiency of nerve conduction (Fig. 6.10).

At the node of Ranvier the myelinating cells form paranodal loops of cytoplasm in continuity with the cell body.

In the central nervous system the axons in the nodes of Ranvier are bare while those in the peripheral nervous system are partly covered by tongues of cytoplasm from adjacent Schwann cells.

The axon at the node of Ranvier is slightly thicker than in the internodal regions and contains most of the Na^+ gated channels of the axonal cell membrane, which is reflected ultrastructurally as a fuzzy thickening of the membrane. These gated channels are anchored via the link protein ankyrin to the cytoskeleton. There are no gated channels in the internodal region beneath the myelin sheath.

Depolarization at a node of Ranvier is followed by rapid passive spread of the depolarization current along the axon beneath the myelin to the next node because leakage of current is minimized by the insulation. As the membrane capacitance is low, which is also the result of the myelin, only a small change is required to cause a significant voltage difference.

When such passively spread conduction encounters the zone of highly concentrated gated channels in the next node of Ranvier along the axon, there is further local depolarization. Thus the depolarization progresses in a series of jumps, with passive spread of charge in between.

Depolarization in a myelinated nerve is much more efficient metabolically than in a non-myelinated nerve, because the restricted entry of Na^+ ions to small areas, instead of to the whole axonal surface, reduces the demand for energy to pump the ions back out again.

MYELIN

- is formed by Schwann cells in the PNS and oligodendrocytes in the CNS

- ultrastructurally is seen as a spiral of membrane wrapped around an axon

- contains special cell adhesion proteins and lipids which differ between the CNS and PNS

- functions to increase the speed of conduction along axons

- occurs in small units with a space between termed the node of Ranvier

CENTRAL NERVOUS SYSTEM

The central nervous system comprises the brain and spinal cord. These contain nerve cells and their processes together with a series of specialized support cells.

The specialized support cells of the CNS are collectively called glia.

The central nervous system (CNS) contains numerous non-neural support cells. These are astrocytes, oligodendrocytes, ependyma, and microglial cells (Fig. 6.11), which are collectively called the **glia**.

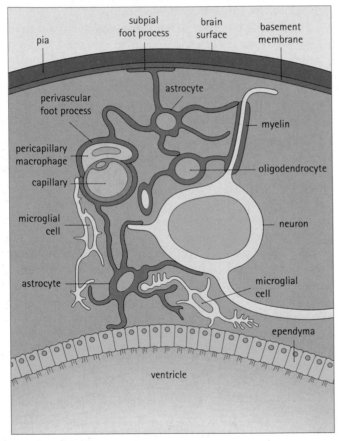

Fig. 6.11 Support cells of the CNS.
The support cells of the CNS are called glia and have several roles.

Astrocytes not only form a scaffolding for the other cells, but also extend foot processes around capillaries to maintain a blood-brain barrier. At the surface of the brain, astrocytes line a basement membrane and form the glia limitans, which surrounds the whole CNS.

Oligodendrocytes myelinate the axons of the nerve cells, while a vast network of antigen-sensing microglial cells is present throughout the CNS. Phagocytic macrophages, which also have an immune defense role, reside in the perivascular space, outside the CNS substance.

The ependymal cells form an epithelial sheet, which, unlike other epithelia, does not lie on a basement membrane. This sheet lines the fluid-filled ventricular cavities of the brain and the central canal of the spinal cord.

Astrocytes are stellate cells with roles in embryogenesis, fluid transport, and structural support.

Astrocytes are large, multi-processed cells with several functions:
- in embryologic development, they form a structural framework to guide the migration of developing nerve cells;
- in the developed brain, they form a structural scaffolding for the more specialized neural elements;
- certain astrocytes transport fluid and ions from the extracellular space around neurons to blood vessels.

Astrocytes are characterized by oval or slightly irregular nuclei with an open chromatin pattern, and a spectacular stellate morphology with numerous fine processes radiating in all directions. These processes contain a specific form of cytoskeletal intermediate filament (see page 26) called **glial fibrillary acidic protein** (GFAP).

The stellate morphology is not evident in conventional H&E section because the processes merge with the processes of other cells, but is seen with special staining methods (Fig. 6.12).

Two types of astrocyte have been identified. **Fibrous astrocytes** are most evident in the white matter and have long cell processes which are rich in bundles of GFAP. **Protoplasmic astrocytes** are most evident in the gray matter of the brain and have long thin processes containing few bundles of GFAP.

One important structural adaptation of astrocytes is seen in their interaction with the blood vessels of the brain, which they surround by forming flat plates termed end feet (Fig. 6.11). The interaction induces changes in the structure of the cerebral vascular endothelium, rendering it highly impermeable, so that it acts as a barrier to diffusion between the blood and brain.

Fig. 6.12 Astrocytes.
Micrograph stained by an immunoperoxidase method to show glial fibrillary acidic protein (GFAP), the intermediate filament of astrocytes. The astrocyte is stained brown and shows the characteristic stellate morphology.

GLIOSIS

When neurons die, the dead cells are removed by macrophages by phagocytosis. The damaged area is then repaired by proliferation of astrocytic cells, which fill the defect and form an astrocytic scar in a process termed **gliosis**.

Fig. 6.13 Oligodendrocytes.

(a) Oligodendrocytes myelinate several adjacent axons within the CNS.
(b) Ultrastructurally, the oligodendrocyte (O) has abundant mitochondria and Golgi but few cytoskeletal elements. Note processes (P) myelinating nearby axons (A).
(c) Oligodendrocytes can be identified by immunochemical staining for specific proteins, in this instance highlighting oligodendrocytes (brown), but not other cells such as microglia or astrocytes.

Oligodendrocytes are the myelin-forming cells of the CNS.

Oligodendrocytes produce myelin within the CNS, each cell sending out several cell processes and myelinating several nearby axons (Fig. 6.13).

In routine histologic preparations of oligodendrocytes, their branching morphology is not seen, but they do show a rounded nucleus with moderately dense-staining chromatin and, in most preparations, a cytoplasm containing a clear 'halo' around the nucleus. Such a halo is an artifact of preparation because oligodendrocytes are fragile and contain few cytoskeletal elements.

Immunohistochemical staining for myelin-related proteins, for example myelin basic protein, can be used specifically to identify oligodendrocytes (Fig. 6.13c).

DISEASES AFFECTING MYELIN

Multiple sclerosis.

The myelin of the CNS is the target for attack by the immune system in multiple sclerosis (Fig. 6.14), which is of unknown cause.

Myelin is vital for the CNS to function effectively and its destruction in multiple sclerosis results in severe functional deficits, such as paralysis, loss of sensation and/or loss of coordination. The nature of the deficit depends on the area of the CNS affected.

Fig. 6.14 Multiple sclerosis.

Low-power micrograph of the pons region of the brain, which has been prepared using a method that stains myelin blue. Large patches of myelin have been destroyed, leaving pale-stained spaces and only a little blue-stained myelin remains.

LEUKODYSTROPHY

Several inherited diseases of metabolism result in defective production of myelin within the nervous system. Such disorders are called leukodystrophies. Affected children have severe neurologic deficits and progressive degeneration of myelin. Some of these diseases are due to lysosomal defects preventing normal metabolism of myelin lipids.

Ependymal cells are epithelial-like and have cilia.

Ependymal cells are epithelial in type and line the cavities in the brain (ventricles) and the central canal of the spinal cord, forming a sheet of cuboidal cells in contact with the cerebrospinal fluid.

Each ependymal cell has a small oval basal nucleus with dense chromatin, and many are ciliated (Fig. 6.15).

Fig. 6.15 Ependyma.
ⓐ Micrograph showing ependymal cells (E) lining the lateral ventricle (V) of the brain. They are cuboidal epithelial cells and rest on underlying glial processes in the brain, (B).
ⓑ Scanning electronmicrograph showing that many of the ependymal cells bear tufts of surface cilia.

Ultrastructurally the cells are bound to each other by prominent desmosomal junctions and have apical microvilli in addition to cilia.

Unlike other epithelial cells, the ependymal cells do not lie on a basement membrane, but have tapering processes which merge with the processes of underlying astrocytic cells.

Microglia are specialized immune cells in the CNS.

The CNS has its own unique set of immune cells, the main type being the microglial cells which are specialized macrophages.

In conventional H&E preparations microglial cells are not easily seen, appearing only as rod-shaped nuclei with no discernible cytoplasmic borders. Immunohistochemical staining (Fig. 6.16), however, shows that they have extensive fine ramifying processes and form a widespread network of cells throughout the brain.

The phenotype of microglia suggests that they are similar to dendritic antigen-presenting cells (see page 123), having a low level of phagocytic activity, and expressing class II major histocompatibility molecules.

In disease states microglial cells become activated and increase in size and number. Under these circumstances they are usually supplemented by monocytes, which enter the brain from the blood and form macrophagic cells.

In addition to the microglial cells, which are intrinsic to the brain, there are large numbers of macrophages in the perivascular spaces outside the brain substance, and these cells can also act as immune effector cells.

The brain appears to have only a very small traffic of lymphoid cells in the normal state.

Fig. 6.16 Microglia.
Micrograph of brain stained by a lectin technique using *Ricinus communis* agglutinin, which binds to a sugar on the surface of microglial cells and endothelial cells in the brain.

Microglial cells (brown) have a rod-shaped or elliptical dark-staining nucleus and a fine ramified dendritic morphology consisting of numerous extremely fine cell processes. They can also be immunocytochemically stained by many of the antisera which react with surface markers expressed by macrophages.

The meninges are membrane systems covering and supporting the CNS.

The CNS is invested by three protective coats, the meninges, which are composed of fibrocollagenous support tissue and epithelial cells (Fig. 6.17). There are three meningeal layers: the dura, the arachnoid and the pia.

The **dura** is a tough fibrocollagenous layer, which forms the outer coat of the CNS. It blends with the periosteum of the skull and is attached to the periosteum of the vertebral canal by the dentinate ligaments. It is covered on its internal surface by an incomplete layer of flat epithelial cells.

The dura is reflected down from the skull to form sheets of tissue, the tentorium cerebelli and the falx cerebri, which separate the structures of the brain. The venous sinuses of the brain run at the base of these sheets of dura.

The **arachnoid** is a layer of fibrocollagenous tissue covered by inconspicuous flat epithelial cells and is located beneath, but not anchored to, the dura. Web-like strands of fibrocollagenous tissue extend down from the arachnoid into the subarachnoid space, which contains the cerebrospinal fluid. The main arteries and veins to and from the brain run in the subarachnoid space.

The **pia** is a delicate layer of epithelial cells associated with loose fibrocollagenous tissue. It lies external to a basement membrane which completely invests the CNS. This basement membrane is formed by a special set of astrocytes, termed the **limiting glia (glia limitans)**.

Fig. 6.17 Meninges and glia limitans.
ⓐ The meninges cover the CNS and are divided into three layers: dura, arachnoid, and pia. Below the pia there is a basement membrane giving rise to a set of astrocytic cells which form a barrier around the CNS termed the glia limitans. The subarachnoid space contains the cerebrospinal fluid.
ⓑ Micrograph showing the arachnoid (A), subarachnoid space (SAS) and underlying brain (B). Blood vessels (BV) run in the subarachnoid space.

ⓒ Meningothelial cells are normally flat, inconspicuous cells, which line the dura, arachnoid and pia, but with age some of these cells become histologically prominent; in this micrograph from the arachnoid of a 60-year-old man, the meningothelial cells (M) form a small aggregate (A).
ⓓ Electronmicrograph showing the glia limitans (GL) which forms an outer barrier investing the whole of the CNS. It is composed of a basement membrane, which is seen just beneath the pia collagen (P), and is produced by a sheet of closely adherent foot processes from astrocytic cells in the underlying brain.

MENINGEAL SPACES IN DISEASE

There are several spaces defined by the meninges of clinical importance. These are the subdural space, the subarachnoid space and the extradural space.

Extradural hematoma
Fracture of the skull causes an accumulation of blood outside the dura in the extradural space.

Subdural hematoma
Following trauma bleeding may occur from venous channels into the space between the dura and the arachnoid (subdural space).

Subarachnoid hemorrhage
Rupture of arteries running outside the brain causes bleeding into the subarachnoid space between the arachnoid and pia.

Meningitis
The cerebrospinal fluid in the subarachnoid space is the site of infection in meningitis.

Fig. 6.18 Choroid plexus.
ⓐ Micrograph showing a portion of choroid plexus covered with a columnar epithelium (E) which is arranged as papillae over vascular stromal cores, (C).
ⓑ Scanning electronmicrograph showing the convoluted surface of the choroid plexus, which is thrown into deep folds, and the fine microvilli on the apical surface of the covering epithelium.

The choroid plexus is responsible for production of cerebrospinal fluid.

The choroid plexuses are located in the ventricular system of the brain and produce cerebrospinal fluid. Each choroid plexus consists of a vascular stroma covered by columnar epithelial cells, which form large frond-like masses (Fig. 6.18). The epithelial cells are anchored by junctional complexes, rest on a basement membrane, have apical microvilli, and are adapted for secretion (see page 42).

The cerebrospinal fluid produced in the ventricles flows out through exit foramina at the base of the brain, and circulates in the subarachnoid space. It is reabsorbed by the venous sinuses in the dura.

TUMORS OF THE NERVOUS SYSTEM

Gliomas
Primary brain tumors are most commonly derived from the glial cells and are collectively termed **gliomas**.

The most common glioma is derived from astrocytes (**astrocytoma**), and varies from a slow-growing lesion, which diffusely infiltrates the brain over many years, to a rapidly growing lesion that soon compresses vital structures.

Ependymomas commonly arise in the region of the ventricles and are recognized histologically by their epithelial characteristics. **Oligodendrogliomas** are most common in the temporal lobe, where they may be a cause of temporal lobe epilepsy.

Certain tumors of the CNS resemble the primitive embryonic cells of the developing brain and are grouped together as **Primitive Neuroectodermal Tumors** (PNET). These are commonest in childhood and may show differentiation towards neuronal, astrocytic, or ependymal cells.

Meningiomas
The epithelial cells of the meninges (meningothelial cells) may form tumors termed meningiomas. These tumors appear macroscopically as rounded nodules, typically 3-4 cm in size, but can be much larger. Histologically meningiomas are made up of sheets of meningothelial cells which characteristically form spherical whorls.

Confirming the diagnosis
The diagnosis of CNS tumors must be confirmed by histology of tumor biopsies, and immunohistochemistry is used increasingly in the laboratory to identify cell types within a tumor. Finding glial fibrillary acidic protein (GFAP) is a strong indication that a tumor is of glial origin.

Blood vessels entering the CNS are surrounded by a perivascular space.

The brain is supplied with blood from major arteries that form an anastomotic link around the base of the brain. From this region, the arteries run in the subarachnoid space before turning and dipping down into the brain.

Around the large vessels within the brain is a perivascular space, called eponymously the **Virchow-Robin space**. In man this space is sealed from the subarachnoid space by reflections of the pia onto the blood vessels as they enter the brain (Fig. 6.19), and is therefore continuous with the potential subpial space.

The perivascular space is bounded externally by the basement membrane of the glia limitans (Fig. 6.17d) and extends as far as the capillaries, where the vascular and glial basement membranes fuse.

A blood-brain barrier prevents diffusion of materials into the CNS from the blood.

The microvascular system in the nervous system is highly specialized. The endothelial cells of brain capillaries are joined by occluding junctions and are not fenestrated, thus they form a barrier to the diffusion of substances from the blood to the brain. The brain endothelial cells have systems for active transport of substances such as glucose into the brain.

External to the capillary endothelium is a basement membrane and external to this is a layer composed of the foot processes of astrocytes (Fig. 6.11).

These three layers (endothelium, basal lamina, astrocyte foot processes) form a functional **blood-brain barrier** which is important in the physiology of CNS function. There is considerable evidence that in embryogenesis it is the interaction of astrocyte foot processes which is responsible for induction of the special properties of the cerebral capillary endothelial cells (see page 86).

Fig. 6.19 Vascular arrangement in the brain.
ⓐ Arteries running in the subarachnoid space penetrate the pia, which is reflected up onto the wall of the vessel, thus isolating the perivascular space from the subarachnoid space. The layer of pia reflected onto the vessel is composed of a single layer of flat meningothelial cells anchored by junctional complexes. The perivascular space is continuous with the potential subpial space.
ⓑ Micrograph showing vessels (V) penetrating the surface of the brain (B) from the subarachnoid space (SAS). The pia (P) is reflected onto the vessel wall and separates the subarachnoid space from the perivascular space (PVS).
ⓒ Scanning electronmicrograph showing the subarachnoid space (SAS) with an artery (A) becoming invested by pia (P). Note the underlying subpial space, (SPS) and brain (B).

PERIPHERAL NERVOUS SYSTEM

The peripheral nervous system is made up of nerve cells and support cells.

The peripheral nervous system is described in terms of nerves and ganglia.

A **nerve** is a collection of axons, linked together by support tissue into an anatomically defined trunk. The axons may be either motor or sensory, myelinated or non-myelinated.

A **ganglion** is a peripheral collection of nerve cell bodies together with efferent and afferent axons, and support cells. Ganglia may be sensory (e.g. spinal sensory ganglia) or contain the cell bodies of autonomic nerves (i.e. sympathetic or parasympathetic ganglia).

Peripheral nerves are bundles of axons associated with support tissues.

A peripheral nerve is composed of:
- axons;
- Schwann cells, which make myelin;
- spindle-shaped fibroblast support cells, which produce fibrocollagenous tissue;
- blood vessels.

The endoneurium, perineurium and epineurium are composed of support tissues.

There are three types of support tissue in a nerve trunk, the endoneurium, perineurium and epineurium (Fig. 6.20).

ENDONEURIUM is composed of longitudinally orientated collagen fibers, extracellular matrix material rich in glycosaminoglycans, and sparse fibroblasts. It surrounds the individual axons and their associated Schwann cells, as well as capillary blood vessels.

PERINEURIUM surrounds groups of axons and endoneurium to form small bundles (fascicles). It is composed of 7–8 concentric layers of epithelium-like flattened cells separated by layers of collagen. The cells are joined by junctional complexes and each layer of cells is surrounded by an external lamina.

EPINEURIUM is an outer sheath of loose fibrocollagenous tissue, which binds individual nerve fascicles into a nerve trunk. The epineurium may also include adipose tissue, as well as a main muscular artery supplying the nerve trunk.

Schwann cells support both myelinated and non-myelinated axons.

Within a peripheral nerve there are both myelinated and non-myelinated axons which are both supported by Schwann cells. Each Schwann cell has a well-defined external lamina which separates the cell from the endoneurium.

The myelin of peripheral nerve differs from that in CNS as it has a different set of myelin-related proteins. Each Schwann cell produces myelin for one axon and this contrasts with oligodendrocytes in the CNS (page 87).

In addition to producing myelin, Schwann cells also support non-myelinated axons which bury themselves into the Schwann cell cytoplasm (Fig. 6.21).

Nerves vary in their relative composition of myelinated and non-myelinated fibers from one anatomic site to another. Myelinated fibers in a typical peripheral nerve in the lower limb of an adult vary in diameter from 2–17 μm (including myelin), there being a bimodal distribution with peaks around 5 μm and 13 μm.

Fig. 6.20 **Support tissue of peripheral nerve.**
(a) Diagram showing the arrangement of support tissue in a peripheral nerve. Individual axons and their associated Schwann cells are surrounded by endoneurium, and bound into fascicles by the epithelial-like perineurium. The epineurium binds individual fascicles into a nerve trunk, and may contain the main muscular artery supplying the nerve trunk.
(b) Micrograph showing nerve fascicles (F) surrounded by perineurium (P) and grouped into a nerve trunk by epineurium (E). Note blood vessels (BV).

Ganglia are neuronal relay centers in the peripheral nervous system.

A ganglion is composed of:
- neuron cell bodies;
- support cells (satellite cells and Schwann cells);
- axons;
- loose fibrocollagenous support tissue (Fig. 6.22).

The neuron cell bodies are large; they have abundant cytoplasm containing Nissl substance and large nuclei with prominent nucleoli.

Satellite cells are small support cells resembling Schwann cells which surround the neuron cell bodies.

Fig. 6.21 Peripheral nerve.
ⓐ Micrograph of the edge of a single fascicle from a peripheral nerve stained with osmium, which stains myelin black. The perineurium (P) surrounds the fascicle. The myelinated axons appear as circular profiles with the central non-staining area occupied by axon. Non-myelinated fibers are not visible.
ⓑ Micrograph of a small nerve fascicle embedded in resin and stained with toluidine blue. The increased resolution allows myelinated axons (M), to be seen with associated Schwann cell nuclei (S), and endoneurial support tissue (E). The perineurium (P) is visible as 2–3 thin cell and collagen layers.
ⓒ Non-myelinated fibers are buried into and thereby supported by the cytoplasm of Schwann cells.
ⓓ Electronmicrograph showing non-myelinated axons (A) of a peripheral nerve embedded in the cytoplasm of Schwann cells, (S).

Fig. 6.22 Ganglion.
Micrograph showing a peripheral sensory ganglion containing neurons (N) with large nuclei and prominent nucleoli, surrounded by small darkly-stained satellite support cells. Axons running to and from the ganglion are supported by Schwann cells and a loose fibrocollagenous stroma.

REPAIR IN THE PERIPHERAL NERVOUS SYSTEM

The axons of neurons can regenerate following damage if the cell body remains alive.

Following section of a nerve supplying a muscle, the axons and myelin beyond the area of damage degenerate and are removed by Schwann cell lysosomes and by macrophages which migrate into the nerve (Wallerian degeneration). The neuron cell body accumulates large amounts of neurofilaments, and the Nissl substance and nucleus migrate peripherally, so that it appears pale and swollen with an eccentric nucleus (chromatolysis).

The Schwann cells proliferate and form longitudinal columns of cells in the distal damaged nerve. At the proximal end the damaged axons re-grow by sprouting, the sprouts growing down the cords of Schwann cells at 2–5 mm/day. One fiber eventually connects with the muscle, becomes remyelinated and reestablishes innervation (Fig. 6.23). The cell body then resumes a normal appearance.

Fig. 6.23 Repair in the peripheral nervous system.
Following damage to a myelinated neuron innervating a muscle fiber, the distal axon and myelin are phagocytosed by proliferating Schwann cells.

The muscle fiber, devoid of innervation, undergoes wasting, while the cell body of the neuron undergoes chromatolysis, with swelling, lateral migration of the nucleus, and loss of Nissl substance.

Axons then sprout from the damaged end of the nerve and grow down the column of Schwann cells, eventually restoring innervation of the muscle.

The Schwann cells remyelinate the axon, but the myelin segments are much shorter than before damage.

Fig. 6.24 Cerebral hemispheres.

(a) Micrograph of a section through the temporal lobe of the brain at low magnification. The cerebral hemisphere is thrown into a series of convolutions, the gyri (G) which are separated by intervening sulci, (S).

The arachnoid covers the brain and is just visible at this magnification over the subarachnoid space (SAS). The white matter (W) contains the axons of nerve cells which run to and from the cortex (C). The cortex is composed of nerve cells and does not contain myelin.

In H&E preparations the white matter stains more intensely with eosin (pink) than the cortex.

(b) Micrograph of the same section shown in (a) after staining with a dye with an affinity for myelin. Such a dye delineates the white matter (W) but does not stain the cortex (gray matter).

Fig. 6.25 Cerebral cortex.

High-power micrograph of cerebral cortex. Neurons (N) vary in size and shape according to their function, which is specific for different levels in the cortex, and in most of the cerebral cortex there are six distinct layers of different neuronal types. Capillary vessels (C) are plentiful.

The small densely stained nuclei belong to a mixture of glial cells, of which oligodendrocytes (O) are most prominent. Cortical oligodendrocytes do not make myelin, but act as support cells for axons and neurons. The oligodendrocytes adjacent to neurons are called satellite cells.

The pink-stained background is a mat of neuronal and glial cell processes (neuropil).

Fig. 6.26 White matter.

High-power micrograph of white matter, in which it is generally not possible to perceive individual nerve fibers or cell processes because they merge into the pink-staining background of the neuropil.

The nuclei of glial cells are prominent but again details of the cytoplasm merge into the neuropil. Different glial types can be distinguished by the character of their nuclei.

Oligodendrocytes (O) are most numerous and have rounded nuclei, which are often surrounded by an ill-defined clear perinuclear halo. Astrocytes (A) are fewer in number and are characterized by larger polygonal nuclei, which commonly contain central nucleoli. The nuclei of microglial cells (M) are frequently rod-shaped or comma-shaped and stain more densely than those of the other glia.

Fig. 6.27 Cerebellum.

ⓐ Micrograph of cerebellum, which is a distinct part of the brain and is characterized by complex folding of cerebellar cortex, generating a pattern of pleats (**cerebellar folia**). The folia contain the nuclei of nerve cells, which produce a purple staining ribbon at this low magnification. The centre of the cerebellum is composed of white matter (W) in which a serpiginous aggregate of nerve cells, termed a **nucleus (N)** is seen.

ⓑ Higher-power micrograph of cerebellum showing that the outer part of the cerebellar cortex is composed of nerve cell processes with scanty glial cells (the **molecular layer, M**) while the bulk of the purple staining ribbon is formed by a band of small nerve cells with dark-staining rounded nuclei (the **granular layer (G)**. Below the granular layer is the white matter, (W) which contains myelinated fibers. At the junction of the molecular layer with the granular layer is a row of large nerve cells (**Purkinje cells, P**) which are characterized by a vast branching pattern of dendrites in the molecular layer, but this is only visible by special staining methods.

Fig. 6.28 Motor neurons of spinal cord.

Micrograph of spinal motor neurons (MN) which send axons (Ax) out to supply voluntary muscles and lie in the anterior part of the spinal cord. These neurons are large because they maintain an axon that may be up to 1 m long. The nucleus is large with a prominent nucleolus and the cytoplasm is packed with purple staining Nissl substance (NS).

Motor neurons make multiple connections with the axons of other neurons via large dendrites (D). The axon of a motor neuron passes out through the spinal nerve roots and eventually forms part of a peripheral nerve.

The background in this micrograph is composed of a neuropil of nerve cell and glial processes and cannot be resolved with this type of preparation. The nuclei of oligodendrocytes (O) and astrocytes (A) are visible.

Fig. 6.29 Neuromelanin-containing neurons.

Micrograph of neurons containing brown neuromelanin pigment (M). Such cells are part of the substantia nigra, so named because of its black color imparted by the melanin, and contain transmitter substance dopamine, which is responsible for coordination and fluidity of movement.

Destruction of these neurons results in Parkinson's disease, which is characterized by rigid, slow movement and a tremor.

Fig. 6.30 Central canal of spinal cord.

Micrograph showing the central canal of the spinal cord. It is lined by ependymal cells (E) and contains cerebrospinal fluid, (CSF).

Fig. 6.31 Peripheral nerve.

In this micrograph of a longitudinally sectioned peripheral nerve, myelin (M) is just visible as long tapering profiles with a granular or foamy texture. The nuclei of the Schwann cells, which make the myelin, are the most conspicuous feature, and are typically long and tapering.

1. IN A NEURON

(a) dendrites carry signals away from the cell body
(b) there are few lysosomes
(c) the smooth endoplasmic reticulum is termed Nissl substance
(d) slow anterograde transport down the axon is mediated by microtubules
(e) the terminal bouton is located at the end of the axon

2. IN A SYNAPSE

(a) synaptic vesicles are derived solely from transport down the axon
(b) release of neurotransmitter is mediated by voltage-sensitive calcium channels in the nerve terminal
(c) release of transmitter substance is via diffusion through the presynaptic membrane
(d) the post synaptic membrane is fused to the presynaptic membrane by cell adhesion proteins
(e) membrane from synaptic vesicles becomes transiently incorporated into the presynaptic membrane

3. MYELIN

(a) completely ensheathes myelinated axons throughout their length
(b) is formed by Schwann cells in the central nervous system
(c) may regenerate after damage in the peripheral nervous system
(d) reduces the conduction speed in very large diameter axons
(e) in the PNS has a different biochemical composition to that in the CNS

4. IN THE PERIPHERAL NERVOUS SYSTEM

(a) the perineurium surrounds a group of nerve fascicles
(b) the epineurium is composed of flattened, epithelial-like cells
(c) axons are all myelinated
(d) nodes of Ranvier are areas of bare axon between segments of myelination
(e) ganglia contain neuronal cell bodies, axons, Schwann cells and satellite cells

7. Blood Cells

The blood is a mixture of cellular elements, fluid, proteins and metabolites.

Blood has four major elements:

- **red blood cells** (erythrocytes) transport oxygen from the lungs to the peripheral tissues;
- **white blood cells** (leukocytes) have a defensive role, destroying infecting organisms such as bacteria and viruses, as well as assisting in the removal of dead or damaged tissues;
- **platelets** (thrombocytes) are the first line of defense against damage to blood vessels, adhering to defects and participating in the blood clotting system;
- **plasma** is the proteinaceous solution in which the above-mentioned cells circulate, and carries nutrients, metabolites, antibodies, hormones, proteins of the blood clotting system and other molecules throughout the body.

In post-natal life, under normal circumstances, the cellular elements in the blood are formed in tissue lying within the center of bones termed the **bone marrow**. Most of the proteins in the plasma are made by the liver.

METHODS OF STUDYING THE BLOOD

Blood is readily accessible by sampling with a needle and syringe. The name for the two main types of cell in blood derives from what is seen if blood is prevented from clotting and left to stand in a tube. Blood settles into several layers; a thick layer of clear plasma is seen at the top of the tube, beneath which is a very thin layer of white material on top of a thick layer of red material. The cells in the white material are called white cells and the cells in the red material red cells.

The usual way to look at blood is to make a very thin smear on a glass slide. The names applied to the white cells are largely derived from the stains used to examine blood smears. The main staining method used (Romanovsky stain) involves applying several dyes which have affinity for different cellular constituents (Fig 7.1).

Under the microscope it is possible to count the proportion of different cell types in blood and since it has been found that this reflects disease processes, a blood count is a valuable clinical investigation. In modern laboratory practice routine counting of cells in blood is done electronically on preparations of cells in suspension. Smears of blood are still examined for morphologic abnormalities of cells.

Fig. 7.1 Blood film.
A blood film is made by smearing a sample of peripheral blood, which has been previously mixed with an anticoagulant, on a slide and staining with a mixture of dyes. Four white blood cells (nucleated) of various types are seen against a background of numerous smaller anucleate red blood cells.

RED BLOOD CELLS

Red blood cells are highly deformable and are specialized for carrying oxygen.

The red blood cells are responsible for oxygen transport. Red cells in peripheral blood smears (Fig 7.2 a, b) appear as rounded bright pink-stained cells. They are 6.5–8.5 μm in diameter and have a biconcave shape, appearing paler in the center and darker at the periphery. The biconcave shape maximizes their surface area/volume ratio and thereby maximizes oxygen exchange. The bright pink color (acidophilia) is due to the content of oxygen-carrying hemoglobin which binds the acidic eosin dye used in staining. Red cells do not have a nucleus as this is lost during formation (page 114). In wax-processed tissue sections, red cells appear smaller and the biconcave shape is generally not discernible.

Ultrastructurally, red cells have a cell membrane which surrounds an electron-dense cytoplasm. There are no discernible organelles as these have been degraded during differentiation. Despite a lack of organelles, red cells are metabolically active and derive energy by anaerobic metabolism of glucose and through ATP generation by the hexose monophosphate shunt.

Functionally, red cells are highly deformable and are able to squeeze through small blood vessels down to 3–4 μm in diameter. The cell membrane is braced by an actin/spectrin-containing cytoskeletal meshwork which is largely responsible for maintaining the distinctive biconcave shape (Fig 7.2c).

Red cells have a limited life span and are eventually destroyed in the spleen.

Red cells have a short life span of 100–120 days in the circulation. The mature red cell is unable to synthesize new enzymes to replace those lost during normal metabolic processes. Diminishing efficiency of ion pumping mechanisms is probably the main factor in red cell aging, the cell becoming progressively less deformable until it is unable to negotiate the splenic microcirculation and is removed by phagocytosis. The spleen, liver and bone marrow all dispose of aged and defective red cells, but their relative contributions under normal conditions is uncertain; the spleen appears to be the most active.

cell membrane   band 3 protein

band 4 protein   ankyrin   actin link piece

spectrin filament

Fig. 7.2 Mature red cell.
(a) Typical appearance of a mature red cell in a stained smear of the peripheral blood. It is a biconcave-disk 1.8 μm thick and ranges from 6.5–8.5 μm in diameter, the size decreasing slightly with age. Its main cytoplasmic constituent is the protein complex hemoglobin, which results in its characteristic acidophilic staining property. Due to its biconcave shape which facilitates oxygen exchange, the centre of the cell appears pale.
(b) Scanning electronmicrograph showing the typical biconcave structure of a mature red cell.
(c) Diagram to illustrate the red cell cytoskeleton, which maintains its distinct shape. A filamentous skeleton of the protein spectrin is anchored to the cell membrane by three main proteins (band 3 protein, ankyrin, and band 4 protein), with short actin pieces, about 15 actin monomers long, linking spectrin to the band 4 protein. Other proteins are also involved, but have been omitted for clarity.

HEREDITARY SPHEROCYTOSIS

Hereditary spherocytosis is caused by an abnormal arrangement of the internal cytoskeleton of red cells. Normally the internal surface of the cell membrane is braced by cytoskeletal proteins via interactions between ankyrin and spectrin (Fig. 7.2c). In hereditary spherocytosis, the ankyrin binding of spectrin is absent. As a result the red cell membrane is not braced and is easily deformed.

In hereditary spherocytosis red cells do not form their normal biconcave disk shape, but appear round and convex (Fig. 7.3). They are abnormally fragile and do not resist changes in osmotic pressure. This abnormally rapid breakdown of red blood cells is called hemolysis.

Fig. 7.3 Hereditary spherocytosis.
Micrograph showing the abnormal round convex-shaped blood cell of hereditary spherocytosis. Compare with Fig. 7.2a.

ANEMIA

The most common blood disorder is anemia in which an inadequate hemoglobin supply causes weakness, pallor and, sometimes, breathlessness. It may be the result of either impaired red cell formation or excessive red cell destruction.

The most common cause is deficiency of iron, which is essential for the formation of hemoglobin. Red cells are released into the circulation containing much less hemoglobin than normal, and are therefore pale-staining (hypochromic) and small (microcytic) (Fig. 7.4).

Excessive red cell destruction usually occurs because the red cells are structurally abnormal and therefore more liable to damage while circulating. Such cells are removed prematurely and in excess by the spleen, causing hemolytic anemia. This can be due to a genetic abnormality of red cell structure, and occurs in hereditary spherocytosis (Fig 7.3). Point mutations in the hemoglobin gene may cause abnormal red cells. Sickle cell anemia is caused by such a mutation leading to precipitation of hemoglobin in red cells subject to hypoxia which causes a sickle-shape instead of the biconcave disk. Sickled cells become disrupted and can also block blood vessels.

Fig. 7.4 Hypochromic, microcytic anemia.
Micrograph of blood smear showing the hypochromic, microcytic red cells of iron deficiency anemia. Compare with Fig. 7.2a.

RED CELLS

- biconcave shape for high surface area/volume ratio

- main function is oxygen carriage

- contain hemoglobin

- have no cell organelles

- cell membrane is braced by an actin-containing cytoskeleton which maintains shape

WHITE BLOOD CELLS

There are five main types of white blood cell.

White cells use the blood for transport from the bone marrow to their major sites of activity. The majority of the functions of white blood cells take place when they leave the circulation to enter tissues. The total number of white cells in peripheral blood is normally 4.0–11.0 $\times 10^9$/liter.

There are five types of white cell, and their names and relative proportions in the circulation are as follows:
- neutrophils 40–75%;
- eosinophils 5%;
- basophils 0.5%;
- lymphocytes 20–50%;
- monocytes 1–5%.

If there is a requirement for increased activity of any one cell type in the peripheral tissues, the number and proportion of that cell type rises accordingly.

Neutrophils, eosinophils and basophils are known as **granulocytes** because their cytoplasm contains prominent granules, and may also be referred to as myeloid cells because of their origin from bone marrow. Neutrophils are also commonly called polymorphonuclear leukocytes or polymorphs because of the multilobed nucleus.

Lymphocytes and monocytes are classed as white blood cells because they are a constituent of the blood and ultimately originate from bone marrow. They are found mainly in tissues such as lymph nodes and spleen. In the tissues, monocytes transform into macrophages and basophils become mast cells.

White cell traffic from blood vessels is mediated by cell adhesion molecules.

Normally white cells circulate in an inactive state in the blood. To leave a capillary vessel and enter tissues white cells have first to stick to the endothelium lining capillaries and then pass into the tissues by traversing the vessel wall. The adhesion to endothelium is mediated by complementary cell adhesion molecules expressed on the white cell surface and the surface of the endothelium. Normally such molecules are not strongly expressed and so there is little traffic. In disease states cytokines cause activation of both white cells and endothelium, there is high expression of adhesion molecules, and cells stick firmly to the endothelium. Further cell signals then cause white cells to become motile and gain the ability actively to migrate into the tissues.

Neutrophils are the commonest type of white blood cell.

Neutrophils (Fig. 7.5) are the most abundant of the circulating white cells. They circulate in a resting state but, with appropriate activation, leave the blood and enter tissues where they become highly motile, phagocytic cells. Their primary function is to ingest and destroy invading microorganisms in tissues. They play a central role in the early stages of the acute inflammatory response to tissue injury and are the major constituent of pus.

The neutrophil nucleus has several lobes.

The characteristic neutrophil nucleus is composed of 2–5 distinct lobes, joined to one another by fine strands of nuclear material, the lobulation developing with cellular maturity. The chromatin is highly condensed, reflecting a low degree of protein synthesis.

In females, about 3% of nuclei exhibit a small, condensed nuclear appendage (drumstick chromosome), which represents the quiescent X chromosome (Barr body).

Neutrophils contain three types of granule.

Neutrophil cytoplasm contains three types (i.e. primary, secondary and tertiary) of membrane-bound vesicles (granules) (Fig 7.6).

Primary granules are similar to lysosomes (see page 21) in other cells. They are the first granules to appear during neutrophil formation, but as the cell matures, their

Fig. 7.5 Neutrophil.
ⓐ A mature neutrophil is 12–14 μm in diameter and has a characteristic multilobed nucleus (N), and pale-staining cytoplasm, in which only a few of the many granules it contains can be seen in a routine stain.
ⓑ Electronmicrograph of a neutrophil from the blood, showing its characteristic multilobed nucleus (N), cytoplasmic processes (CP), and mixture of granule types within its cytoplasm. At this magnification, individual granule types cannot be identified.

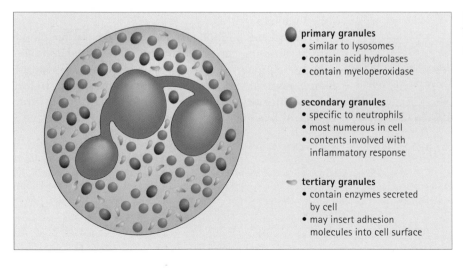

Fig 7.6 Neutrophil granules.
The neutrophil contains three types of granule.

primary granules
- similar to lysosomes
- contain acid hydrolases
- contain myeloperoxidase

secondary granules
- specific to neutrophils
- most numerous in cell
- contents involved with inflammatory response

tertiary granules
- contain enzymes secreted by cell
- may insert adhesion molecules into cell surface

number falls with respect to secondary granules (see below), making them difficult to see with light microscopy. With electron microscopy, they are large and electron-dense. As with lysosomes, primary granules contain acid hydrolases, but in addition they also contain antibacterial and digestive substances, most notably myeloperoxidase, which can be detected by the peroxidase stain. Myeloperoxidase is therefore a useful light microscopic marker not only for these granules, but also in establishing cell lineage in the diagnosis of leukemias (see page 107).

Secondary granules are specific to neutrophils and twice as numerous as primary granules. With a diameter of 0.2–0.8 μm (i.e. smaller than primary granules), they are barely visible with light microscopy.

Ultrastructural studies have shown secondary granules to be of variable size, shape and density and to contain substances involved in the mobilization of inflammatory mediators and complement activation. These substances are secreted into the extracellular environment.

Tertiary granules have only recently been described and contain enzymes (e.g. gelatinase) secreted into the extracellular environment. They also insert some glycoproteins into cell membranes, and this may promote cellular adhesion and hence may be involved in the phagocytic process.

Neutrophils are adapted for anaerobic metabolism.

The neutrophil cytoplasm contains few organelles apart from granules. There are only a few scattered profiles of rough endoplasmic reticulum and free ribosomes, with the remnants of the Golgi complex involved in granule packaging earlier in development. While mitochondria are also few, they provide about 50% of energy needs.

Once activated, neutrophils need to be able to operate in devascularized tissue where oxygen and glucose may be in short supply. They therefore contain abundant glycogen for anerobic metabolism, which occurs mainly via the glycolytic pathway. Energy production may also take place via the hexose monophosphate shunt, but this is used to generate microbicidal oxidants rather than for general cellular upkeep.

Once neutrophils have become activated in tissues, they do not live for long. The neutrophil cytoplasm also contains various antioxidants to destroy potentially toxic peroxides which may be generated during lysosomal activity.

Neutrophils migrate into areas of tissue damage where they have a defensive role.

Phagocytosis (Fig. 7.7) is the process whereby cells ingest extracellular particles for destruction. Neutrophils have a role in the phagocytosis of bacteria and dead cells.

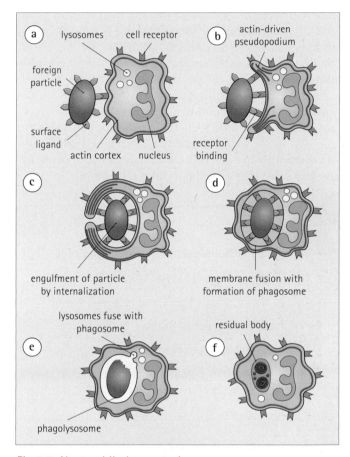

Fig 7.7 Neutrophil phagocytosis.
(a) Neutrophils have membrane receptors, mainly for the Fc portion of antibodies, complement factors bound to foreign particles, and bacterial polysaccharides. Neutrophils do not phagocytose material to which they do not bind.
(b) As the first step in phagocytosis the neutrophil binds to the abnormal particle by its specific receptors. The cell pushes out pseudopodia to surround the particle, driven by assembly and disassembly of actin filaments.
(c) The pseudopodia fuse to enclose completely the abnormal particle and form an endocytotic vesicle. Special proteins probably allow final sealing of the membrane.
(d) The internalized particle in the endocytotic vesicle is called a phagosome.
(e) The phagosome fuses with neutrophil granules, particularly primary granules, which discharge their contents, exposing the particle to a potent mixture of lysosomal enzymes. If the particle is a bacterium, killing is enhanced by hydrogen peroxide and superoxide generated by the enzymatic reduction of oxygen by respiratory burst oxidase (RBO) a membrane enzyme.
(f) Foreign particle destruction is associated with formation of a residual body containing degraded material.

To reach an area of infection or tissue damage, neutrophils leave the circulation by adhering to endothelial cells by adhesion molecules expressed in response to local secretion of cytokines, and move through the endothelium and basement membrane.

Once in the support tissue, neutrophils respond to chemicals (chemotaxins), moving towards the highest concentration. Chemotaxins include degradation products of complement, products leaking from dead cells, and bacterial-derived polysaccharides in the extracellular space. Neutrophil motility is derived from assembly and disassembly of cellular actin filaments.

Neutrophils typically die soon after phagocytosis as this highly energy-dependent process uses up their glycogen reserve. When they die their lysosomal enzymes are released in the extracellular space, causing liquefaction of adjacent tissue. The collection of dead neutrophils, tissue fluid and abnormal material is termed pus.

NEUTROPHILS

- one of the myeloid series of white blood cells

- one of the granulocyte type of white blood cells

- main role in phagocytosis and bacterial killing

- contains three types of granule in cytoplasm

- cells marked by myeloperoxidase

- increase in number in blood in bacterial infection and inflammation ('neutrophilia')

Eosinophils have a bilobed nucleus and acidophilic granules.

Eosinophils have a bilobed nucleus and contain strongly eosinophilic granules (Fig. 7.8). They are phagocytic, with a particular affinity for antigen–antibody complexes, but have less microbicidal activity than neutrophils.

After production in the bone marrow eosinophils are stored for several days before release into the circulation, where they remain for 3–8 hours before preferentially migrating to the skin, lungs and gastrointestinal tract. They may enter lung and gut secretions via lymphatics or by direct migration.

Circulating eosinophil numbers show a marked diurnal variation, being maximal in the morning and minimal in the afternoon. They increase greatly in many types of parasitic infestation, and protection against parasitic disease appears to be one of their main functions.

Tissue (and sometimes blood) eosinophil numbers are also increased in certain allergic states, for example in the nasal and bronchial mucosae in hay fever and asthma, and in adverse reactions to drugs. Eosinophils do not usually re-enter the circulation after tissue migration, and their life span is uncertain.

Fig. 7.8 Eosinophil.
(a) The eosinophil is 12–17 μm in diameter in blood films, and is easily recognizable by its large granules, which stain bright red. Most have a bilobed nucleus, but nuclear detail is often obscured by the numerous overlying, densely packed granules.
(b) Electronmicrograph of an eosinophil from blood showing its characteristic bilobed nucleus (N) scattered mitochondria (M) and cytoplasmic glycogen.

The characteristic granules (LG) are large and ovoid in shape (0.15–1.5 μm long and 0.3–1.0 μm wide), and contain a central electron-dense crystalloid (C) surrounded by a less dense matrix. In humans, the crystalloid has a cubic lattice structure and consists of an extremely alkaline (basic) protein called major basic protein, as well as other basic proteins, hydrolytic lysosomal enzymes and peroxidase, which has a different substrate specificity to the neutrophil myeloperoxidase.

Smaller granules (G) 0.1–1.5 μm in diameter, are also present in mature eosinophils and contain acid phosphatase and aryl sulfatase, which is eight times more concentrated than in other white cells and appears to be secreted in the absence of phagocytosis and degranulation.

Eosinophil phagocytosis and degranulation

Like neutrophils, eosinophils move chemotactically in response to bacterial products and complement components. They are preferentially attracted by substances released from mast cells, notably histamine and eosinophil chemotactic factor of anaphylaxis (ECF-A), as well as by activated lymphocytes (see Chapter 8).

All eosinophils have surface receptors for IgE (not found on neutrophils), which may be involved in the destruction of parasites. Only a few eosinophils have IgG Fc receptors, but these increase markedly in eosinophilia.

Phagocytosis involves the usual endocytotic process, but if the object is too large to be engulfed (e.g. a parasite), the eosinophil appears to release its granule contents into the external environment.

Eosinophils may function to localize the destructive effect of reactions causing secretion of mast cell granules (hypersensitivity allergic reactions) by:

- neutralizing histamine;

- producing a factor (eosinophil-derived-inhibitor), which is probably composed of prostaglandins E1 and E2, and is thought to inhibit mast cell degranulation.

Activated eosinophils inhibit vasoactive substances (e.g. leukotriene 3, formerly called SRS-A), which are produced by basophils and mast cells.

Basophils leave the circulation to form mast cells in tissues.

Basophils are the least common white cell in the blood. They are characterized by large, intensely basophilic, cytoplasmic granules, and are probably the precursors of tissue mast cells with which they have many structural and functional similarities (Fig. 7.9).

The granules of basophils and mast cells contain the sulfated proteoglycans, heparin and chondroitin sulfate, together with histamine and leukotriene 3.

Both basophils and mast cells have highly specific membrane receptors for the Fc segment of IgE produced in response to allergens (see Chapter 8). Exposure to allergen results in rapid exocytosis of their granules, thereby releasing histamine and other vasoactive mediators, and

resulting in an **immediate hypersensitivity (anaphylactoid)** reaction. Such a reaction causes allergic rhinitis (hay fever), some forms of asthma, urticaria, and anaphylaxis. Mast cells reside in support tissues, especially those beneath epithelia, around blood vessels, and lining serous cavities. They are long lived and can proliferate in the tissues. In mucosae, but not in other sites, proliferation appears to depend on interaction with T lymphocytes.

Monocytes are part of a cell network, the monocyte-macrophage system.

Monocytes are the blood and bone marrow-located precursors of the macrophages found in tissues and lymphoid organs, and are members of a single functional unit, the monocyte-macrophage system (mononuclear phagocyte system). This system consists of the bone marrow precursors (monoblasts and promonocytes), circulating monocytes, and tissue macrophages, both free and fixed (histiocytes). Also included in this system are:

Fig. 7.9 Basophil and mast cell.
(a) The basophil is 14–16 μm in diameter. Its nucleus (N) is bilobed, the two lobes exhibiting marked chromatin condensation. The cytoplasmic granules are large, dark-blue staining, and often obscure the nucleus.
(b) Mast cells in tissues are ovoid or elongated spindle cells with a non-segmented nucleus. Their granule content imparts a diffuse purplish color to the cytoplasm in H&E paraffin sections, unless special stains are used to demonstrate individual granules (as here). In thin resin H&E sections, the granules can be resolved by light microscopy.
(c) Ultrastructurally, mast cell granules (BG) are round or oval, membrane-bound and contain dense particles and less dense matrix. There is also a small population of smaller uniform granules found near the nucleus. Mast cell cytoplasm also contains free ribosomes, mitochondria and glycogen, while the cell membrane exhibits blunt, irregularly spaced surface projections.

- Kupffer cells of the liver;
- sinus lining cells of the spleen and lymph nodes (see Chapter 8);
- pulmonary alveolar macrophages;
- free macrophages in synovial, pleural and peritoneal fluid;
- dendritic antigen-presenting cells (see Chapter 8).

Monocytes are large motile, phagocytic cells. In blood films they often show vacuolated cytoplasm (Fig. 7.10).

Ultrastructurally monocyte cytoplasm contains numerous small lysosomal granules and cytoplasmic vacuoles. The granules are electron-dense, homogeneous and membrane-bound, and are of two types. One type represents primary lysosomes, contain acid phosphatase, aryl sulfatase and peroxidase, and are analogous to the primary granules of neutrophils. The content of the other group of granules is less certain. Numerous small pseudopodia extend from the monocyte, reflecting its phagocytic ability and ameboid movement.

Monocytes respond chemotactically to the presence of necrotic material, invading microorganisms, and inflammation, and leave the blood to enter the tissues, where they are called macrophages.

Monocyte numbers are depressed by corticosteroid administration.

Monocytes express high levels of MHC class II molecules on their surface. They are an important site for the formation of the cytokine IL-1, which has an important role in mediating systemic responses in acute inflammation.

Lymphocytes are responsible for generating specific immune responses.

In adults and older children lymphocytes are the second most numerous white cell in the blood, their numbers increasing in response to viral infections; they are the most numerous white cell in young children. Most circulating lymphocytes are small (Fig. 7.11), but about 3% are large, with a diameter of 9–15 μm. Their nuclei are ovoid or kidney-shaped, with the dense chromatin typical of cells with little biosynthetic activity. There are two main types of lymphocyte, termed B and T cells, which perform different but linked roles in generation of specific immune responses (see Chapter 8).

The small mature lymphocytes circulating in the blood emigrate into tissues and into special organs of the immune system. They are responsible for immune surveillance, constantly sampling their environment for foreign material. Lymphocytes then transform into active cells, mediating the immune responses, particularly in specialized lymphoid tissues (see Chapter 8). Large lymphocytes may be seen in the blood, representing such activated lymphocytes en route to the tissues.

Plasma cells are formed from B lymphocytes and secrete immunoglobulin.

Plasma cells are a differentiated form of B lymphocyte (Chapter 8) and actively synthesize immunoglobulin.

Plasma cells form a small population in normal marrow and are usually seen in support tissues and specialized lymphoid organs. In health, they are not found in the blood.

Plasma cells are large and have an eccentrically located, round or oval nucleus with the chromatin coarsely clumped in a characteristic cartwheel or clockface pattern, reflecting active transcription.

Their cytoplasm is moderately basophilic due to its large content of ribosomal RNA in abundant rough endoplasmic reticulum required to manufacture the immunoglobulin protein. A well-developed Golgi complex displaces the nucleus and is visible as a paranuclear halo, termed a hof (Fig 7.12)

Fig. 7.11 Lymphocyte.
(a) In small lymphocytes, which have a diameter of 6–9 μm, the nucleus (N) occupies about 90% of the cell. The cytoplasm (C) appears only as a narrow rim and is slightly basophilic due to the presence of free ribosomes (RNA); rough endoplasmic reticulum is minimal.
(b) Ultrastructurally, lymphocyte cell membrane shows small cytoplasmic projections (CP) which appear as short microvilli with the scanning electron microscope, and are most numerous on B lymphocytes. Cytoplasm is sparse and contains only a few mitochondria (M) and occasional aggregates of glycogen.

Fig. 7.10 Monocyte.
This monocyte is a large cell, up to 20 μm in diameter, with a pale staining vacuolated cytoplasm (C) and an irregular nucleus (N) often with a deep indentation on one side.

Fig 7.12 Plasma cell.
Plasma cells (P) have a rounded nucleus, with a speckled chromatin pattern and a central nucleolus, which is often likened to a clock-face. The cytoplasm is deeply purple staining reflecting the RNA content. Note the clear, pale-stained area next to the nucleus which is the area occupied by the Golgi complex.

WHITE BLOOD CELL ABNORMALITIES

Increased numbers of white cells appear in the peripheral blood in a variety of disorders and provide a useful clue to underlying disease. For example, while in both cases the white cells are qualitatively normal, there is:

- a considerable and sustained increase of circulating neutrophils in bacterial infections;
- an increase of circulating eosinophils in parasitic infestations and some allergies.

The most important and life-threatening disorders of white cells are the leukemias, in which there is a malignant proliferation of the white cell precursors in the bone marrow. This produces vast numbers of white cells and their precursors, many of which spill over into the blood.

Leukemias are classified according to the cell line involved (i.e. granulocytic, monocytic, lymphocytic) and also according to their degree of malignancy.

In **chronic leukemias** (Fig. 7.13a), the proliferating cells are partly or completely differentiated, for example, myelocytes, metamyelocytes, band forms and neutrophils in granulocytic leukemias. The diseases are slowly progressive.

In **acute leukemias** (Fig. 7.13b), the proliferating cells are the virtually undifferentiated precursor cells, for example, myeloblasts in acute granulocytic leukemia and lymphoblasts in acute lymphoblastic leukemia. Acute leukemias are rapidly progressive.

Fig 7.13 Leukemia.
ⓐ In this blood film from a patient with chronic granulocytic leukemia there are increased numbers of mature white cells, mainly neutrophils (N) as well as precursor cells, mainly myelocytes (Mc) and metamyelocytes (Mm) which have escaped from the marrow into the blood.

ⓑ In this typical blood film from a patient with an acute granulocytic leukemia the malignant cells are immature granulocyte precursors, mainly myeloblasts (Mb). Very few mature neutrophils (N) are being formed.

PLATELETS AND MEGAKARYOCYTES

Platelets are small cell fragments derived from megakaryocytes and are important in hemostasis.

Platelets (thrombocytes) are small, disk-shaped, anuclear cells (Fig. 7.14), and are formed by the cytoplasmic fragmentation of huge precursor cells (megakaryocytes) in the bone marrow. Platelets contain mitochondria, microtubules, glycogen granules, occasional Golgi elements and ribosomes, as well as enzyme systems for aerobic and anaerobic respiration. Their most conspicuous organelles,

however, are their granules of which there are four types:
- α granules are variable in size and shape and contain three important groups of proteins (platelet exclusive proteins, coagulation factors and other proteins);
- dense granules (δ granules) are electron-dense and appear to contain serotonin, which is not synthesized by platelets but absorbed from the plasma;
- lysosomes are membrane-bound vesicles containing lysosomal enzymes (e.g. acid hydrolases);
- peroxisomes are few in number and have peroxidase (probably catalase) activity.

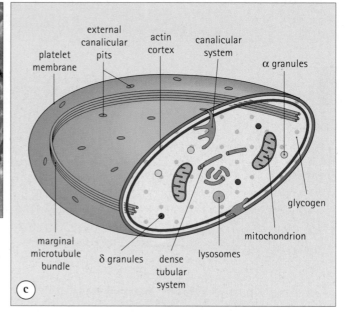

Fig. 7.14 Platelets.

ⓐ Platelets (P) are 1.5–3.5 μm in diameter in peripheral blood.

ⓑ Scanning electronmicrograph showing the smooth disk shape of an inactive platelet. The surface canalicular pores (see below) cannot be seen at this magnification.

ⓒ Diagram to illustrate platelet structure. Platelet cell membrane, which has a prominent glycocalyx that includes cell adhesion molecules for platelet adhesion, contains many external pits which connect a system of interconnected canalicular membrane channels with the external environment.

The cytoplasmic aspect of these membranes is associated with an actin cortex (see page 24). This canalicular system secretes the contents of the α granule, while the contractile proteins in the actin cortex (previously called thrombosthenin), are involved in clot retraction and extrusion of granule contents.

A well-developed cytoskeleton incorporates a marginal band of microtubules arranged beneath the cell periphery; these polymerize into component filaments at the onset of platelet aggregation.

Deep to the marginal band of microtubules and also scattered throughout the cytoplasm is the dense tubular system (DTS) consisting of narrow membranous tubules containing a homogeneous electron-opaque substance. Although histochemical studies have shown a platelet-specific isoenzyme of peroxidase within the DTS, the function of this system is poorly understood; there is some evidence that it may be the site of prostaglandin synthesis.

ⓓ Electronmicrograph of a platelet. The circumferential band of microtubules (MT) and elements of the (DTS), and canalicular system (CS) can be seen, as well as a selection of granules, including α and δ granules and some lysosomes (L).

Platelets aggregate together and degranulate in hemostasis.

Platelets are essential to normal hemostasis, undergoing aggregation in the process (Fig. 7.15). Hemostasis is achieved by the following steps.

After loss of the lining endothelium of blood vessels, platelets adhere to exposed collagen by interacting with glycoprotein receptors for Von Willebrand factor attached to it.

Platelet actin, myosin and microtubules cause reversible platelet moulding and adhesion along a broad surface. They then irreversibly release the contents of their granules through the canalicular system, in a secretion reaction, and synthesize thromboxane.

Thromboxane, ADP and Ca^{++} ions mediate adhesion of other platelets. Platelet phospholipids (with Ca^{++} ions) activate the blood clotting cascade, leading to the formation of fibrin.

PLATELET DISORDERS

Severe reduction in the number of platelets in circulating blood is called **thrombocytopenia**. It causes spontaneous bleeding because of the failure of platelets to seal over microscopic breaches in vessel walls resulting from minor trauma.

In the skin, this manifests as a reddish-purple blotchy rash, either small blotches (purpura) or larger, bruise-like patches (ecchymoses).

Severe thrombocytopenia may be a stand-alone condition, for example idiopathic thrombocytopenic purpura. It may also be part of a wider failure of hemopoietic bone marrow, when it is associated with a reduction in the number of circulating neutrophils (neutropenia) and red cells. This may arise, for example, when normal hemopoietic marrow is suppressed by tumor invasion in acute leukemia (Fig. 7.13b) or caused by drugs such as the cytotoxic drugs used in cancer therapy.

Megakaryocytes are large multinucleate cells which give rise to the platelets.

Megakaryocytes (Fig. 7.16) are the largest cells seen in bone marrow aspirates, and produce platelets by cytoplasmic fragmentation.

The precursor of the megakaryocyte in bone marrow is the megakaryoblast, which duplicates its nuclear and cytoplasmic constituents up to seven times without cell division, each causing increased ploidy, nuclear lobulation and cell size.

Cytoplasmic maturation involves the elaboration of granules, vesicles and demarcation membranes (see page 110), and progressive loss of free ribosomes and rough endoplasmic reticulum.

Fig. 7.15
Aggregating platelets.
ⓐ Scanning electronmicrograph of platelets in the early stages of aggregation. They show extensive alteration in shape, becoming spherical. They also develop numerous long thin cytoplasmic processes (CP). Compare with Fig. 7.14b.
ⓑ Transmission electron micrograph of aggregating platelets. Note the interlinking of some cytoplasmic processes and the decrease in granule numbers in some platelets. Compare with Fig. 7.14d.

Fig. 7.16 **Megakaryocyte.**
Megakaryocytes are huge polyploid cells 30–100 μm in diameter, with a large irregular, multilobular nucleus (N) which contains dispersed chromatin, and is devoid of nucleoli. Their extensive cytoplasm (C) is filled with fine basophilic granules reflecting their profusion of cytoplasmic organelles.

With light microscopy, the cell margin is often difficult to define clearly due to the presence of numerous disaggregating platelets, cytoplasmic processes, ruffles and blebs.

Megakaryocyte cytoplasm is divided into three zones. Firstly, the perinuclear zone contains the Golgi and associated vesicles, rough and smooth endoplasmic reticulum, developing granules, centrioles and spindle tubules. It remains attached to the nucleus after platelet shedding. Secondly, the intermediate zone contains an extensive system of interconnected vesicles and tubules (the demarcation membrane system, DMS), which is in continuity with the cell membrane and has the function of delineating developing platelet fields (i.e. potential platelets) which, like platelets, are uneven in size. Finally, the marginal zone is filled with cytoskeletal filaments and traversed by membranes connecting with the DMS.

Fig 7.17 Hemopoiesis in fetal liver.
Micrograph showing hemopoietic cells (H) in the sinusoidal spaces (S) between plates of liver cells (L) in a fetus.

HEMOPOIESIS

Blood cells are made in the bone marrow in adult life.
The site of blood cell formation (hemopoiesis) changes several times during fetal development, the earliest sites being the yolk sac and then the liver (Fig. 7.17) and spleen. At 5 months, the fetal bone marrow begins to produce white cells and platelets, while red cell production by bone marrow starts later, at around 7 months.

At birth, the bone marrow is the main site of red cell production and almost all bones in the body are involved.

Over the next few years, with the rapid increase in bone size, the hemopoietic capacity of the bone marrow expands far beyond even emergency requirements, and so the hemopoietic bone marrow occupies less of the marrow space available. By skeletal maturity only the marrow of the vertebrae, ribs, skull, pelvis and proximal femurs is hemopoietic, the rest having been replaced by adipose tissue, although retaining its capacity to resume hemopoiesis should the need arise.

In adult life, cell formation from the bone marrow is enough to meet normal requirements. If there is disease of the bone marrow, such that it can no longer make adequate numbers of blood cells, then hemopoietic activity may develop once again in the liver and spleen; this is termed **extramedullary hemopoiesis.**

Pluripotential stem cells give rise to all of the different types of blood cell.
All cellular elements of the blood originate from a common pluripotential progenitor stem cell (hemopoietic stem cell, HSC, Fig 7.19). These pluripotential stem cells are in very small numbers in sites of blood cell formation and even smaller numbers can be found in the peripheral blood. Histologically they resemble lymphocytes but can be identified by use of immunohistochemical techniques as they have distinctive cell-surface antigens. The pluripotential cells divide and give rise to cells with a more restricted line of growth.

Hemopoietic progenitor cells

The different types of progenitor cell and their relationship to each other are shown in Fig 7.19. The nomenclature that applies to stem cells is with reference to their ability to form differentiating colonies of committed cells in culture, termed **colony forming units** (CFU): the stem cells being termed **colony forming cells** (CFC).

Two main types of multipotential progenitor cells derive from the pluripotential hemopoietic stem cell:

- lymphoid progenitor cells which give rise to the different types of lymphocyte (B and T cell types);
- granulocyte/erythroid/monocyte/megakaryocyte (CFU-GEMM or CFU-MIX) progenitor cells which give rise to the main types of blood cell.

The types of committed progenitor cell derived from the multipotential CFU-GEMM (CFU-MIX) cells are:

- erythroid (CFU-E), which give rise to red cell precursor cells;
- granulocyte/monocyte progenitors cells (CFU-GM), which give rise to granulocytes and monocytes by forming further subsets of specific progenitor cells (CFC-G and CFC-M);
- eosinophil (CFU-Eo), which give rise to eosinophils;
- basophil (CFU-Bas), which give rise to basophils;
- megakaryocytic (CFC-Meg), which give rise to megakaryocytes (and so platelets).

It is possible to divide blood-forming cells into four groups depending on capacity for self-renewal, cell division, and ability to form different cell types (Fig 7.18). **Pluripotential stem cells** are capable of forming any type of blood cell, **multipotential progenitor cells** are capable of forming a specific but wide range of blood cells, **committed progenitor cells** are capable of forming only 1 or 2 types of blood cell, and **maturing cells** are undergoing structural differentiation to form one cell type and so are incapable of division.

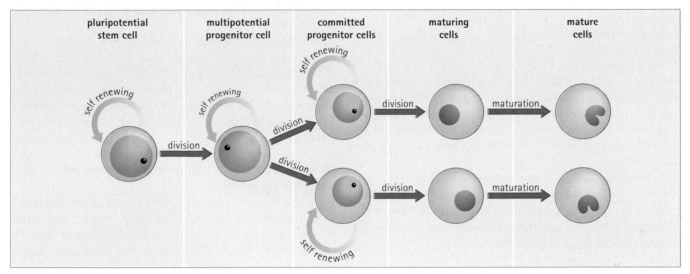

Fig 7.18 Hemapoietic precursor cells.
The precursor cells of the blood can be divided into four main classes according to their ability to differentiate into different cell types and their capacity for self renewal.

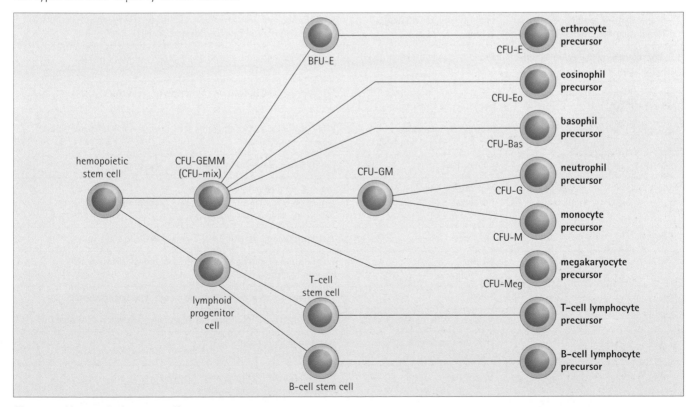

Fig 7.19 Hemapoietic stem cells.
All of the cellular blood elements are formed from one multipotential stem cell. The progenitor cells are termed colony-forming units (CFU) after the ability of cells to form colonies in cell culture. Red cell precursors are capable of rapid bursts of cell growth in culture and a 'burst-forming-unit' (BFU-E) precursor can be identified.

Growth control of blood stem cells is through secreted growth factors and local cell contacts.

The best understood mechanism of control of growth of the different types of hemopoietic stem cells is through the action of growth factors. These substances are secreted systemically or locally and modulate three aspects of cell growth:

- proliferation;
- differentiation;
- maturation.

The names and activities of the main factors are listed in Fig 7.20. It is apparent that each factor has more than one activity, some acting in synergy to promote a specific aspect of cell development. Many of these substances can now be synthesized and are being used in the treatment of diseases of the blood.

Less well understood in the control of blood cell formation is the role of local cell/cell contacts. Stromal cells in the bone marrow appear to be important in control of differentiation and maturation; however, the signals involved are at present unknown.

BONE MARROW

The bone marrow is the main site of hemopoiesis.

Bone marrow occupies the spaces between the trabeculae of medullary bone (see Chapter 13), and consists of highly branched vascular sinuses and a reticulin scaffolding, with the interstices packed with hemopoietic cells (Fig. 7.21).

In addition to its hemopoietic function the bone marrow, along with the spleen and liver, contains fixed macrophagic cells which remove aged and defective red cells from the circulation by phagocytosis. It also plays a central role in the immune system, being the site of maturation of B lymphocytes, which produce antibodies (see Chapter 8).

Bone marrow has a highly developed set of vascular sinusoids.

Bone marrow is supplied by medullary branches derived from the nutrient artery of the bone, which pierces the cortical bone through a nutrient canal, giving off a series of small branches to the cortical and medullary bone.

Cytokine	Cells of origin	Activity
Granulocyte–macrophage colony stimulating factor (GM-CSF)	Endothelium, macrophages, T-cells	Proliferation and activation of granulocyte and monocyte precursors Proliferation of multilineage progenitor cells
Granulocyte colony stimulating factor (G-CSF)	Monocytes, endothelium, fibroblasts	Proliferation and maturation of precursors of granulocytes
Macrophage colony stimulating factor (M-CSF)	Endothelium, monocytes, fibroblasts, endometrium	Proliferation and activation of monocyte precursors
Stem cell factor	Marrow stromal cells, endothelial cells, fibroblasts	Proliferation of early and committed progenitor cells in synergy with other cytokines
Erythropoietin	Kidney, liver	Proliferation of erythroid and megakaryocyte precursors
IL-1	Monocytes, endothelium, fibroblasts	Induces stem cells to enter cycle Induces G-CSF, GM-CSF, M-CSF, IL-3 production Release of neutrophils from marrow
IL-2	T-cells	Proliferation and activation of T-cells, NK-cells, monocytes
IL-3	T-cells	Proliferation of early and committed hemopoietic stem cells especially megakaryocytes
IL-5	T-cells	Proliferation and activation of eosinophil and basophil precursors
IL-6	Monocytes, fibroblasts, T-cells	Induces stem cells proliferation especially megakaryocyte progenitors
IL-8	Endothelium, monocytes, fibroblasts	Neutrophil activation
IL-9	Monocytes	Proliferation of erythroid and mast cell precursors Maturation of megakaryocytes
IL-11	Fibroblasts	Proliferation of monocyte progenitors and early committed progenitor cells

Fig 7.20 Growth factors involved in hemopoiesis. IL, interleukin.

This is augmented by smaller vessels from the muscle and periosteum surrounding the bone, which similarly penetrate the cortical bone. A capillary network opens into a well-developed series of thin-walled sinusoids which empty into a large central sinus. Blood leaves the bone in the emissary vein via the nutrient canal.

The bone marrow sinusoids are lined by flat cells (endothelial cells), which normally line blood vessels (see page 138), and these lie on a discontinuous basement membrane. In places, cytoplasm of endothelial cells is so thin that the endothelial barrier is little more than the inner and outer layers of endothelial cell membrane. Mature blood cells probably adhere to the marrow sinusoidal endothelium before being released into the circulation.

The bone marrow support cells have important roles in hemopoiesis.

Outside the endothelium and basement membrane of the marrow sinusoids is a discontinuous layer of fibroblast-like support cells (reticular cells) which synthesize collagenous reticulin fibers (Fig. 4.5), extracellular matrix materials, and certain growth factors. Reticular cells have extensive branched cytoplasmic processes, which enclose well over 50% of the outer surface area of the sinusoid wall. The reticular cells also ramify throughout the hemopoietic spaces forming a regular sponge-like matrix, a meshwork to support the hemopoietic cells.

By accumulating lipid, the reticular support cells may transform into the adipocytes found in bone marrow.

The extracellular matrix in the hemopoietic compartment contains coarse collagen fibers, as well as laminin and fibronectin, which facilitate adhesion of the hemopoietic cells to the marrow stroma. The associated proteoglycans, chondroitin sulfate, hyaluronic acid and heparan sulfate, may also bind growth factors, which control hemopoiesis.

Fig. 7.21 Bone marrow.
Micrograph of decalcified vertebra showing hemopoietic bone marrow (H) in the spaces between the bony trabeculae (T) of the ilium. Some of the space is also occupied by adipocytes (A).

There is an intimate contact between developing blood cells and stromal cells in the marrow. It is believed that such cell/cell contacts are important in the control of hemopoiesis.

Erythropoiesis is associated with formation of distinct precursor cells termed erythroblasts.

Red cells are the terminal differentiated progeny of one cell line of pluripotent bone marrow stem cells which is committed to erythropoiesis only.

CFU-GEMM (CFU-Mix) cells give rise to progenitor cells that form 'bursts' of erythroid cells in culture (BFU-E), and these give rise to cells (CFU-E) responsive to the growth factor erythropoietin. The erythroid stem cells are few in number and cannot be identified in routine bone marrow smears. Immunochemical techniques have allowed characterization of erythroid progenitor cells which have large nucleoli, many polyribosomes and large mitochondria. Differentiation of these stem cells into mature red cells is associated with:

- decreasing cell size;
- hemoglobin production;
- gradual decrease and eventual loss of all cell organelles;
- changing cytoplasmic staining, from intense basophilia due to large numbers of polyribosomes to eosinophilia due to hemoglobin;
- condensation and eventual extrusion of the nucleus.

Along the path of red cell differentiation, certain morphologic cell types can be distinguished in routine marrow smears: proerythroblast, basophilic erythroblast, polychromatic erythroblast, orthochromatic erythroblast and reticulocyte (Fig. 7.22).

Red cell formation occurs in small cellular islands in the marrow.

Red cells are formed in small erythroblastic islands consisting of one or two specialized macrophages surrounded by red cell progenitor cells. The macrophages have long cytoplasmic processes and deep invaginations to accommodate the dividing erythroid cells, which migrate outwards along the cytoplasmic process as they differentiate.

When mature, the red cell contacts nearby sinusoidal endothelium and passes out to enter the circulation.

Red cell production is controlled by erythropoietin.

The term **erythron** describes the whole mass of mature red cells and their progenitors. It functions as a dispersed organ, the number of red cells in the circulating blood being regulated to meet oxygen-carrying needs, and the rate of red cell production varying with changing rates of their removal from the circulation.

This behavior is mediated by a number of factors, but particularly by the growth factor **erythropoietin**, which adjusts red cell production to match oxygen demand. Erythropoietin is secreted mainly by the kidneys in adults and by the liver in the fetus.

	Proerythroblast	Basophilic erythroblast (early normoblast)	Polychromatic erythroblast (intermediate normoblast)	Orthochromatic erythroblast (late normoblast)	Reticulocyte
diameter	20–25µm	16–18µm	12–15µm	10–12µm	–
nucleus	large (80% of cell)	more condensed	condensed	extremely condensed, eccentrically located	absent
chromatin	fine and in clumps	in wheel spoke or clock face arrangement	clumps with more regular distribution	pyknotic	–
nucleoli	one or more, pale	variably identifiable	absent	–	–
cytoplasm	intensely basophilic (due to polyribosomes)	basophilic (due to polyribosomes)	polychromatic (combination of basophilia due to polyribosomes and eosinophilia due to hemoglobin)	more eosinophilic (due to increased hemoglobin content)	eosinophilic (due to hemoglobin)
organelles	plentiful, particularly polyribosomes	plentiful, particularly polyribosomes	reduction in number of organelles; hemoglobin formation commences	elimination of most, especially polyribosomes and mitochondria	remnants of organelles not easily visible with conventional stains, but can be demonstrated by supravital methods*
other features	contain ferritin (free and in lysosomes), divide into 8–16 cells	characteristic pale staining perinuclear halo	perinuclear halo still evident, cell replication complete	divides into smaller part containing nucleus (phagocytosed by macrophages), and larger part (passes through sinusoidal endothelium to enter circulation as a reticulocyte)	matures into red cell in 24–48 hours. Form 1% of circulating red cells, the proportion increasing when red cell demand increases, eg, after blood loss, as shown in micrograph above

* To demonstrate organelle remnants, fresh blood is incubated with brilliant cresyl violet or methylene blue dye (supravital staining); the remnants precipitate as blue reticular strands, hence the name reticulocyte

Fig 7.22 Morphologic stages in erythropoiesis.

Certain factors are required by the bone marrow for the formation of red cells, notably iron (as a component of hemoglobin), folic acid and vitamin B12. Lack of any of these factors leads to defective red cell formation and development of anemia (page 101).

RETICULOCYTES

A reticulocyte is an immature red cell which still contains some cellular RNA and organelles undergoing degradation. These immature forms are not detected on normal blood films but can be detected by incubating blood cells in the dye Cresyl violet, which stains the RNA as a fine blue stippling. Reticulocytes are not normally seen in peripheral blood except in very small numbers (<1% of red cells). If there is rapid demand for red cell formation then increased numbers of reticulocytes are released from the bone marrow and can be detected in the blood. A reticulocyte count can therefore be used as an estimate of rate of red cell formation.

Granulopoiesis occurs with formation of distinctive cell types in marrow.

The formation of granulated white cells is termed granulopoiesis. This takes place under the influence of cytokines. The first recognizable precursor of neutrophil formation is the myeloblast. The stages of subsequent maturation through promyelocyte, myelocyte, metamyelocyte and band cell are shown in Fig. 7.23.

Maturation from myeloblast to neutrophil takes about 7–8 days, and involves five cell divisions between myeloblast and metamyelocyte stages, after which no further multiplication divisions take place, and chemotactic ability, complement and Fc receptors are acquired.

Structurally mature neutrophils remain in the marrow for about 5 days and are then released into the blood. After circulating for about 6 hours, they migrate into the peripheral tissues where they survive for 2–5 days, unless destroyed earlier as a result of their phagocytic activity.

Increase in numbers of circulating neutrophils may occur by two mechanisms.

A huge pool of stored neutrophils is maintained, loosely adherent to the sinusoidal endothelium in the bone marrow. This pool can be mobilized rapidly when there is a disease process. Stimuli cause a sudden outpouring of granulocytes from the bone marrow, leading to an increase in number of blood neutrophils (neutrophil leukocytosis). This mechanism copes with a sudden demand for neutrophils.

If it is necessary to maintain a high blood neutrophil count, for example during bacterial infection, there is increased proliferation of the granulocyte precursors in the marrow. This is regulated by systemic secretion of cytokines, especially IL-1, GM-CSF and G-CSF.

Eosinophil and basophil formation morphologically resembles neutrophil granulopoiesis.

Eosinophils are derived from CFU-Eo progenitor cells under the influence of cytokines. Eosinophil myeloblasts resemble neutrophil myeloblasts, and there are comparable subsequent developmental stages. Eosinophils are readily distinguishable from neutrophils at the early myelocyte stage by the appearance of their larger granules, most of which are eosinophilic, but a few are initially basophilic.

Fig 7.23 Morphologic stages in neutrophil granulopoiesis. Micrograph showing granulocyte precursors at various stages of maturation.

The myeloblast (Mb) is a large cell largely occupied by a nucleus in which nucleoli are prominent; its scanty cytoplasm contains a few granules.

The promyelocyte (Pm) contains more abundant cytoplasm and more primary granules; nucleoli are still present.

The myelocyte (Mc)shows early flattening or invagination of one face of the nucleus from which the nucleoli have disappeared. Its cytoplasm contains a mixture of a few primary granules and smaller secondary granules.

The metamyelocyte (Mm) shows more advanced invagination of the nucleus to a reniform shape, and a later stage, the band or stab form (B) has a horseshoe-shaped nucleus.

Increasing lobation of the nucleus produces the mature neutrophil (N) which features a multilobed nucleus and abundant cytoplasm containing small secondary granules.

Basophils are formed from CFU-B progenitor cells. Basophil myeloblasts resemble neutrophil myeloblasts; development then proceeds through analogous stages to those of neutrophils and eosinophils. Basophil granules are distinguishable at the early myelocyte stage.

Monocytes leave the marrow soon after formation, with no marrow pool.

Monocytes are derived from CFC-M cells under the influence of cytokines. Two morphologic monocyte precursors are recognized: the monoblast and the promonocyte. At least three cell divisions occur before the mature monocyte stage is reached. Mature monocytes leave the bone marrow soon after their formation and there is no reserve pool. They spend about 3 days in the blood before migrating into the tissues in an apparently random fashion; they are then unable to re-enter the circulation.

Lymphoid precursors migrate to peripheral lymphoid tissues.

The bone marrow is the site of formation of primitive lymphocyte precursors which subsequently give rise to both T and B lymphocytes at different sites.
- B cells undergo initial maturation in the bone marrow and move on to colonise peripheral lymphoid tissues.
- T cells migrate to the thymus gland where they undergo initial maturation before moving on to colonise peripheral lymphoid tissues.

Lymphoid cells are capable of division in adult life, when expansion of selected clones is desirable to mount a specific immune response. **Lymphoblasts** are recognizable dividing lymphocytes, having a large open nucleus, prominent nucleolus, and small amount of cytoplasm. This cell division takes place in the specialized peripheral lymphoid tissues, discussed in Chapter 8.

HEMOPOIESIS

- takes place in liver and spleen in early life and bone marrow later

- all blood cells formed from a common stem cell

- controlled by cytokines and local cell/cell interactions in the marrow

- erythropoietin controls red cell production

- red cell formation is through CFU-GEMM progenitor, BFU-E progenitor, CFU-E progenitor, proerythroblast, basophilic erythroblast, polychromatic erythroblast, orthochromatic erythroblast, reticulocyte, red cell

- neutrophil formation is through CFU-G progenitor, myeloblast, promyelocyte, myelocyte, metamyelocyte, band cell, neutrophil

1. RED BLOOD CELLS

   (a) have a biconcave shape which maximizes the surface/volume ratio for gas transfer in capillary vessels
   (b) have no mitochondria
   (c) have a membrane-associated cytoskeleton which maintains their shape
   (d) have a life span in peripheral blood of about 20 days
   (e) are removed, when aged, by cells in the spleen

2. NEUTROPHILS

   (a) have a regular, spherical nucleus
   (b) perform their main functions in the peripheral blood
   (c) contain the enzyme myeloperoxidase, which is important for bacterial killing
   (d) express cell adhesion molecules on their surface to allow them to adhere to endothelium prior to emigration into tissues
   (e) have receptors on their surface which recognize foreign material for internalization by phagocytosis

3. WHITE BLOOD CELLS HAVE SPECIALIZED ROLES

   (a) basophils emigrate into tissues and form plasma cells
   (b) monocytes emigrate into tissues and form macrophages
   (c) lymphocytes of certain types can secrete immunoglobulin
   (d) eosinophils are increased in number in the tissues and blood in allergic reactions
   (e) neutrophils have a long half-life of about 30 days once they are activated and have entered tissues

4. HEMOPOIESIS GENERATES ALL FORMS OF BLOOD CELL

   (a) all blood cells derive from a common hemopoietic stem cell
   (b) both granulocytes and monocytes derive from a common committed progenitor cell
   (c) each of the cytokines which control and modulate hemopoiesis act very specifically on one cell line
   (d) platelets are formed from myeloid cells
   (e) committed progenitor cells are not self-receiving

8. Immune System

INTRODUCTION

The immune system is part of an array of defense systems used to combat disease.

The body must constantly protect itself from invasion by a variety of living organisms and other foreign bodies, which may gain entry via the skin, gut, respiratory tract, and other routes. This protection is provided by the following three mechanisms:

- surface protection;
- acute inflammation;
- immune response.

The nonspecific mechanisms of surface protection are provided by keratin in the skin, mucus in the respiratory and alimentary tracts, and by an acid environment in the vagina.

The organized tissue response, termed acute inflammation, is also nonspecific and proceeds in the same way whatever the initiating factor. Foreign agents are destroyed or neutralized by neutrophils that migrate into the tissues from local blood vessels.

In contrast, the immune response is highly specific and targeted to chemicals on invading organisms or foreign particles.

Lymphocytes are the most important cells in the specific immune response.

The immune response is served by specialized tissues and cells, which form the immune system. This system depends on the recognition of exogenous materials as foreign to the body: any foreign substance so recognized is known as an **antigen**. Such recognition then activates the immune system to neutralize or destroy the antigen, with **lymphocytes** playing the central role. The immune response is highly antigen-specific, but may employ the phagocytic cells of the nonspecific tissue defense system (see page 123) in initial antigen presentation or to effect final antigen destruction.

The two main types of immune response are termed cell-mediated and humoral.

The immune response is served by several types of cell acting synergistically. Exogenous agents (commonly microorganisms) are first recognized by **antigen-presenting cells** (APCs), which constantly patrol their local environment and are similar to macrophages. The exoge-nous agents are broken down within the APCs into key components. These act as antigens which are then presented to specialized effector cells (lymphocytes). Lymphocytes recognize the foreign antigens by specifically binding to them. Such lymphocytes then proliferate and are able to mount an immune response which may be one of two main types:

- **cell-mediated immunity** – characterized by the joint action of lymphocytes and macrophages to destroy or neutralize the foreign agent;
- **humoral immunity** – characterized by the secretion of proteins (antibodies) by one type of lymphocyte. Antibodies neutralize foreign agents by specifically binding to the antigen.

These two systems usually work together in the elimination of a foreign agent.

While the immune response occurs in all body tissues, the growth, maintenance and programming of immune cells takes place preferentially in the lymph nodes, spleen, thymus gland and bone marrow, which are the special organs of the immune system.

ANTIBODIES

- are synthesized by B lymphocytes and bind to specific antigens

- are also known as immunoglobulins, and fall into five different structural classes, IgG, IgA, IgD, IgM and IgE

- have two main components, immunoglobulin light chain (κ or λ) and immunoglobulin heavy chains (γ, α, δ, μ or ε)

- have heavy and light chains with highly variable regions (antigen-binding sites) and constant regions, which form the main part of the molecules

- may circulate in the blood and body fluids, or remain bound to the B lymphocyte surface where they activate the B cell on meeting the appropriate antigen

Different cells of the immune system can be identified by characteristic markers.

Many markers are cell-surface receptors or their ligands and have roles in signaling or cell adhesion. The many cytoplasmic and cell membrane proteins that characterize cells of the immune system have been given names according to an international system, which relates them to proteins (antigens) expressed at different phases of cell maturation. These are called CD (cluster designation) molecules (Fig. 8.1). Antibodies to the different CD molecules can be used to identify specific subtypes of lymphoid cell using immunohistochemical staining.

CD molecules can be considered in three main groups:
- markers which are expressed by a cell line throughout its life;
- markers which are expressed transiently during one phase of differentiation;
- markers which are expressed when cells are activated.

LYMPHOCYTES

The three main types of lymphocyte are termed B cells, T cells and natural killer (NK) cells.

B cells turn into plasma cells and secrete antibodies.

B lymphocytes (B cells) are mainly concentrated within the specialized lymphoid organs. They also circulate in the peripheral blood – accounting for between 5% and 15% of blood lymphocytes – and migrate through body tissues. Thus the constant movement of this type of lymphoid cell means they are readily available for immune defense. When stimulated by an appropriate antigen, B cells undergo proliferation and convert into plasma cells, which then secrete specific proteins called immunoglobulins. B cells, plasma cells and antibodies in the blood and body fluids are the basis of the **humoral response**.

CD	Function/identity	Expression
CD-1		cortical thymocytes, Langerhans cells, some B cells
CD-2	LFA-3 receptor	T cells, some NK cells
CD-3	T cell receptor complex	T cells
CD-4	MHC class II receptor	some T cells (T helper) monocytes
CD-5		T cells and some B cells
CD-8	MHC-class I receptor	some T cells (T cytotoxic)
CD-10	CALLA	pre-B cells
CD-16	FcγRIIIA	NK cells and monocytes
CD-19		B cells
CD-20		B cells
CD-21	CR2	mature B cells
CD-22		B cells
CD-35	CR1	B cells, monocytes
CD-40	cell signaling	B cells
CD-45	leukocyte common antigen	lymphocytes, granulocytes, macrophages
CD-45RA	restricted leukocyte common antigen	TS cells, monocytes, B cells
CD-45RO	restricted leukocyte common antigen	TH cells, monocytes, B cells
CD-45	leukocyte common antigen	lymphocytes, granulocytes, macrophages
CD-56	NCAM	NK cells
CD-79a	Igα	B-cells
CD-79b	Igβ	B-cells

Fig. 8.1 CD markers.
Table showing the most common CD markers in routine diagnostic laboratory use.

All developing B cells have common genes coding for the production of immunoglobulins. At this stage they are called germ line B cells. During B cell maturation, and after antigen stimulation, these genes undergo rearrangement to produce different unique immunoglobulin proteins, which can specifically interact with antigen. In this way the diversity of the humoral immune response is generated. Cells that produce an immunoglobulin recognizing a normal body (self) antigen are eliminated during development. Some activated cells become dormant and remain as so-called 'memory cells'. These can rapidly proliferate on repeated encounter with the same antigen.

B cell antigen receptor complex

B cells recognize antigen by expressing IgM antibody on their surface as part of a B cell antigen receptor complex. The other proteins which form the receptor complex are detected by antibodies to CD79a and CD79b.

B cells originate in hemopoietic tissues and later colonize lymphoid tissues.

B cells mature from small inactive cells to large immunoglobulin-secreting cells. Their cytologic appearance varies according to their activity.

Originating in the hemopoietic tissues of the liver and bone marrow, B cells develop from lymphoid stem cells. They leave their site of development and populate specialized lymphoid tissues (lymph nodes, spleen and gut mucosa in particular). In birds, B cells develop in a structure called the bursa of Fabricius, hence the origin of the term B (bursal) cells.

Inactive B cells are small cells, 6–8 μm in diameter, with barely discernible cytoplasm. The nucleus is rounded with compact chromatin reflecting a lack of DNA transcription.

When B cells become activated and proliferate they develop large nuclei with prominent nucleoli and moderate amounts of cytoplasm. These cells are termed **lymphoblasts**, **centroblasts** and **immunoblasts**.

The fully differentiated immunoglobulin-secreting B cell is termed a plasma cell, and has cytologic features that reflect its function as a protein-secreting cell (see Fig. 7.12). The cytoplasm is basophilic because of a high content of rough endoplasmic reticulum, and there is a clear area near the nucleus corresponding to the Golgi complex. The nucleus has an open chromatin pattern, said to resemble a clock face, and a large central nucleolus.

T cells are responsible for cell-mediated immunity.

T lymphocytes (T cells) are found concentrated within the specialized lymphoid organs but they also circulate in the peripheral blood and migrate through body tissues. When

Markers of B cells

- Pre-B cells express CD10. This is lost with maturation.

- B cells in blood express IgM and IgD on their surface as well as class II major histocompatability (MHC) antigens.

- CD19, CD20, CD22 are the main markers used in identification.

- CD21 and CD35 (complement receptors) are expressed when cells are activated

- CD40 is expressed and is involved in activation signaling with helper T (TH) cells.

- B cells in tissues may express IgG, IgA, IgE, IgM and IgD.

stimulated by an appropriate antigen, T cells undergo proliferation. They become able to direct and recruit other cells of the immune system, as well attacking diseased cells directly. T cells have cell-surface receptors which recognize specific antigen in a similar way to that of antibodies. Activated T cells also secrete cytokines (lymphokines), (Fig. 8.2). T cells, T cell receptors and cytokines are the basis of the **cell-mediated immune response** as well as being essential for organizing many aspects of the humoral response.

The T cell receptor proteins are assembled with proteins of CD3 to form a complex which sits on the T cell surface (T cell receptor complex). During maturation, genetic mechanisms (somatic mutation and T cell receptor gene rearrangement) generate the diversity of T cells needed to respond to different antigens. Cells that recognize a normal body (self) antigen are eliminated during development.

T cells can be divided into two types depending upon the type of antigen receptor.

All developing T cells have common genes coding for the production of T cell receptor proteins. At this stage they are called germ line T cells. The T cell receptors have variable regions which, like antibodies, can bind to different antigens. The receptors are assembled as pairs (dimers) of antigen-binding peptides. There are two types of resulting T cell receptor (TCR) termed TCR-1 and TCR-2:

- TCR-2+ cells express α and β chain together (αβ T cell receptor) and account for about 90% of lymphocytes in the blood;
- TCR-1+ cells express γ and δ chains together (γδ T cell receptor) and account for about 10% of lymphocytes in the blood.

Cytokine	Cells of origin	Activity
Granulocyte macrophage colony stimulating factor (GM-CSF)	endothelium, macrophages, T cells	proliferation and activation of granulocyte and monocyte precursors proliferation of multilineage progenitor cells
Granulocyte colony stimulating factor (G-CSF)	monocytes, endothelium, fibroblasts	proliferation and maturation of precursors of granulocytes
Macrophage colony stimulating factor (M-CSF)	endothelium, monocytes, fibroblasts, endometrium	proliferation and activation of monocyte precursors
Stem cell factor	marrow stromal cells, endothelial cells, fibroblasts	proliferation of early and committed progenitor cells in synergy with other cytokines
Erythropoietin	kidney, liver	proliferation of erythroid and megakaryocyte precursors
IL-1	monocytes, endothelium, fibroblasts	induces stem cells to enter cycle induces G-CSF, GM-CSF, M-CSF, IL-3 production release of neutrophils from marrow
IL-2	T cells	proliferation and activation of T cells, NK cells, monocytes
IL-3	T cells	proliferation of early and committed hemopoietic stem cells especially megakaryocytes
IL-5	T cells	proliferation and activation of eosinophil and basophil precursors
IL-6	monocytes, fibroblasts, T-cells	induces stem cell proliferation especially megakaryocyte progenitors
IL-8	endothelium, monocytes, fibroblasts	neutrophil activation
IL-9	monocytes	proliferation of erythroid and mast cell precursors maturation of megakaryocytes
IL-11	fibroblasts	proliferation of monocyte progenitors and early committed progenitor cells.

Fig. 8.2 Cytokines.
A major function of T cells is to synthesize proteins called cytokines (lymphokines), which mediate interactions between cells. Cytokines, however, are not unique to lymphoid cells and are secreted by other cell types to influence the growth and differentiation of cells. (IL, interleukin).

TCR-1+ cells are present in large numbers in mucosal tissues.

T cells undergo maturation in the thymus gland.

T cells originate from stem cells in the hemopoietic tissues of the liver and bone marrow and are so named because they undergo maturation in the thymus gland. From the thymus gland, T cells leave to populate specialized lymphoid tissues (lymph nodes, spleen, and gut mucosa in particular).

T cells have a varied morphology.

The histologic appearance of T cells depends on their activity.

Inactive T cells can be of two morphologic types. The commonest form in peripheral blood, accounting for between 60% and 90%, is called a **small lymphocyte**. This is 6–7 μm in diameter with barely discernible cytoplasm and a rounded nucleus with compact chromatin (see Fig. 7.11a). Ultrastructurally, such cells contain a so-called **Gall body** which is a small cluster of lysosomes associated with a small lipid droplet. This structure may be seen as a paranuclear spot using enzyme histochemical methods for lysosomal enzymes. The second type of inactive T cell is called a **large granular lymphocyte** (Fig.

Fig 8.3 Large granular lymphocyte.
Blood film showing a large granular lymphocyte. Note that the nucleus is larger than in a small lymphocyte and that there is a moderate amount of cytoplasm with small numbers of pink-staining (azurophilic) granules.

8.3). These cells are 7–10 μm in diameter; they have a moderate amount of cytoplasm which contain small numbers of granules which stain with azure dyes (**azurophilic granules**). T cells that have been stimulated to divide as part of an immune response are larger than the inactive cells and have a moderate amount of basophilic cytoplasm. The nucleus is large with a convoluted appearance (in contrast to that of B cells) and an open vesicular chromatin pattern and a visible nucleolus, reflecting gene transcription.

Lymphokine-secreting activated T cells have basophilic cytoplasm due to their high content of rough endoplasmic reticulum (ER), and a large nucleus with a convoluted contour.

The three functional subsets of T lymphocyte are termed helper, cytotoxic and suppressor types.

There are several subsets of T cells which can be defined by their expression of specific markers and their functional activity. TCR-2+ cells can be divided into three groups:
- **helper T cells** or TH cells;
- **cytotoxic T cells** or TC cells;
- **T suppressor cells** or TS cells.

TH cells, which express the CD4 molecule, help other lymphocytes perform their effector functions. Their assistance is necessary to induce B cells to produce antibody and to activate macrophage defense systems (see page 122). This type of cell recognizes antigen when it is presented on cells which also express class II MHC molecules (class II MHC).

TC cells, which express CD8 molecule, are able to kill target cells. This type of cell recognizes antigens when presented on cells in association with class I MHC molecules (Class I MHC).

TS cells, which express either CD8 or CD4 molecules, are capable of inhibiting the response to TH cells and thus modulate the immune response.

TCR-1+ cells generally do not express CD4 or CD8, although some may express CD8. These types of lymphocyte are particularly abundant in mucosal-associated lymphoid tissues (MALT, page 134) and generally have cytotoxic functions. The relationships between these forms of T cell are shown in Figure 8.4.

HIV INFECTION AND THE IMMUNE SYSTEM

The virus which causes the acquired immune deficiency syndrome (AIDS), HIV-1, gains entry to cells by using the CD4 surface protein as a receptor. One of the most important markers of progression in HIV infection is reduction in the number of CD4+ cells in the blood.

Helper T cells

Subtypes of TH cell have been identified according to the cytokines they secrete.

- THP cells are unstimulated and secrete IL-2.

- TH0 cells are cells which have just been stimulated by antigen and secrete IL-2, IL-4, IL-10 and IFNγ.

- TH1 cells secrete IL-2, IL-3, granulocyte macrophage colony stimulating factor (GM-CSF) and IFNγ.

- TH 2 cells secrete IL-3, IL-4, IL-10 and GM-CSF.

- TH M cells are inactive memory cells that secrete IL-2.

The TH cell population can also be divided into two subtypes based on the expression of different CD molecules.

- A subtype that promotes the activity of both T cells and B cells expresses CD29 and CD45RO.

- A subtype that induces CD8 cells to become suppressor/cytotoxic cells expresses CD45RA.

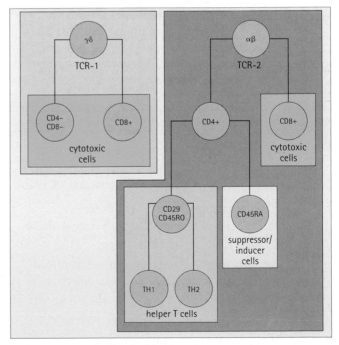

Fig 8.4 T cell subtypes.
T cells may be grouped according to their T cell receptor into TCR-1 and TCR-2 types. Cytotoxic cells, helper cells and suppressor cells are associated with the expression of other surface markers.

Natural killer cells are activated to become cytotoxic lymphocytes.

NK cells are the third main type of lymphocyte and in the peripheral blood have the morphology of large granular lymphocytes (see Fig 8.3). As well as forming a population in the blood they are also present in the spleen. This type of cell is capable of activation by IL-2, as it carries an IL-2 receptor, and has the ability to kill other cells (**cell-mediated cytotoxicity**). The main role of this type of cell is in the elimination of virus-infected cells and some tumor cells. When activated, NK cells may also release cytokines such as IL-1 and GM-CSF to modulate other immune responses.

NK cells can be recognized by immunochemical techniques as they do not express CD3 (part of the T cell receptor complex). However, they do express CD16 (a

Cytotoxic lymphocytes

Cytotoxic lymphocytes may be artificially stimulated to enhance their activity. When lymphocytes from blood or spleen are incubated *in vitro* with IL-2, a population of cells develops with enhanced cellular cytotoxicity. These are termed lymphokine-activated killer cells or LAK cells. They are believed to develop from large granular lymphocytes, which are a mixture of TCR-1+, TCR-2+ and CD8+ cells and NK cells.

This technique of enhancing immune function is being tested in patients with cancer. Patients' own blood lymphocytes are cultured with IL-2 and then returned to the bloodstream in the hope that the host will develop immunity to the disease and the LAK cells will kill cancer cells.

LYMPHOCYTES

- there are three main types: T cells, B cells and NK cells

- there are two morphologic types of inactive lymphocyte: small lymphocytes and large granular lymphocytes

- the different types of lymphoid cell are identified using immunochemical techniques to detect specific markers

- B cells mature into plasma cells and secrete immunoglobulin

- T cells have several roles as cytotoxic cells, helper cells and suppressor cells

- NK cells have a primary cytotoxic role

surface receptor involved in activation) and CD56 (a cell adhesion molecule). Many NK cells express CD2.

MACROPHAGES AND DENDRITIC CELLS

Macrophages and dendritic cells are part of the mononuclear phagocyte system.

Macrophages and dendritic cells are derived from monocytes (see page 105) which become resident in tissues where they may assume a variety of morphologic appearances as they differentiate to serve specialized roles:

- they may form a population of cells adapted mainly for phagocytosis (fixed tissue macrophages or histiocytes);
- they may be stimulated by T cells to secrete cytokines that control local cellular immune responses;
- they may form specialized immune surveillance cells (i.e. dendritic antigen-presenting cells, APCs).

The cells adapted mainly for phagocytosis remove or store material by assuming a rounded morphology with short broad pseudopodia. They contain large numbers of lysosomes (Fig. 8.5).

Secretory-type macrophages are large cells with voluminous pink-staining cytoplasm due to expansion of the Golgi complex and smooth ER. They are seldom seen in normal tissues, but are important in T cell-mediated immune responses, when they are termed **epithelioid cells** because of their superficial resemblance to epithelial cells.

Fig. 8.5 Macrophages.
Macrophages are particularly abundant in the loose fibrocollagenous support tissue found in most organs. In this site they are adapted for major phagocytic activity, which is reflected in their high lysosome content. In H&E sections, normal macrophages are inconspicuous, but they may be detected by histochemical staining for acid phosphatase or immunochemical staining for lysosomal enzymes as here.

APCs are characterized by elongated ramified cell processes and a low content of lysosomal enzymes.

Fixed tissue macrophages, secretory macrophages, epithelioid cells and APCs are often grouped together with blood monocytes to form the **mononuclear phagocytic system**.

Macrophagic cells are widely distributed in most tissues.

The morphology of macrophages is variable according to their site and function.

Specialized macrophages are seen in the lung (alveolar macrophages, see page 170), liver (Kupffer cells, see Fig. 12.3), brain (microglial cells, see Fig. 6.16) and skin (Langerhans cells, see Fig. 18.9).

Macrophages are an important component of the specialized organs of the immune system. They are also particularly abundant in loose fibrocollagenous support tissue, which is found in most parts of the body (Fig. 8.5).

Most antigen-presenting cells are a special form of macrophage.

APCs phagocytose antigenic material, process it and present the fragments to lymphocytes.

Most APCs are monocyte-derived and express markers of white cell lineage (leukocyte common antigen). Some non-monocyte-derived cells also function as antigen-presenting cells, for example the follicular dendritic cells of lymph nodes.

APCs have fine ramifying cytoplasmic processes which increase the surface area of cell membrane interacting with other cells and antigen. These give rise to their descriptive name, dendritic antigen-presenting cells (Fig. 8.6).

Although actively pinocytotic, APCs have low levels of lysosomal enzymes, unlike other monocyte-derived cells specialized for phagocytosis. They have high levels of class II MHC molecules (HLA-Dr);. this feature is essential for presenting new antigen to T cells. The follicular dendritic cells differ in this respect as they present antigen to B cells and lack class II MHC expression.

Cells that can be classified as dendritic APCs are:
- Langerhans cells of the skin;
- dendritic reticulum cells of lymph nodes;
- follicular dendritic cells;
- interstitial dendritic cells, which form a population of dendritic cells in the support tissues of most organs;
- veiled cells of the blood, which are thought to be circulating forms of dendritic APCs in transit between tissues;
- microglia of the central nervous system (see Fig. 6.16).

Despite certain common attributes, each of these cell types is microenvironmentally specialized, and each has slightly different cell-surface receptors and proteins which adapt them to antigen presentation in different sites.

In addition to this group of cells, which have a primary role in antigen presentation, several other cells, particularly the nonspecific phagocytic macrophages, can present antigen.

THE IMMUNE RESPONSE

- occurs in specialized tissues and organs of the immune system, particularly lymph nodes and spleen

- is initiated when antigen interacts with lymphocytes; this usually involves APCs

- activates lymphocytes to proliferate; some will mature to become memory T and B cells which respond rapidly to the antigen by proliferation and activation on re-exposure

BONE MARROW

The bone marrow is the site of origin of B and T cell precursors, and of macrophages, and is discussed in detail in Chapter 7.

THYMUS

The thymus is the site of T cell development.

Immunologically naive lymphocytes from bone marrow differentiate into mature T cells in the thymus. During this process, the immune system distinguishes self from foreign antigens and develops self-tolerance.

Fig. 8.6 Dendritic antigen–presenting cells.
Micrograph showing the ramifying cell processes of dendritic antigen-presenting cells from one area (paracortex) of a lymph node. This section is stained by an immunoperoxidase method which detects a protein specific to this cell type.

The thymus is also an endocrine organ, secreting hormones and other soluble factors which not only control T cell production, differentiation, and maturation in the thymus, but also regulate T cell function and interactions in peripheral tissues.

The thymus is the first lymphoid organ to develop, and is derived from the endoderm and a small ectodermal element of the ventral wing of the third pharyngeal pouch on each side.

The thymus is a soft lobulated organ located in the superior and anterior mediastinum.

At birth, the thymus is pinkish gray in color and weighs 10–15 g, increasing to 30–40 g by puberty. Thereafter it undergoes progressive involution and extensive fatty infiltration, and assumes a yellowish color.

In the child, the thymic parenchyma is divided into an outer, highly cellular cortex and a pale-stained central medulla. The cortex is divided into irregular lobules 0.5–2.0 mm in diameter by fine septa extending in as far as the corticomedullary junction from a loose fibrocollagenous capsule. The less cellular medullary tissue forms a continuous central core. The main cell types in the thymus are epitheliocytes, lymphocytes, and macrophages (Fig. 8.7).

The thymic epitheliocytes are true epithelial cells.

The epitheliocytes form the stromal meshwork of the thymus, and have a variety of ultrastructural and immunohistochemical features. At least four distinct cell types are recognizable, the subcapsular cortical, inner cortical, medullary and Hassall's corpuscle cells.

Fig. 8.7 Thymus.
(a) In the child the cortex (C) of the thymus is divided into lobules by fibrocollagenous septa (S) and is surrounded by adipose tissue of the mediastinum. The medulla (M) is less cellular.
(b) In the adult there is involution of the thymus with replacement by adipose tissue (A). The division into a cellular cortex (C) and less cellular medulla (M) is still apparent.
(c) The dominant feature of the thymic cortex is its vast number of densely packed lymphocytes, which range in size from small to large, depending on their activity.

Most if not all of the lymphocytes are in direct contact with epitheliocytes (E), which permeate the whole gland and act as a supporting framework. They are difficult to identify in the sea of lymphoid cells, but are visible where they surround blood vessels entering the gland.

Numerous macrophages (M) are scattered throughout the cortex and contain the phagocytosed debris of eliminated lymphocytes.
(d) The dominant feature of the thymic medulla is its epithelial component, the cells having large pale nuclei and abundant eosinophilic cytoplasm. Lymphocytes are less densely packed,than in the cortex; most are T cells probably *en route* to the general circulation.

Hassall's corpuscles (H) are derived from epitheliocytes which first appear during fetal development and form continuously thereafter. The process begins with the enlargement of a single medullary epitheliocyte which undergoes progressive degenerative changes characterized by nuclear disintegration and increasing cytoplasmic eosinophilia. Vacuoles appear in the cytoplasm, taking up the nuclear debris.

This process is repeated in nearby epithelial cells which form concentric lamellae around a central hyalinizing mass.

Hassall's corpuscles may grow as large as 100 μm in diameter and undergo a variety of degenerative changes, becoming infiltrated by lymphocytes, macrophages and eosinophils; they may also show cystic change or calcification.

Beneath the **capsule**, the epitheliocytes form a continuous layer, which is carried deeply into the thymus to invest the septa and vessels entering and leaving the organ.

Within the **cortex**, the epitheliocytes form a sponge-like structure containing an extensive network of spaces which becomes colonized by lymphocytes (see Fig. 8.7c).

In the medulla, sheets of epitheliocytes converge to form a coarser, more solid structure with smaller interstices accommodating much smaller numbers of lymphocytes.

Deep in the medulla, the epitheliocytes form bulky cords and whorls, some of which contain lamellated structures (**Hassall's corpuscles**, see Fig. 8.7d).

Thymic epitheliocytes have pale-staining oval nuclei and eosinophilic cytoplasm and can be readily identified in the medulla. In the cortex, however, their fine cytoplasmic extensions make them difficult to identify within the mass of lymphocytes.

With the electron microscope, typical desmosomes (see Fig. 3.11) are seen to bind the epithelial cells, which contain bundles of intermediate (cytokeratin) filaments.

Epitheliocytes in the cortex are in close contact with thymic lymphocytes and are called nurse cells.

In much of the thymic cortex, the epitheliocytes are in intimate contact with the lymphocytes, and completely enclose them by deep infolding of surface membrane. Described as **thymic nurse cells**, these cells are thought to eliminate immature T cells that recognize self antigens.

Epitheliocytes also promote T cell differentiation, proliferation, and subset maturation. In addition, they secrete hormones and other substances which regulate T cell maturation and proliferation within the thymus and other lymphoid organs.

The thymic lymphocytes are T cells undergoing development.

Most thymic lymphocytes are T cells in various stages of differentiation. B cells are also present, but in smaller numbers. Although the term thymocyte is often used as a generic term for thymic lymphocytes, it strictly applies to immature lymphocytes of T cell lineage.

Clones of T cells are produced by cell division in the outer part of the thymic cortex and undergo maturation as they are pushed deep into the cortex toward the medulla.

In the medulla, the maturing T cells enter blood vessels and lymphatics to join the pool of circulating T cells. They subsequently populate peripheral lymphoid tissues, where they reach full immunologic maturity.

Only a small minority of lymphocytes generated in the thymus are believed to reach maturity. These are clones of T cells with the ability to recognize foreign antigens.

The rest of the lymphocytes are thought to recognize self antigens and are eliminated: this results in immunologic self-tolerance.

The thymus has a rich vascular supply which allows migration of lymphoid cells.

The thymus receives its arterial supply via many small branches of the internal thoracic and inferior thyroid arteries, which enter the thymus mainly via the interlobular septa.

In the region of the corticomedullary junction the vessels give rise to small radially arranged arterioles and capillary loops to supply the cortex and medulla.

The cortical capillaries have continuous endothelium (see Chapter 9), whereas those of the medulla and septa may be fenestrated.

At the corticomedullary junction, which is the site of lymphocyte migration into the thymus, the postcapillary venules have a taller endothelium with features of high endothelial venules.

Venous tributaries follow the course of the arterial vessels in the septa, some forming a plexus within the thymic capsule before draining via the thymic veins into the left brachiocephalic, internal thoracic and inferior thyroid veins.

The thymus receives no afferent lymphatics, but the medulla and corticomedullary area give rise to efferent lymphatics which follow the course of the arteries and veins.

The thymus undergoes involution after puberty.

The thymus reaches its maximum weight at puberty, declining thereafter, so that in old age it may be so small as to be unrecognizable. Involution involves replacement of the gland by adipose tissue (fatty infiltration) and a decline in its lymphocyte content.

Fatty infiltration begins at birth, but accelerates after puberty. Adipocytes increase in number in the perivascular compartment. Initially this is most apparent in the septa, thus the cortex is involved first and then the process is extended into the medulla (see Fig. 8.7b).

Lymphocyte depletion begins after one year of age and thereafter continues at a constant rate independent of puberty. It results in progressive collapse of the sponge-like epitheliocyte framework, which nevertheless remains intact, so that cords of epitheliocytes can be seen histologically even in the most atrophic thymic remnants. Such cells probably continue to secrete thymic hormones into old age.

Despite the progressive decrease in their number with involution, thymic lymphocytes continue to differentiate and proliferate, thus maintaining a supply of T cells throughout life.

THE THYMUS

- functions for development and maturation of T cells

- is composed of lymphoid cells, thymic epithelial cells, macrophagic cells, and stromal cells

- is divided into cortex and medulla

- undergoes involution after puberty

LYMPH NODES

The lymph nodes are an important site for generation of immune responses.

Lymph nodes are small organs found in groups or chains at sites where lymphatic vessels draining an anatomic region converge to form larger lymphatic vessels, for example in the neck, axillae, groins and para-aortic area. They have two main functions.

Phagocytic cells within the nodes act as nonspecific filters for particulate matter such as microorganisms and carbon, preventing them from reaching the general circulation.

They provide an elegant mechanism whereby lymphocytes can interact with new antigens and APCs at an interface between lymph and the blood. Starting with only a small number of lymphocytes recognizing an antigen, lymph nodes facilitate proliferation of activated cells and consequently amplification of the immune response by forming clones of lymphocytes.

When relatively inactive, each lymph node is only a few millimeters in length, but they may become greatly enlarged when functional demands are increased.

The cells of the lymph node can be divided into three functional types: lymphoid cells, immunologic accessory cells, and non-immunologically active stromal cells.

Lymphoid cells in lymph nodes include lymphocytes of all types and their derivatives. Most of the lymphocytes enter the node via the blood, while a few enter via lymph draining from the tissues.

Immunologic accessory cells comprise a variety of macrophages, including those with phagocytic antigen processing, antigen presenting and nonspecific effector functions.

Non-immunologically active **stromal cells** comprise the lymphatic and vascular endothelial cells, and fibroblasts, which elaborate the stromal reticular framework. Many of the endothelial cells are highly specialized for interaction with lymphoid cells.

Each lymph node is divided into several functional compartments.

The lymph node is a bean-shaped organ with a fibrocollagenous capsule from which fibrous trabeculae extend into the node to form a supporting framework (Fig. 8.8).

The convex surface of the gland is penetrated by a number of afferent lymphatic vessels, which drain into the node, while at the hilum there is an efferent lymphatic vessel, which transports lymph toward larger collecting lymphatic vessels. In turn these vessels drain into more proximal nodes or chains of nodes, before entering the blood via either the thoracic duct or right lymphatic duct.

Lymph nodes contain three functional compartments (Fig. 8.9):

- a network of endothelial-lined **lymphatic sinuses** continuous with the lumina of the afferent and efferent lymphatic vessels;

- a network of small blood vessels, where circulating lymphocytes enter the node;

- a parenchymal compartment composed of superficial cortex, paracortex and medulla.

The structural integrity of the lymph node is provided by a framework of reticulin fibers (see page 51), which are linked to the fibrous trabeculae. These fibers are most dense in the parenchymal compartment, although some fibers do traverse the lymphatic compartment where they are completely invested by endothelial cells.

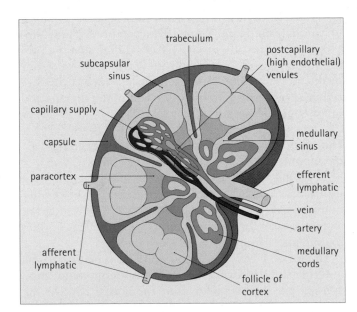

Fig. 8.8 Lymph node structure.
The bean-shaped lymph node has a hilum into which blood vessels enter, and from which efferent lymphatics emerge. It has an investing capsule.

Afferent lymphatic vessels penetrate the convex surface of the gland and drain into the subcapsular and medullary sinus system.

The lymphoid parenchyma is divided into cortex, paracortex and medulla. The most prominent structures in the cortex are the lymphoid follicles.

Lymph node sinuses carry lymph throughout the nodal structure.

Afferent lymphatics drain into a major subcapsular sinus running around the periphery of the lymph node. From this sinus, cortical sinuses pass down toward the medulla through the cortical cell mass.

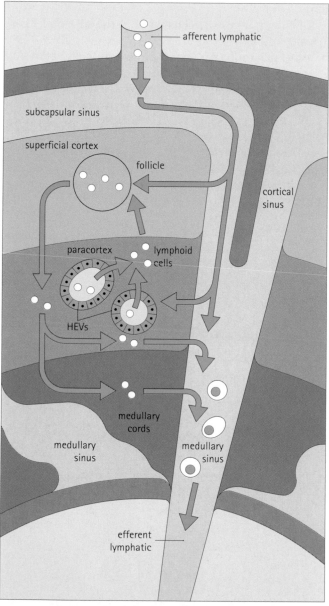

Fig. 8.9 Functional compartments of the lymph node.
Antigens, accessory cells and lymphocytes enter the lymph node via the afferent lymphatics, which drain into the subcapsular sinus and thence into the cortical sinuses.

These antigens, accessory cells and lymphocytes may then enter the superficial cortex (composed of diffuse sheets of T cells) or remain in the sinuses and leave the lymph node via the efferent lymphatic vessel.

The majority of lymphocytes enter the node from the blood via the high endothelial venules (HEVs), which are lined by a special endothelium bearing lymphocyte homing receptors.

Within the medulla the dominant feature is a network of interconnected lymphatic channels called the medullary sinuses, which converge upon the efferent lymphatic vessel at the hilum.

Only the larger channels of the lymphatic compartment can be visualized by light microscopy. The cortical sinuses are generally difficult to see because of their highly convoluted shape and numerous fine extensions, which penetrate the cellular mass of the cortex.

The extremely thin and pale-staining endothelial lining cells of the sinuses are almost impossible to identify with ordinary staining methods.

The blood supply of lymph nodes is the main route of entry of lymphocytes into the node.

The blood supply also provides the metabolic needs of the lymph node. One or more small arterial vessels enter the node via the hilum and then divide in the medulla into branches, which ramify into a capillary network corresponding to the cortical follicles and paracortex.

Within the paracortex, the postcapillary venules (see Chapter 9) have a cuboidal endothelium bearing specialized cell receptors (lymphocyte-homing receptors), which are recognized by circulating lymphocytes and facilitate the passage of lymphocytes from the blood and into the lymph node. The postcapillary venules are often described as **high endothelial venules** (HEVs).

The blood vessels of the superficial cortex and medullary cords are thought to be nonspecialized and do not appear to allow the exit of lymphocytes. Small veins draining the node leave via the hilum.

The superficial cortex of the lymph node contains the densely staining spheroidal aggregations of lymphocytes (lymphoid follicles).

Some of the follicles (**primary follicles**) are of fairly uniform staining density; however, most of the follicles responding to antigen have less densely staining **germinal centers** and are described as **secondary follicles**.

The lymphocyte population of the follicles consists predominantly of B cells, but there are smaller populations of TH cells, macrophages and accessory cells.

The main cells of the lymphoid follicles are B cells.

B cells enter a lymph node via the HEVs of the paracortex. Within a few hours many have migrated to the superficial cortex. If activated they proliferate and remain in the lymph node for an extended period as memory cells or plasma cells. In contrast, non-activated cells re-enter the general circulation within a matter of hours via the efferent lymph.

The primary follicles contain mainly naive B cells and some memory cells. The secondary follicles, in contrast, contain small naive B cells peripherally and activated B cells in their germinal centers.

It is possible to identify several stages in the maturation of B cells in the follicles (Fig. 8.10). Activated B cells proliferate and mature and thereby produce an expanded population of identical cells recognizing the same antigen.

The activated B cells in the germinal center are collectively called **follicle center cells**. They are characterized by open nuclei, and have more cytoplasm and are less densely packed than the smaller, more peripheral follicular B cells; this explains the lower staining intensity of the germinal centers.

The proliferation and differentiation of antibody-secreting plasma cells is thought to result from T cell–B cell interaction in the paracortex. The plasma cells then migrate directly to the medullary cords, where they are conveniently sited to secrete antibody into the efferent lymph.

Accessory cells in the superficial cortex are involved in antigen processing.

A variety of immunologic accessory cells are found in the superficial cortex. These are derived from bone marrow and reach the lymph node via the afferent lymph. These cells all appear to play some role in antigen processing; this also applies to the accessory cells of the paracortex and medulla.

The main accessory cells types in the superficial cortex are:

* **sinus macrophages**, highly phagocytic cells of the subcapsular and cortical sinuses;
* **veiled cells**, monocyte-derived cells so named because of their veiled appearance on scanning electron microscopy; they are located mainly in the subcapsular sinuses;

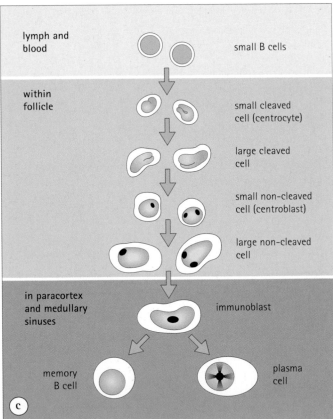

Fig. 8.10 Follicular B cells.

ⓐ Micrograph of an H&E-stained secondary lymphoid follicle, which consists mainly of B cells. Small naive B cells and a few T cells form the dark mantle zone (M), while the paler germinal center (G) contains B cells in various stages of maturation. Accessory cells (see Fig. 8.11) are present, but are barely discernible at this magnification.

ⓑ Micrograph of lymph node cortex stained to show B cells by an immunoperoxidase method. The follicle (F) is densely stained brown, being composed of B cells. The paracortex (P) is not stained, being composed of T cells.

ⓒ The maturation of B cells from small naive cells to dividing cells responding to a specific antigen is associated with a distinct series of morphological changes.

From the small lymphocyte, the cell changes first into a centrocyte with a cleft nucleus, and then into a centroblast. This cell enlarges, leaves the follicle and migrates to the paracortex and medullary sinuses as an immunoblast, ultimately transforming into a plasma cell or a memory B cell.

- **tingible body macrophages**, so named because they contain cellular debris, and are found within the germinal centers with an abundance of lysosomal enzymes;
- **marginal zone macrophages**, which constitute a morphologically diverse group of phagocytic cells located within the follicular interstitium immediately beneath the subcapsular sinus;
- **follicular dendritic cells**, which have numerous fine branching surface projections covered by electron-dense material.

Follicular dendritic cells retain antigen on their surface for many months. These cells present antigen directly to B cells and lack the class II MHC expression normally seen on other antigen-presenting cells.

These immunologic accessory cells cannot be readily distinguished in H&E sections, but may be stained by immunochemical techniques for special macrophage markers (Fig. 8.11).

The main cells of the lymph node paracortex are T cells.

The cell population of the paracortex consists of lymphocytes and accessory cells, which constantly move in and out of the region.

T cells dominate the paracortex (Fig. 8.12), entering the node from the blood via the HEVs and leaving 6–18 hours later via the efferent lymphatic.

When activated, T cells enlarge to form lymphoblasts. These then proliferate to produce an expanded clone of activated T cells. In a T cell-dominated immunologic response, the paracortex may expand into the medulla, producing a so-called **paracortical reaction**. Activated T cells are then disseminated via the circulation to peripheral sites where much of their activity occurs.

Accessory cells of the paracortex act as antigen-presenting cells.

Interdigitating cells are prominent in the paracortex and are one form of dendritic APC, being so named because of their numerous cytoplasmic processes which interdigitate with those of other cells. These cytoplasmic processes also make numerous contacts with other cell types in the vicinity.

Macrophages are also found in the paracortex. Their cytoplasm is often observed packed with lipid (possibly engulfed cell membrane) and nuclear debris.

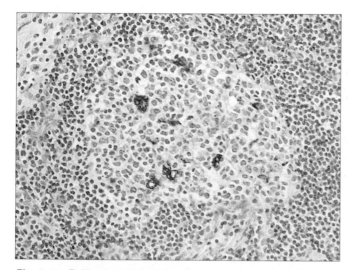

Fig. 8.11 Follicular accessory cells.
The follicular accessory cells are not easily distinguished in H&E sections, but can be stained by immunochemical techniques. This micrograph shows the tingible body macrophages stained brown by localizing a lysosomal enzyme, cathepsin D.

Fig. 8.12 Lymph node paracortex.
(a) Micrograph of lymph node paracortex showing sheets of T cells, which vary in morphology from small inactive cells to large cells representing activated proliferating T cells. The high endothelial venules (HEV) are prominent, but accessory cells are inconspicuous even at high magnification.
(b) Micrograph of lymph node stained by an antibody technique that detects T cells. The paracortex stains brown (i.e. is T cell in nature), while the adjacent portion of cortical follicle (C) is not stained, being composed of B cells.

The lymph node medulla is composed of a series of sinuses separating cords of cells.

The medulla of the lymph node contains mainly:

* cell-rich medullary cords;
* wide medullary sinuses (separating the medullary cords) through which lymph percolates toward the hilum from the cortex;
* larger blood vessels and their supporting trabeculae.

As in the cortex, the interstitial compartment of the medulla is supported by a framework of reticulin fibers, a small number of which traverse the sinuses.

The medulla contains plasma cells and macrophages.

The most common cells in medullary cords are plasma cells and their precursors. Plasma cells synthesize antibody, which is carried from the node to the general circulation via the efferent lymph. In addition, some mature plasma cells probably migrate from the node.

Classical macrophages are the main accessory cell type in the medulla. They are located in the sinuses and derive support from the traversing reticulin fibers.

Lymph entering the node is filtered and antigens are presented to lymphoid cells.

Lymph draining into a lymph node via afferent lymphatics first enters the subcapsular sinus and then percolates through the cortical sinusoidal maze to drain into the medullary sinuses before leaving the node via the efferent lymphatics.

Some particulate matter is probably taken up from the lymph and disposed of by the phagocytic activity of the endothelial cells without evoking any immune response.

Antigens are phagocytosed and processed by various types of APC exposed to the lymph. They are then transferred via the APC cytoplasmic extensions to sites where they may be encountered by lymphocytes.

Lymphocytes entering a lymph node in the afferent lymph constitute less than 10% of all of the lymphocytes entering the node, except in the case of mesenteric nodes where they may constitute up to 30%. The rest of the lymphocytes gain entry via the high endothelial venules.

Activated lymphocytes pass through the endothelium of the subcapsular sinus and enter the germinal centers of the cortical follicles.

SPREAD OF CANCER TO LYMPH NODES

Cancerous cells may break off from primary tumours and enter lymphatic vessels, from where they migrate to lymph nodes. Once in the node they adhere to and proliferate in the sinuses (Fig. 8.13).

Fig. 8.13 Spread of cancer to lymph nodes.
Micrograph showing clumps of cancer cells from a carcinoma of the stomach in the subcapsular (S) and cortical (C) sinuses of a lymph node.

LYMPH NODES

* function to allow interaction between antigen and lymphoid cells
* main site for expansion of lymphoid cells in an immune response
* follicles are composed of B cells (follicle center cells)
* paracortex is composed of T cells
* medulla contains plasma cells and macrophages.
* most lymphocytes enter the node from specialized high endothelial venules
* antigen from tissues enters the node in lymph which circulates around a series of sinuses

SPLEEN

The spleen lies in the left upper abdomen and weighs around 150 g in the adult.

The two principal functions of the human spleen are:

* to mount a primary immune response to antigens in the blood;
* to act as a filter to remove particulate matter and aged or abnormal red cells and platelets from the circulation.

The following description is specific to **human** spleen.

The spleen contains vascular sinusoids supported by a reticulin scaffold.

The spleen has a thin fibrocollagenous capsule from which short septa extend into the organ. These septa support an extensive meshwork of reticulin fibers which serve as a scaffold for the splenic parenchyma.

The reticulin framework is also attached to fibrocollagenous tissue associated with a branching arterial and venous network emanating from the splenic hilum. Such perivascular tissue does not form septa; it forms a sheath around the larger vessels.

Most of the spleen is composed of a vast array of sinusoids and vascular sinuses filled with blood (**red pulp**). A branching array of arteries (central arteries) associated with aggregates of lymphoid tissue is called **white pulp** (Fig. 8.14), and accounts for 5–20% of the total mass of the spleen.

The splenic red pulp is composed of cords of cells separated by sinusoids.

The red pulp consists of loose support tissue supported by reticulin fibers with several functional areas:

- **capillaries**, which terminate by draining into a fusiform-shaped macrophage-lined space, forming the ellipsoidal (sheathed) capillaries;
- a **parenchyma** composed of stellate reticular support cells, which surrounds sponge-like cavities, through which blood from the sheathed capillaries slowly percolates;
- **venous sinuses**, which run adjacent to columns of parenchymal tissue and drain blood that has filtered through the parenchyma, as well as blood that has come directly from the sheathed capillaries (Fig. 8.15).

The sinuses are lined by flattened endothelial cells resting on a discontinuous basement membrane, which is interrupted by numerous narrow slits through which red cells squeeze. Phagocytic cells are closely associated with the walls of these sinuses.

Fig. 8.15 Splenic red pulp.
(a) Micrograph of red pulp, which is composed of parenchymal areas (P), termed splenic cords, and sinusoids (S). The endothelial cells protrude into the sinuses.
(b) Micrograph of an ellipsoidal sheathed capillary (C), seen here in cross-section.
(c) Micrograph of splenic red pulp venous sinusoids, which have been immunostained for the lysosomal enzyme cathepsin-D. This technique highlights in brown the abundant network of phagocytic macrophages associated with the walls of the venous sinusoids (S).

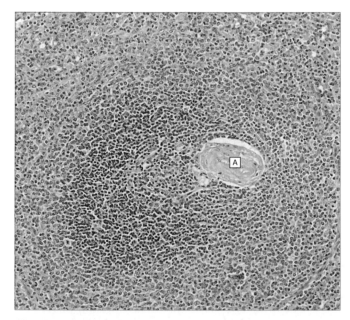

Fig. 8.14 Spleen.
Micrograph of an H&E-stained section of spleen. The white pulp is seen as dense-staining aggregates of lymphoid cells adjacent to central arteries (A). The red pulp is less densely stained as it has fewer nuclei, and at this magnification it is not possible to distinguish between the various sinuses and parenchymal components.

The splenic white pulp is composed of lymphoid cells.

The white pulp or splenic lymphoid masses are of two types: T cell and B cell. The functions of these two types of lymphoid tissue appear to be similar to those of the paracortex and superficial cortex of the lymph nodes.

White pulp T cells belong mainly to the TH subset and form irregular masses around the central arteries. The central arteries are generally located at one side of the T cell area (Fig. 8.16).

At the periphery of the T cell zone is a narrow mantle zone of small lymphocytes enclosed by a broader marginal zone, in which less densely packed larger lymphocytes and dendritic APCs surround fine vascular channels with a reticulin scaffold.

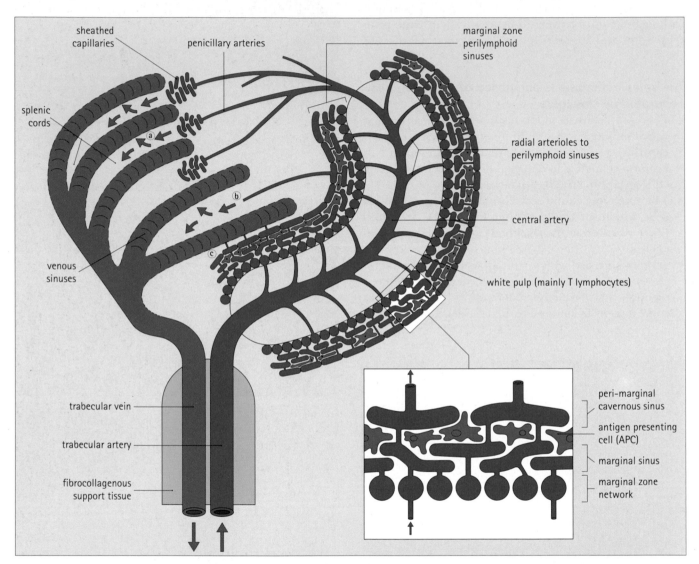

Fig. 8.16 Vascular anatomy of the spleen.
The spleen has two main functions: it removes aged and effete red cells from the circulation, and it mounts an immune response to antigens, particularly bacteria, circulating in the blood.

Blood enters the spleen in the splenic artery; this branches to form the trabecular arteries which give rise to a series of central arteries surrounded by T cells of the white pulp.

In order for red cells to be removed, blood passes along the central arteries and then enters the red pulp through a series of specialized vessels (penicillary arteries and sheathed capillaries) to drain into the splenic parenchyma (splenic cords). The blood then percolates through spaces between the reticular cells forming the splenic cords, and squeezes through narrow slit spaces to enter the splenic venous sinuses. Normal red cells are deformable and survive this passage, but aged red cells have rigid membranes and are lysed. Fragments of destroyed red cells are removed by phagocytic cells along the sinus walls.

Red cells leave the system via trabecular veins and enter the splenic vein. This pathway is the open circulation (a).

A proportion of the splenic circulation enters small arterioles to reach a series of marginal sinuses which run around the lymphoid sheaths. In this area blood comes into contact with dendritic antigen-presenting cells, and foreign antigens can be trapped and presented to appropriate lymphoid cells.

Most of the blood from the marginal sinuses enters the red pulp and then drains into the venous sinuses (b), but a small proportion passes directly into the sinuses and forms a closed circulation (c).

White pulp B cells form follicles which are usually located near an arteriole. In young people, many of the follicles have germinal centers; the proportion of such follicles diminishes with age.

In addition to these lymphoid areas associated with the central arteries, a significant number of B cell, T cell and plasma cell aggregates are present in the splenic parenchyma.

The perilymphoid zones of the red pulp are adapted for antigen presentation.

The zone of red pulp immediately surrounding the T and B lymphoid masses is composed of a sparse reticulin scaffold and anastomosing fine vascular channels surrounded by dendritic APCs (marginal zone).

About 10% of blood entering the spleen is believed to pass into this perilymphoid parenchyma from where it drains into the sinusoids or directly into the venous sinuses of the red pulp.

The function of the sinuses in the perilymphoid zones is not clearly understood, but they may be a means of enhancing the interaction of APCs and splenic lymphoid immune responsive tissue with antigens that are blood-borne rather than tissue-based (e.g. circulating bacteria in septicemia).

The splenic vasculature is arranged to filter blood through the red pulp.

Central arteries run eccentrically in the white pulp of the spleen and lead to:
- strands of arterioles and capillaries which supply the white pulp;
- arterioles and capillaries that run directly into a system of marginal zone fine vascular sinusoids (Fig. 8.16).

The marginal zone sinusoids are arranged concentrically around the white pulp in the perilymphoid zone. In human spleen, perfusion studies have defined three concentric systems:
- the marginal zone network;
- the marginal sinuses;
- the perimarginal cavernous sinus.

The central arteries terminate in a series of straight arterial vessels which are traditionally called **penicillary arteries**. These arteries are devoid of an investing layer of lymphoid cells and run in the red pulp. In turn, they give rise to arterioles and capillaries which tend to leave the arterioles at right angles.

The splenic capillaries of the red pulp have a standard endothelial cell structure which terminates abruptly in a fusiform arrangement of mononuclear phagocytes. They are described as ellipsoid sheathed capillaries (see Fig. 8.15b).

Most of the sheathed capillaries drain into the splenic parenchyma proper, which consists of a sponge-like network of spaces between stellate reticular cells (splenic cords). A small proportion of the sheathed capillaries also drains directly into the perimarginal cavernous sinuses.

SPLENECTOMY

Removal of the spleen is necessary:
- when it is ruptured following abdominal trauma;
- in some diseases, for example lymphomas;
- as part of major surgery, for example removal of the stomach for cancer.

Effects of splenectomy

The effects of removing the spleen highlight its main functions.

CHANGES IN THE BLOOD The blood film (Fig. 8.17) from a patient who has had a splenectomy shows increased numbers of platelets and abnormal red cells with deformed shapes. In addition, aged red cells contain blue-staining particulate inclusions of degenerate cell material (Howell–Jolly bodies). These cells would normally be removed by percolation through the splenic cords and into the splenic sinuses.

INFECTION Patients who have had a splenectomy are at risk of developing life-threatening bacterial septicemia. The commonest organism involved is *Streptococcus pneumoniae*. The presence of *S. pneumoniae* in blood would normally excite an immune response and prevent the development of an overwhelming infection, but in a person without a spleen the organism can circulate in the blood and reproduce.

Because the organism is in the blood it does not reach the immune surveillance systems provided by the lymph nodes. It is therefore recommended that anyone undergoing a splenectomy should be immunized against *S. pneumoniae*.

Fig. 8.17 Postsplenectomy blood film.
Micrograph of blood film from a patient following splenectomy. The red cells have bizarre shapes and in this field some of the cells contain small particulate dark-staining inclusions (Howell–Jolly bodies). Platelets are increased in number.

Splenic blood circulation

Blood can be filtered by percolation through the parenchyma (splenic cords) and then into the sinusoids – **open** circulation – the main route of blood flow in the human spleen.

The **closed** circulation appears to be a minor component of human splenic blood flow. Blood from the perimarginal cavernous sinuses bypasses the slow route through the splenic parenchyma and enters the splenic venous sinus instead. This provides a system for blood to pass rapidly through the spleen without filtration. In man a small number of capillaries arising from the central arteries also open directly into the venous sinuses.

THE SPLEEN

- destroys aged red cells
- filters antigens circulating in the blood
- is composed of red pulp and white pulp

MUCOSA-ASSOCIATED LYMPHOID TISSUE

Lymphoid cells may concentrate in mucosal surfaces to provide defense.

In addition to the mass of the peripheral lymphoid tissue encapsulated in the lymph nodes and spleen, the body contains an equally large amount of non-encapsulated lymphoid tissue which is located in the walls of the gastrointestinal, respiratory and urogenital tracts.

This tissue is known as **mucosa-associated lymphoid tissue (MALT)** and takes the form of diffuse infiltrates or more discrete nodules; it provides immunologic protection against invasion by pathogens via vulnerable exposed absorptive surfaces.

The **gut-associated lymphoid tissue (GALT)** includes:
- the palatine, lingual and pharyngeal tonsils (adenoids);
- mucosal nodules in the esophagus;
- **Peyer's patches** in the small intestine (see Chap. 11);
- lymphoid aggregations in the large intestine and appendix;
- a vast number of lymphocytes and plasma cells scattered throughout the lamina propria of the small and large intestines.

The bronchus-associated lymphoid tissue (BALT) is located beneath the mucosa of the large respiratory passages (bronchi) and shows close structural similarities with other forms of MALT.

In large aggregations of MALT, which are seen mainly in the tonsils and Peyer's patches, the lymphoid tissue is arranged into follicles which often contain germinal centers, and are similar to those of the lymph nodes.

With immunohistochemical techniques, discrete B and T cell zones containing typical antigen-processing accessory cells can be identified and have functions analogous to those of the superficial cortex and paracortex of the lymph node, respectively. The T cells found in mucosal tissues are mainly of the TCR-1+ type.

The scattered lymphocytes in the lamina propria of the gut and respiratory tract include B cells, some of which mature into antibody-secreting plasma cells. All classes of antibody are produced, but IgA predominates.

IgA is secreted into the gut lumen in a form called secretory IgA, which is resistant to enzymatic digestion and provides protection against pathogens before they breach the tissues.

IgG and IgM are secreted into the lamina propria to deal with organisms eluding the surface protective mechanisms.

IgE mediates the release of histamine from mast cells, which are present in large numbers in the lamina propria.

The recirculation of lymphoid cells from mucosal-associated lymphoid tissues is to local lymph nodes rather than to lymph nodes which drain non-mucosal tissues.

Peyer's patches are large aggregations of lymphoid tissue found in the small intestine.

Peyer's patches number about 200 in the human. They extend through the lamina propria and submucosa, and often bulge into the gut lumen. The overlying epithelium of a Peyer's patch (dome epithelium) is characterized by cuboidal rather than tall columnar cells (see Fig. 11.26), and contains large numbers of intraepithelial lymphocytes. Goblet cells are absent.

Some of the epithelial cells exhibit numerous surface microfolds instead of the usual microvilli and have been designated **M cells**. These cells migrate from the mucosal crypts and function in the transfer of antigen between the lumen and the Peyer's patch.

Tonsils are lymphoid tissues in the oropharynx.

Waldeyer's ring of pharyngeal lymphoid tissue comprises four groups of tonsillar tissue. The largest is the palatine tonsils, which contain 12 to 15 deep tonsillar crypts lined by stratified squamous epithelium (Fig. 8.18). These crypts frequently contain plugs of lymphocytes, bacteria and epithelial debris, which may become calcified.

The tonsils contain numerous lymphoid follicles with germinal centers, and the lymphoid tissue as a whole appears to have a similar cellular make-up to that of

Fig. 8.18 Tonsil.
Medium power micrograph of a tonsil showing a tonsillar crypt (C) lined by squamous epithelium and surrounded by tonsillar lymphoid tissue (L). The crypt contains colonies of oral commensal bacteria, which is a normal finding.

Peyer's patches. The epithelium overlying the tonsillar tissue contains T cells as well as dendritic APCs.

Bronchus-associated lymphoid tissue is encountered in the lung.

The lymphoid aggregates of the respiratory tract are similar to those of the gut (i.e. Peyer's patches), but are generally smaller. They are covered by similar antigen-sampling and transport M cells as in the gut. There are no afferent lymphatics; however, efferent lymphatics drain lymph to the regional nodes.

Activated lymphocytes derived from the respiratory tract aggregations tend to home specifically in on the respiratory mucosa.

1. B LYMPHOCYTES

(a) turn into plasma cells and secrete immunoglobulin
(b) are derived from cells which originate in the bone marrow
(c) are the main cell type in the paracortex of lymph nodes
(d) have receptors for antigen on their surface
(e) can be seen as small lymphocytes in peripheral blood

2. T LYMPHOCYTES

(a) may be seen as large granular lymphocytes in peripheral blood
(b) may express CD4, or CD8
(c) secrete antibodies as well as cytokines
(d) may be divided into two main groups on the basis of expression of distinct types of T cell receptors
(e) are the main cell responsible for the cell-mediated immune response

3. THE THYMUS GLAND

(a) is divided into red and white areas
(b) contains epithelial cells which interact with developing T cells
(c) contains structures called Hassall's corpuscles which are vessels wrapped by surrounding macrophagic cells
(d) undergoes involution after puberty
(e) becomes replaced by adipose tissue in adult life

4. IN LYMPH NODES

(a) the germinal centers are found in the superficial cortex and are predominantly composed of B cells
(b) the majority of lymphocytes gain entry via the high endothelial venules in the paracortex
(c) antigen-presenting cells are not found in germinal centers but are concentrated in the paracortex
(d) lymph enters the subcapsular sinus via afferent lymphatics
(e) plasma cells are mainly concentrated in the medullary sinuses

9. Blood and Lymphatic Circulatory Systems and Heart

INTRODUCTION

The main transport systems are the circulatory systems, in which substances are dissolved or suspended in liquid and carried from one part of the body to another in a system of tubes (vessels). There are two main circulatory systems: the blood circulatory system and the lymphatic system.

The **blood circulatory system** is the main method of transporting oxygen, carbon dioxide, nutrients and metabolic breakdown products, cells of the immune and other defense systems, chemical messengers (hormones), and many other important substances (e.g. clotting factors).

The **lymphatic system** drains extracellular fluid from the tissues, returning it to the blood circulatory system after passage through lymph nodes. This system is also involved in absorption of nutrients from the gut.

BLOOD CIRCULATORY SYSTEM

The three main blood circulatory systems are the systemic, pulmonary and portal systems.

There are three types of blood circulatory system, two of which (systemic and pulmonary circulations) depend on a central pump, the heart, to push the blood around (Fig. 9.1).

The systemic circulation transfers oxygenated blood from a central pump (the heart) to all of the body tissues (systemic arterial system) and returns deoxygenated blood with a high carbon dioxide content from the tissues to the central pump (systemic venous system).

The pulmonary circulation transfers deoxygenated blood with a high carbon dioxide content from a central pump (the heart) to the lungs (pulmonary arterial system) and transfers reoxygenated blood from the lungs back to the central pump (pulmonary venous system).

The **portal systems** are specialized vascular channels that carry substances from one site to another, but do not depend on a central pump. The largest portal system (hepatic portal venous) runs between the intestines and the liver (see Chapter 12).

SYSTEMIC BLOOD VESSELS

There are two main types of blood vessels:
- arteries, which carry blood away from the heart at relatively high pressure;
- veins, which carry blood back to the heart at relatively low pressure.

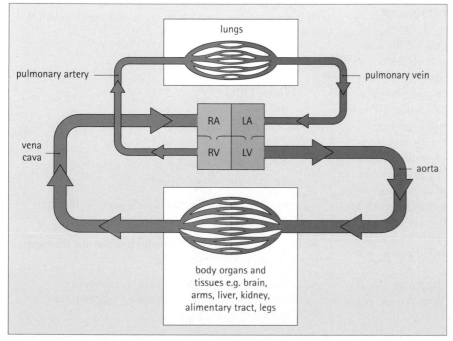

Fig. 9.1 Systemic and pulmonary blood circulations.
Diagram illustrating the main components and interrelationships of the systemic and pulmonary blood circulations.

The heart is a four-chambered pump central to both systems. The direction of blood flow is indicated by arrows.

Blood vessels that transport blood away from the heart are called arteries (arterial systems) and those that take blood to the heart are called veins (venous systems). The systemic venous and pulmonary arterial vessels carry deoxygenated blood; the pulmonary venous and systemic arterial vessels carry oxygenated blood.

In organs and tissues other than the lung the oxygenated blood gives up much of its oxygen and becomes deoxygenated; in the lungs deoxygenated blood is oxygenated. Gaseous exchange takes place in small, thin-walled vessels called capillaries.

Blood vessels are composed of three layers which vary in prominence in different vessel types.

The walls of blood vessels are made up of three identifiable layers: **intima**, **media** and **adventitia**.

The intima is composed of a lining layer of highly specialized multifunctional flattened epithelial cells termed **endothelium**. This sits on a basal lamina; beneath this is a very thin layer of fibrocollagenous support tissue.

The media is the middle layer in a blood vessel wall and is composed predominantly of smooth muscle reinforced by organized layers of elastic tissue which form elastic laminae. The media is particularly prominent in arteries, being relatively indistinct in veins and virtually nonexistent in very small vessels. In vessels which are close to the heart, receiving the full thrust of the systolic pressure wave, elastic tissue is very well developed, hence the term **elastic arteries**. In muscular arteries and arterioles the prominent elastic lamina just below the intima is termed the **internal elastic lamina**.

The adventitia is the outer layer of blood vessels. It is composed largely of collagen, but smooth muscle cells may be present, particularly in veins. The adventitia is often the most prominent layer in the walls of veins. Within the adventitia of vessels with thick walls are small blood vessels, the **vasa vasorum**, which send penetrating branches into the media to supply it with blood. These are not seen in thinner vessels, which obtain their oxygen by diffusion from the lumen. The adventitia also carries autonomic nerves which innervate the smooth muscle of the media.

The differences between the layers in the wall of a small artery and a small vein are illustrated in Figure 9.2.

The endothelium is highly specialized with endocrine, exocrine, cell adhesion, clotting and transport functions.

The endothelium is composed of flattened cells with diverse functional roles. In routine histologic sections the cytoplasm of most endothelial cells is barely visible and only the small flattened nuclei are seen. Ultrastructurally, each cell can be seen to be anchored to an underlying basal lamina; individual cells are anchored together by adhesion junctions, including prominent tight junctions which prevent diffusion between cells. A prominent feature of endothelial cells is the presence of many pinocytotic vesicles which are involved in the process of transport of substances from one side of the cell to the other. In small blood vessels of the nervous system the endothelial cells express transport proteins which are responsible for active transport of all substances, for example glucose, into the brain.

Endothelial cells are able to sense changes in blood pressure, oxygen tension and blood flow by as yet unknown mechanisms. In response to changes in local factors they respond by secreting substances which have powerful effects on the tone of vascular smooth muscle (endothelins, nitric oxide and prostacyclin, PGI_2). Substances which cause relaxation of vascular smooth muscle increase local blood flow by causing vasodilation.

Endothelial cells are important for control of blood coagulation and under normal circumstances the endothelial surface prevents blood clotting. This is done by high expression of factors which prevent blood clotting and low expression of factors which activate this process (Fig. 9.3).

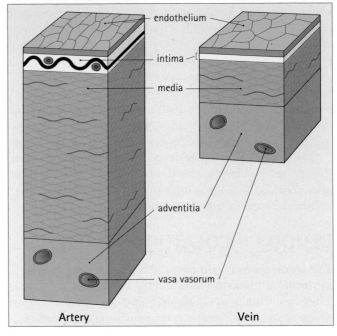

Fig 9.2 General structure of blood vessel wall.
The wall of a vessel is divided into intima, media and adventitia. In an artery, the intima contains elastic lamina and myointimal cells. In an artery, the media is much more developed than in a vein of the same diameter.

ENDOTHELIUM

- cells are bound together by junctional complexes and have many pinocytotic vesicles

- cells have many functional roles despite their apparent structural simplicity

- normally secretes factors which prevent blood clotting

- normally secretes factors which maintain the tone of vascular smooth muscle

- can be activated by cytokines to express cell adhesion molecules which allow white blood cells to stick

Factor secreted by endothelium	Activities
prostacyclin	vasodilation, inhibits platelet aggregation
nitric oxide	vasodilation, inhibits platelet adhesion and aggregation
tissue plasminogen activator (tPA)	regulates fibrinolysis
thrombomodulin	anticoagulant activity
thromboplastin	promotes blood coagulation
platelet activating factor (PAF)	activation of platelets and neutrophils
von Willebrand factor	promotes platelet adhesion and activation of blood coagulation

(a)

(b)

Fig 9.3 (a) Substances produced by endothelial cells that modulate blood coagulation and vasodilation.

(b) High-power electron micrograph of part of an endothelial cell showing characteristic Weibel-Palade bodies (W) close to the surface contacting the vessel lumen (L).

Activated endothelium

The endothelium can adapt rapidly to changes in its environment. Under certain circumstances, especially in response to adverse stimuli, the endothelium may become activated and change its function.

Endothelium may become activated by cytokines and develop specialization for **emigration of lymphoid cells**. The endothelial cells become cuboidal in shape and express surface adhesion molecules which facilitate lymphocyte adhesion and migration. This type of endothelium is normally seen in the specialized venules in the lymph node paracortex (high endothelial venules).

Endothelium may become activated by cytokines and express cell adhesion molecules for neutrophils. This normally occurs after any form of tissue damage and **allows neutrophils to migrate into local tissues** in the process of acute inflammation. The substance P-selectin, a cell adhesion molecule, is stored in special vesicles (Weibel–Palade bodies) inside the endothelium (Fig. 9.3b). With appropriate stimulation, these vesicles dock with the endothelial cell membrane. P-selectin is then available on the cell surface for neutrophil adhesion.

Endothelium is normally locally impermeable to substances in the blood. Under the effects of certain factors, for example histamine, endothelial cells lose attachment to each other and retract. This allows fluid and proteins to diffuse out into the local tissues causing tissue swelling termed **edema**. This reorganization of cell–cell junctions is rapid and reversible and takes place in the space of a few minutes.

The systemic vascular system is composed of arteries, arterioles, capillaries, venules and veins.

The systemic arterial circulation is an extensive high-pressure system. The structure of its vessels reflects the high pressures to which they are subjected.

The output of the left ventricle is carried in large-diameter vessels with a high component of elastic tissue in their walls which smooths the systolic pressure wave. These are called the **large elastic arteries** (i.e. the aorta and its large branches such as the carotid, subclavian and renal arteries).

Distal to these large elastic arteries are smaller vessels in which the artery walls become proportionately more muscular. These **muscular arteries** gradually decrease in size as they branch within tissues until they form **arterioles**. The arterioles then open into a system of very fine vessels termed **capillaries**.

From capillaries blood moves into **venules** and then into **veins,** which become progressively larger as they approach the heart. The large veins carry blood at low pressure and hence have a small amount of muscle in their wall compared with arteries.

The pulmonary vasculature is discussed in Chapter 10.

Elastic arteries are characterized by multiple elastic laminae in the media.

Elastic arteries are the largest arteries and receive the main output of the left ventricle: thus they are subjected to the high systolic pressures of 120–160 mmHg. Furthermore, these large vessels are adapted to smooth out the surges in blood flow, since blood is impelled through them only during the systolic phase of the cardiac cycle. The elastic tissue in their walls provides the resilience to smooth out the pressure wave.

The intima of large elastic arteries is composed of endothelium with a thin layer of underlying fibrocollagenous tissue.

Elastic arteries have a thick, highly developed media of which elastic fibers are the main component. These are gathered together in sheets arranged in concentric layers throughout the thickness of the media. In the largest artery, the aorta, there are often 50 or more layers (Fig. 9.4).

The elastic fibers are arranged so that they run circumferentially rather than longitudinally in order to counteract the tendency for the vessel to over-distend during systole. Return of the elastic fibers from their stretched to unstretched state during diastole maintains a diastolic pressure within the aorta and large arteries of about 60–80 mmHg. Interposed between the elastic layers are smooth muscle cells and some collagen.

The adventitia of the large vessels carries vasa vasorum and nerves.

Muscular arteries have a media composed almost entirely of smooth muscle.

The large elastic arteries gradually merge into muscular arteries by losing most of their medial elastic sheets, usually leaving only two layers, an internal elastic lamina and an external elastic lamina, at the junction of the media with the intima and adventitia, respectively. The general structure of a muscular artery is shown in Figure 9.5a.

In a muscular artery the media is composed almost entirely of smooth muscle. These arteries are therefore highly contractile, their degree of contraction or relaxation being controlled by the autonomic nervous system

as well as by endothelium-derived vasoactive substances. A few fine elastic fibers are scattered among the smooth muscle cells, but are not organized into sheets. These are most numerous in the large muscular arteries, which are a direct continuation of the distal end of the elastic arteries (Fig. 9.5b, c).

Muscular arteries vary in size from about 1 cm in diameter close to their origin at the elastic arteries, to about 0.5 mm in diameter. In the larger arteries there may be 30 or more layers of smooth muscle cells, whereas in the smallest peripheral arteries, there are only 2 or 3 layers. The smooth muscle cells are usually arranged circumferentially at right angles to the long axis of the vessel.

The internal elastic lamina is commonly a distinct prominent layer, but the external elastic lamina is less well defined, and is often incomplete.

Fig. 9.4 Elastic artery.
Low power view of elastic Van Gieson-stained large elastic artery (aorta). The predominant layer is the media (M), which is composed of elastic fibers (black) arranged as concentric sheets and separated by smooth muscle fibers and collagen.

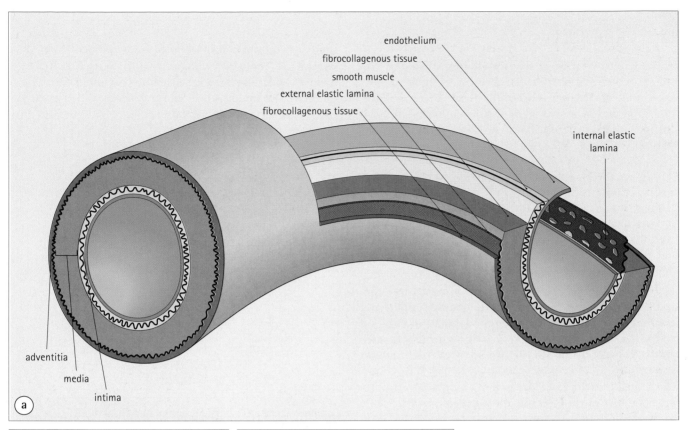

endothelium
fibrocollagenous tissue
smooth muscle
external elastic lamina
fibrocollagenous tissue

internal elastic lamina

adventitia
media
intima

a

b

c

Fig 9.5 Muscular artery

(a) The most prominent layer of a muscular artery is the media. Composed of smooth muscle, it is bounded by an internal and an external elastic lamina.

(b) Elastic Van Gieson-stained longitudinal section through a muscular artery. The intima is scarcely visible, the predominant layer being the muscular media (M) situated between an internal elastic lamina (IEL) and an external elastic lamina (EEL), which are composed of condensed sheets of elastic fibers (black). The outer adventitia stains red, being composed largely of collagen.

(c) Medium power view of the same artery showing the intima (I) and the fine black-staining elastic fibers running through the muscular media (arrows). In this large muscular artery the collagenous adventitia (A) is thick.

ATHEROMA

Atheroma is a disease of arteries which starts in the intima. It is characterized by infiltration of the intima by fatty material which accumulates in macrophages, accompanied by increased deposition of collagen. Such intimal thickening forms a so-called atheromatous plaque.

There are three common consequences of atheroma.

IMPAIRED BLOOD FLOW In small-bore arteries atheromatous change leads to reduction in the size of lumen of the vessel so that blood flow is decreased.

THROMBUS FORMATION Another complication of atheroma is that it damages the smooth internal lining of endothelial cells, exposing circulating blood to the underlying intimal collagen. This can trigger coagulation of blood to form a mass of blood clot, termed a thrombus, within the vessel. Thrombus further reduces the lumen of the vessel, and may block it completely (Fig. 9.6), resulting in death of the tissue (infarction) supplied by the vessel. The myocardium of the left ventricle is particularly vulnerable to infarction (see Fig. 9.24), as is the brain (stroke) and the feet and toes (gangrene).

ANEURYSM FORMATION As a plaque of atheroma enlarges, elastic and smooth muscle are lost from the underlying media. In the large elastic arteries such as the aorta, these specialized components become replaced by non-contractile, inelastic collagen and the vessel dilates to form an abnormally wide sac termed an aneurysm. The danger of an aneurysm is that the vessel wall is greatly weakened and is prone to burst.

Fig. 9.6 Coronary artery atheroma and thrombosis.
Micrograph showing a transverse section from the coronary artery supplying the area of dead muscle shown in Figure 9.24. The lumen has been greatly reduced by thickening of the intimal layer (I) by atheroma. The media (M) and adventitia (A) are normal. The intimal thickening and irregularity have led to the formation of a thrombus (T), which has blocked the vessel lumen.

Arterioles are the smallest branches of the arterial tree.

Arterioles vary in diameter ranging from 30 μm to 400 μm (0.4 mm).

The intima of an arteriole is composed of endothelial cells lying on a basement membrane with an underlying fine internal elastic lamina in the larger arterioles.

The arteriolar media is composed of one or two layers of smooth muscle cells (Fig. 9.7). As the arterioles get smaller, the continuous layers of smooth muscle become progressively discontinuous. In the smallest arterioles, the endothelial cells have basal processes which pierce the basement membrane and make junctional contacts with the smooth muscle cells. The adventitia of arterioles is insignificant.

Arterioles are very responsive to vasoactive stimuli and make a major contribution to the vascular resistance.

Fig. 9.7 Arteriole.
Micrograph of a thin epoxy resin toluidine blue-stained section of two arterioles showing basement membrane (BM) as a pale-staining membrane surrounded by a number of smooth muscle cells (SM). The inner endothelial cells (E) in the larger vessel appear rather cuboidal because it has contracted during the biopsy process. Note that the two arterioles differ not only in size, but also with regard to the number of muscle cells.

ARTERIAL SYSTEM

- large elastic arteries have a media composed of concentric layers of elastic and smooth muscle (for example, aorta and subclavian arteries)

- muscular arteries have a prominent media composed of smooth muscle which is bounded by internal and external elastic laminae (for example, coronary arteries)

- arterioles are the smallest part of the arterial tree and have 3–4 complete layers of smooth muscle in their media

The microvasculature starts at the level of the arterioles.

The microvasculature (Fig. 9.8) is composed of small-diameter blood vessels with partly permeable thin walls that permit the transfer of some blood components to the tissues and vice versa. Most of this exchange between blood and tissues occurs in the extensive capillary network, the smallest arterioles (metarterioles) emptying into the capillary system. The capillary networks drain into the first components of the venous system, the venules.

Capillaries are specialized for diffusion of substances across their wall.

Capillaries are the smallest vessels of the blood circulatory system (5–10 μm in diameter) and form a complex interlinking network.

Capillaries have the thinnest walls of all blood vessels and are the major site of gaseous exchange, permitting the transfer of oxygen from blood to tissues, and carbon dioxide from tissues to blood. Fluids containing large molecules pass across the capillary wall in both directions.

The capillary wall (Fig. 9.9) is composed of endothelial cells, a basement membrane, and occasional scattered contractile cells called pericytes.

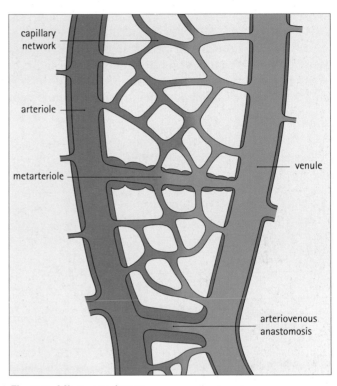

Fig. 9.8 Microvasculature.
Diagram showing the microvasculature. Blood flows from arteriolar to venular vessels through a complex network of capillaries, arising either directly from the arteriole or from the smaller metarteriole. Opening of the arteriovenous anastomosis directs blood flow out of the capillary network.

Fig. 9.9 Capillary.
(a) An epoxy resin section stained with toluidine blue of a capillary in longitudinal section. The wall is composed almost entirely of thin basement membrane (BM), the endothelial cytoplasm lining its internal surface not being visible at this magnification. An endothelial cell nucleus (EN) can be seen at one end. A similar but smaller capillary is seen in transverse section (arrow) between individual muscle fibers.

(b) Electron micrograph of the capillary arrowed in a . At this low magnification the endothelial cytoplasm (EC) is just visible, but the basement membrane is indistinct.

(c) High power electron micrograph of part of the capillary wall showing the basement membrane (BM), endothelial cytoplasm (C) and anchoring junction (J) between the cytoplasm of adjacent endothelial cells.

Capillaries may be of two types: continuous or fenestrated.

Capillaries with **continuous** endothelium are the most common type, the endothelial cells forming a complete internal lining to the capillary without any intercellular or intracytoplasmic defects (Fig. 9.10).

Capillaries with **fenestrated** endothelium are seen most commonly in the gastrointestinal mucosa, endocrine glands and renal glomeruli (see Figs 15.7 & 15.13) The endothelial cell cytoplasm is pierced by pores (fenestrations) which extend through its full thickness. In some fenestrations there is a thin diaphragm which is thinner than the cell membrane; its nature is uncertain.

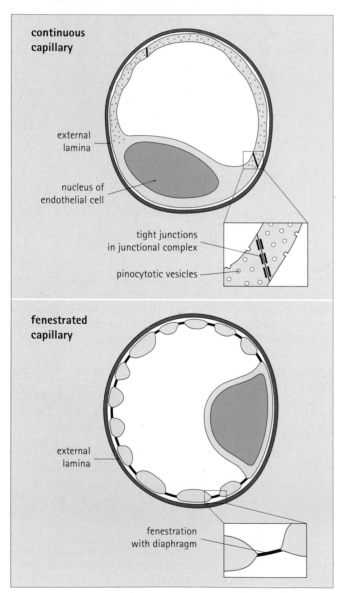

Fig 9.10 Types of capillary.

There are two types of capillary, continuous and fenestrated. In continuous capillaries substances are transported across the wall by pinocytosis.

Sinusoids are large-diameter channels with thin walls.

Highly specialized vascular channels, called sinusoids, are seen in some organs, for example the liver (see Fig. 12.1) and spleen (see Fig. 8.15). They are endothelium-lined channels with a larger diameter than capillaries, and scanty, discontinuous or absent basement membrane.

The endothelial cells in sinusoids are commonly highly fenestrated, often with large pores, and there may be substantial gaps between the cells.

CAPILLARIES

- receive blood from metarterioles

- are composed of a single layer of endothelium attached to a basal lamina

- most have a continuous layer of endothelial cells which are tightly attached (continuous type)

- some have pores which allow free diffusion from the lumen to tissues (fenestrated type)

Blood from capillaries enters a system of venules.

Capillaries drain into **postcapillary venules**, which are the smallest venules (10–25 μm in diameter). They resemble capillaries in structure, but have more pericytes (Fig. 9.11).

Postcapillary venules drain into **large collecting venules** 20–50 μm in diameter, in which the pericyte layer becomes continuous and surrounding collagen fibers appear.

As the collecting venules become larger bore, the pericytes are progressively replaced by smooth muscle cells, which form a layer 1 to 2 cells thick, and a fibrocollagenous adventitia becomes identifiable; these are **muscular venules** and are 50–100 μm in diameter. Muscular venules drain into the smallest veins.

Veins have thin walls and carry blood at low pressure.

Veins vary in size from less than 1 mm to 4 cm in diameter. In comparison with arteries of comparable external diameter, veins have a larger lumen and a relatively thinner wall, and are therefore commonly collapsed in histologic sections unless inflation-fixed.

Although intimal, medial and adventitial layers are present in veins, they are less clearly demarcated than in arteries, and it is often difficult to identify where one layer ends and another begins. Furthermore, there is considerable variation in vein wall structure according to location. The following description of veins of different sizes is therefore a generalization.

Fig. 9.11 Postcapillary venule.

ⓐ Toluidine blue-stained epoxy resin section of a partly collapsed postcapillary venule. The endothelial cell nucleus (EN) and basement membrane (BM) can be identified. There are a few pericyte processes (PP) and a pericyte nucleus (PN) in the wall, but the details are not clearly visible.

ⓑ Electron micrograph of a postcapillary venule showing the endothelial cell cytoplasm (C), basement membrane (BM) and pericytes (P) more clearly. Note that the finer pericyte processes (PP) apparently intervene between layers of the basement membrane (arrow).

Small veins are a continuation of the muscular venules and have a similar wall structure, but are larger, up to 1 mm in diameter, with more clearly defined muscle cell and outer fibrocollagenous layers (Fig. 9.12a).

Medium-sized veins are 1–10 mm in diameter. They have an inner layer of endothelial cells on a basement membrane. This is separated by a narrow zone of collagen fibers from an indistinct condensation of elastic fibers producing a thin, discontinuous internal elastic lamina.

The inner layer is fairly consistent in structure, differing only in quantity of collagen and elastic fibers between the endothelium and the condensation of elastic fibers. However, the outer layers – still called the media and adventitia, but often arbitrarily and with little justification – vary considerably in thickness, proportions of collagen, elastic fibers and smooth muscle, and in the orientation of the muscle fibers in particular.

Large veins have an inner (intimal) layer similar to that of medium-sized veins, but there are usually more collagen and elastic fibers between the endothelial basement membrane and the elastic lamina, which is generally discontinuous. External to the elastic lamina there is a layer of smooth muscle embedded in collagen, and outside this is a thick layer of collagen in which there are bundles of longitudinally oriented smooth muscle fibers. Some elastic fibers intermingle with the collagen (Fig. 9.12b).

Valves in large veins assist the flow of blood to the heart.

Venous circulation of blood is maintained by the contraction of venous smooth muscle, supplemented to varying degrees by external pressure from the contraction of the surrounding skeletal muscle responsible for arm and leg movement. Such assistance from skeletal muscle contraction is particularly important for maintaining the venous circulation of the arms and legs.

Fig. 9.12 Veins.

ⓐ Micrograph showing an elastic Van Gieson (EVG)-stained small vein. The rather variable and irregular arrangement of smooth muscle (yellow), collagen (red) and elastic fibers (black) in its wall is evident.

ⓑ Micrograph showing the wall of the largest vein in the body, the inferior vena cava. There is a distinct intima (I) and internal elastic lamina (EL), a layer of smooth muscle (yellow, SM) and an irregular layer of thick collagen (red, C). This collagen indicates the approximate beginning of the adventitial layer, the thickest layer in large veins, being expanded by the presence of large bundles of longitudinally running smooth muscle (SML) (EVG stain).

The veins in the arms and legs, which carry blood against gravity, are equipped with valves to prevent blood flowing back down the vein. These valves are thin flaps of intima that project into the lumen, the free edges of the valve flaps pointing toward the heart; this allows blood to flow toward the heart, but prevents backflow. Incompetence of the valves in the veins of the legs causes varicose veins.

Valves are also present in other medium and large veins, their number depending on whether or not the vein is carrying blood against gravity.

Arteriovenous anastomoses allow blood to bypass capillary beds.

As well as the microvasculature (i.e. arterioles emptying into a capillary network, which drains into a venular system), there are additional vessels that bypass the capillary bed, allowing arterioles to communicate directly with venules; these are arteriovenous anastomoses (see Fig. 9.8).

At its arteriolar end, an arteriovenous anastomosis is thick-walled, mainly due to an abundant smooth muscle coat which is richly innervated. Contraction of the thick smooth muscle layer closes off the lumen of the anastomosis at its origin and diverts blood into the capillary bed; relaxation opens up the lumen allowing blood to flow directly into a venule, bypassing the capillary network.

Arteriovenous anastomoses are widespread, but are most common in the skin in certain regions such as the fingertips, lips, nose, ears and toes. They are thought to play an important role in the skin's thermoregulatory function (see Chapter 18). Closure of the anastomosis diverts blood into the extensive dermal capillary system and permits heat loss, while opening of the vessel closes the capillary bed and conserves heat.

In the fingertips, there is a highly specialized type of arteriovenous anastomosis, the glomus body, which has a prominent arterial end (Sucquet–Hoyer canal) connecting directly to the venular end. The canal is surrounded by modified smooth muscle cells (glomus cells), which are richly innervated by the autonomic nervous system.

Blood vessels have both an efferent and afferent innervation.

Blood vessels that can significantly alter their lumen size by contraction and relaxation of their smooth muscle fibers have a major supply of adrenergic sympathetic fibers, stimulation of which causes muscle contraction and vasoconstriction.

Some blood vessels in skeletal muscles also have a cholinergic sympathetic innervation capable of producing vasodilation.

In certain areas blood vessels have an afferent innervation, which provides information about the luminal pressure (baroreceptive information) and blood gas (i.e. carbon dioxide and oxygen) levels (chemoreceptive information). These are mainly located in the carotid sinuses, and in the region of the aortic arch, pulmonary artery and large veins entering the heart.

Afferent fibers from the carotid sinus receptors travel in the glossopharyngeal nerve to the cardiorespiratory centers in the brain stem.

PORTAL BLOOD SYSTEMS

A portal system connects two capillary systems.

Portal circulations are venous channels that connect one capillary system with another and do not depend on the central pumping action of the heart.

The nature of portal connecting vessels varies from site to site; for example, the vessels of the hepatic portal system (see Fig. 12.2), which connects capillaries in the intestine to the capillary-like sinusoids in the liver, are venuous in nature, being small venules adjacent to the capillary beds, and medium and large-sized veins in between. In the other main portal system, between the hypothalamus and posterior pituitary (see Fig. 14.3) the connecting vessels are large capillaries and venules.

LYMPHATIC CIRCULATORY SYSTEM

The lymphatic system carries fluid that drains from the intercellular space of tissues.

The intercellular spaces of almost all tissues contain small endothelial-lined tubes which are blind ending but otherwise identical in structure to blood capillaries. These are lymphatic capillaries and are permeable to fluids and dissolved molecules in the interstitial fluid.

In some areas the lymphatic capillaries have a fenestrated endothelium and a discontinuous basement membrane, permitting the entry of larger molecules such as large molecular weight proteins, triglycerides, etc., and also some cells, particularly cells of the immune system.

The lymphatic capillary network acts as a drainage system, removing surplus fluid (lymph) from tissue spaces. Lymph is normally a clear colorless fluid, but lymph draining the intestine during absorption is often milky in appearance because of its lipid high content. This is called chyle.

The lymphatic capillaries merge to form thicker-walled vessels which resemble venules and medium-sized veins.

Lymph moves sluggishly from the capillary network into the larger lymphatic vessels; backflow is prevented by numerous flap-like valves similar to those in veins (Fig. 9.13).

On its way to the larger vein-like lymphatics from the smaller lymphatics, lymph passes through one or more lymph nodes. It enters the lymph node at its convex periphery, and leaves it through one or two lymphatic vessels at the concave hilum (see Fig. 8.8). During this passage, any antigens in the lymph can be processed by the immune system. Activated lymphocytes, which are important to immune defense, are added to the lymph. The larger lymphatic vessels have muscular walls and pump the lymph into the following two main lymphatic vessels:

- the thoracic duct, which empties lymph into the venous system at the junction of the left internal jugular and left subclavian veins;
- a more variable lymphatic vessel, the right main lymphatic duct, which empties into the junction between the right internal jugular and right subclavian veins.

Fig. 9.13 Lymphatic capillary.
Micrograph showing a large lymphatic capillary (LC) containing pale pink-staining lymph. Note the delicate flap-like valves (V) controlling the direction of flow.

SPREAD OF CANCER BY LYMPHATICS

All lymphatic capillaries from a particular area drain into lymph nodes serving that area (regional lymph nodes). Such drainage is particularly important in the spread of cancer, since cancer cells in lymph can enter the lymphatic capillaries and be carried to other sites. Cancer cells may also be trapped in the regional lymph node, where they can multiply and produce secondary tumors at some distance from the site of the primary cancer (see Fig. 8.13).

For example, most cancers that originate in the breast may be carried in the lymph to the regional lymph nodes of the breast, most of which are in the subcutaneous tissue of the axilla. Careful palpation of the axillary lymph nodes is therefore a vital part of the physical examination of any patient with suspected breast cancer.

THE HEART

The heart is a muscular pump with four chambers. Two of these, the **atria**, receive blood from the systemic and pulmonary venous circulations, while the other two, the **ventricles**, pump blood into the systemic and pulmonary arterial circulations. In between the cardiac chambers and at the outflow of the heart are the **heart valves** which prevent backflow of blood.

The wall of the heart is composed of the epicardium, the myocardium and the endocardium.
The three layers of the heart wall are:
- a very thin outer **epicardium** (visceral pericardium) covered with flat mesothelial cells to produce a smooth outer surface (see page 148);
- a middle **myocardium** making up the vast bulk of the heart wall and composed of specialized muscle (cardiac muscle), which is responsible for the pumping action of the heart;
- a very thin, inner smooth lining, the **endocardium**, covered by endothelial cells in direct contact with the circulating blood.

The pericardium surrounds the heart and is lined by mesothelial cells.

The heart is enclosed within the pericardial sac, which is composed of compact fibrocollagenous and elastic tissue, and lined internally by a layer of flat mesothelial cells, termed the **parietal pericardium**. This smooth mesothelial layer reflects over the outer surface of the heart to form the **visceral pericardium,** also termed the **epicardium**.

The pericardial cavity is the space between the parietal and visceral pericardial layers. It contains a small amount of serous fluid to lubricate the surfaces and permit friction-free movement of the heart within the cavity during its muscular contractions.

The epicardium forms the outer covering of the heart and has an external layer of flat mesothelial cells. These cells lie on a stroma of fibrocollagenous support tissue, which contains elastic fibers, as well as the large arteries supplying blood to the heart wall, and the larger venous tributaries carrying blood from the heart wall. The large arteries (coronary arteries) and veins are surrounded by adipose tissue, which expands the epicardium (Fig. 9.14).

The coronary arteries originate from the first part of the aorta just above the aortic valve ring and pass over the surface of the heart in the epicardium, sending branches deep into the myocardium. This superficial location of the arteries is of great practical importance since it permits surgical bypass grafting of blocked arteries.

The myocardium is composed of specialised striated muscle termed cardiac muscle.

The bulk of the heart is myocardium, which is the contractile element composed of specialized striated muscle fibers called cardiac muscle (see Fig. 5.10).

The amount of myocardium and the diameter of muscle fibers in the chambers of the heart varies according to the workload of the chamber (Fig. 9.15).

The left and right atria push blood into empty ventricles against minimal resistance during diastole and therefore have a thin wall composed of cells of small diameter.

The right ventricle pushes blood through the pulmonary valve and through the lungs, to enter the left atrium (see Fig. 9.1). It therefore has a moderately thick muscle layer composed of fibers intermediate in diameter between atrial and left ventricular muscle cells.

The left ventricle pumps blood through the high-pressure systemic arterial system and therefore has the thickest myocardium with the largest diameter muscle fibers (see Fig. 9.15b).

The outer surface of the myocardium beneath the pericardium is smooth, but the internal surface beneath the endocardium is raised into trabeculations, which are most marked in the ventricles. The trabeculations are covered by smooth endocardium and do not interfere with the smooth flow of the blood.

In both ventricles, raised mounds of cardiac muscle (papillary muscles) protrude into the ventricular lumina and point toward the atrioventricular valves. Papillary muscles are the site of attachment of chordae tendinae, narrow tendinous cords that tether the atrioventricular valve leaflets to the wall of the ventricle beneath them.

Fig. 9.14 Visceral pericardium (epicardium).
Section of thin epicardium showing a narrow layer of fibrocollagenous tissue (F) containing elastic fibers (black), covered by flat mesothelial cells (M) identical to those of the inner surface of the parietal pericardium. (Elastic Van Gieson stain.)

Fig. 9.15 Myocardium.
ⓐ Micrograph of left atrial myocardium in approximate transverse section. The myocardial fibers (M) form an interconnecting network separated by loose fibrocollagenous tissue (the endomysium, E).
ⓑ Micrograph of left ventricular myocardium in approximate transverse section at the same magnification as ⓐ. The general structure is the same as left atrial myocardium, but the fibers of the left ventricle are of larger diameter and have larger nuclei.

Cardiac muscle cells secrete atrial natriuretic hormone.

Atrial myocardial fibers are smaller than those of the ventricles and contain small neuroendocrine granules, which are usually sparse and located close to the nucleus; they are most numerous in the right atrium. These granules secrete atrial natriuretic hormone when the atrial fibers are stretched excessively.

Atrial natriuretic hormone increases the excretion of water and sodium and potassium ions by the distal convoluted tubule of the kidney. It also decreases blood pressure by inhibiting renin secretion by the kidneys and aldosterone secretion by the adrenals (see Chapter 14).

The endocardium lines the chambers of the heart and varies in thickness in different areas.

The internal lining of all four heart chambers is the endocardium, which is composed of three layers (Fig. 9.16):
- the layer in direct contact with the myocardium;
- the middle layer;
- the innermost layer.

The outermost layer is composed of irregularly arranged collagen fibers that merge with collagen surrounding adjacent cardiac muscle fibers. This layer may contain some Purkinje fibers, which are part of the impulse conducting system.

The middle layer is the thickest endocardial layer and is composed of more regularly arranged collagen fibers containing variable numbers of elastic fibers, which are compact and arranged in parallel in the deepest part of the layer. Occasional myofibroblasts are present.

The inner layer is composed of flat endothelial cells, which are continuous with the endothelial cells lining the vessels entering and emerging from the heart.

The endocardium is variable in thickness, being thickest in the atria and thinnest in the ventricles, particularly the left ventricle. The increased thickness is due almost entirely to a thicker fibroelastic middle layer (Fig. 9.16). Localized areas of endocardial thickening (jet lesions) are common, particularly in the atria, and result from turbulent blood flow within the chamber.

The heart valves prevent blood flowing back into the heart chambers after emptying.

During contraction of the ventricles (systole), blood is prevented from flowing back into the atria by two valves:
- the right atrioventricular (tricuspid) valve between the right atrium and right ventricle;
- the left atrioventricular (bicuspid or mitral) valve between the left atrium and left ventricle.

Similarly, to prevent blood flowing back into the two ventricles at the end of their contraction, there are valves between the ventricles and the large vessels into which they empty:
- the pulmonary valve between the right ventricle and its outflow vessel, the pulmonary artery;
- the aortic valve between the left ventricle and its outflow vessel, the aorta.

A central fibrocollagenous skeleton anchors the valves and chambers of the heart together.

The heart has a fibrocollagenous skeleton, the main component being the **central fibrous body**, located at the level of the cardiac valves.

Extensions of the central fibrous body surround heart valves to form the **valve rings** which support the base of each valve. The valve rings on the left side of the heart surround the mitral and aortic valves and are thicker than those on the right side, which surround the tricuspid and pulmonary valves.

A downward extension of the fibrocollagenous tissue of the aortic valve ring forms a fibrous septum between the right and left ventricles called the **membranous interventricular septum**. This is a minor component of the septum between the right and left ventricles, most of which is composed of cardiac muscle covered on both sides by endocardium. The membranous part is located high in the septal wall beneath the aortic valve.

Fig. 9.16 Endocardium.
(a) Micrograph of elastic Van Gieson (EVG)-stained right atrial endocardium (AE). The collagenous content stains red, elastic fibers stain black, myocardial muscle fibers (M) stain yellow. The nature of endocardial fibers is not apparent in a routine H&E-stained section. The atrial endocardium is much thicker than that which covers the ventricles.
(b) Micrograph of EVG-stained left ventricular endocardium (VE) at the same magnification. It is a much thinner layer than in the atrium and contains much less elastic tissue; the muscle fibers (M) are large.

The inner mesothelial cell layer is always poorly preserved in post-mortem material, as here.

The aortic and pulmonary valves have three cup-like cusps.

The outflow valves of the right and left ventricles, the pulmonary and aortic valves, are composed of three cup-like cusps that fit closely together when closed. Because of their shape they are sometimes called semilunar valves.

The base of each valve is attached to a fibrocollagenous valve ring. The junctions between the cusps and are called commissures (Fig. 9.17).

The mitral and tricuspid valves are attached to heart muscle by tendinous cords.

The atrioventricular valves are thin flaps attached to their respective valve ring at the base, and tethered on their undersurface (ventricular surface) by the chordae tendinae (Fig. 9.18). This prevents eversion of the valve leaflets into the atrium during ventricular contraction.

A heart valve is composed of fibroelastic tissue and is covered by endothelium.

The heart valves all have the same general structure with a dense fibrocollagenous central plate (the fibrosa), which is an extension of the fibrocollagenous tissue of the central fibrous body and fibrocollagenous valve ring. The fibrosa is covered on both surfaces by a layer of fibroelastic tissue, and is covered by outer layers of flat endothelial cells. The thickness of the layers varies between valves, and between sites within the same valve, and with age (Fig. 9.19).

There are minor modifications to this general structure in the atrioventricular valves. Much of the lower ventricular surface of the atrioventricular valves is roughened, the roughening marking the points of insertion of the chordae tendinae. The chordae are not inserted solely at the free edge of the leaflet; some attach farther back and a few small chordae insert near the base. The chordae fibers merge with the collagenous fibers of the central fibrosa of the valve leaflet. The atrioventricular valves may also have a thin layer of muscle fibers, continuous with those of the atrial wall, on their upper surface.

In addition to the general histologic structure of heart valves, the aortic valve shows prominent fibroelastic thickening at the sites of cusp apposition during valve closure. This is sometimes visible as white lines (linea alba) just below the free edge of the cusps, with a central nodule at the midpoint of each cusp (see Fig. 9.17). These are present but much less prominent on the pulmonary valve cusps because of the less forceful valve closure in the low-pressure pulmonary system.

Fig. 9.17 Aortic valve.
(a) Photograph showing the opened aortic valve between the left ventricle (LV) and its large emptying artery, the aorta (A). The three cusps (C) of the valve, the commissures (arrows), the origin of one of the coronary arteries (CA) and the pale fibrocollagenous valve ring (FR) are clearly seen.

(b) Photograph of the closed aortic valve viewed from above. Note how closely the three cusps (C) fit together. The pressure of blood against the closed valve ensures coronary artery blood flow during diastole.

Fig. 9.18 Mitral valve.

(a) Photograph showing the opened left side of the heart to demonstrate the mitral valve between the left atrium (LA) and the left ventricle (LV). It has two cusps (C), the free edges of which are tethered to the papillary muscles (P) by thin chordae tendinae (CT).

(b) Photograph of the closed mitral valve viewed from above. There are two cusps, one anterior (AC) and one posterior (PC).

Fig. 9.19 Histology of heart valves.

(a) High magnification micrograph of H&E-stained aortic valve. The bulk of the valve leaflet is composed of loose fibrocollagenous tissue with non-staining glycosaminoglycans between the collagen fibers. There is a dense area of elastic tissue (El) on the superior surface. The flat endocardial cells (En) can be seen clearly on both surfaces of the valve.

(b) High magnification micrograph of elastic Van Gieson (EVG)-stained aortic valve. The dense elastic tissue (El) stains black and the collagen (C) stains red.

(c) Micrograph of EVG-stained mitral valve close to its origin at the left atrioventricular valve ring. The leaflet is composed of red-staining collagen with some elastic fibers (black) running through it. The collagen is thickest, densest and most irregular on its inferior (ventricular) surface where the chordae tendinae (CT) are attached. The chordae have a structure similar to that of tendon (see Fig. 13.9).

DISORDERS OF HEART VALVES

There are three important abnormalities of the heart valves, all most commonly affecting the structure of the valves of the left side of the heart.

Rheumatic valve disease

Heart valves are damaged during the acute stage of a childhood illness called rheumatic fever. Healing of such damage results in progressive scarring of the valve leaflets and their elastic content is replaced by irregular masses of collagen scar. The valves therefore become more rigid. The leaflets may also partially fuse, which limits their ability to open (stenosis) or close (incompetence).

Calcific valve disease

Calcific valve disease mainly affects the aortic valve, particularly if it is congenitally abnormal with only two cusps (i.e. bicuspid). The valves become thickened and distorted by fibrous scarring and deposition of calcium nodules (Fig. 9.20). This renders the valve leaflets immobile and impairs blood flow from the left ventricle during systole, leading to heart failure.

Infective valvitis

Heart valves may become colonized by bacteria or fungi, most commonly when the valve has been damaged previously, for example by rheumatic disease. The damaged valve becomes covered in thrombus (blood clot) in which organisms proliferate. This causes signs of infection, the valve may become eroded and badly damaged, and fragments of thrombus may break off and enter the systemic circulation where is can block smaller systemic arteries.

Fig. 9.20 Calcific valve disease.
Micrograph showing a bicuspid aortic valve that has become thickened and distorted by fibrous scarring and calcium nodule (CN) deposition. Compare with normal valve, Figure 9.17b.

The conducting system of the heart is composed of modified muscle fibers.

The heart contracts involuntarily, at a rate of around 70 beats per minute. The rhythmic contractions of atria and ventricles do not depend on nerve stimulation, but result from impulses generated within the heart itself. This is fortunate since cardiac transplantation would otherwise be impossible as there are no nervous connections to the grafted organ. However, the autonomic nervous system can control the rate of heartbeat; stimulation of the parasympathetic (vagus) innervation slows the heart rate, while sympathetic stimulation increases it.

The conducting system of the heart is composed of muscle fibers which are modified to act as transducers rather than contractile cells. The impulse for contraction is initiated at a small body called the **sinoatrial (SA) node**, which acts as a pacemaker and stimulates atrial contraction. The impulse passes through the atrium and arrives at another node, the **atrioventricular (AV) node**. This node then initiates the later contraction of the ventricles, the impulse passing down specialized bundles of cardiac muscle (the main bundle, the right and left bundle branches, and the so-called Purkinje fibers) to the farthest reaches of the ventricular muscle (Fig. 9.21).

Firing of the sinoatrial node regulates the cardiac rate.

The SA node is located where the main vein from the upper part of the body (the superior vena cava) enters the right atrium (Fig. 9.22a & b). Its position is constant, but the curved linear structure is so small that it is not visible to the naked eye, being only 1–1.5 cm long and only 0.1–0.15 cm wide on the outer surface of the vena caval–atrial junction just beneath the pericardium.

The SA node is composed of an irregular meshwork of muscle fibers 3–4 µm in diameter. These are considerably smaller than normal atrial cardiac muscle fibers.

In contrast to normal cardiac muscle cells, SA muscle fibers do not have intercalated discs, but connect with each other by desmosomes. They contain few myofibrils and lack an organized striation pattern.

The cells of the SA node are embedded in a bulky fibro-collagenous support tissue containing numerous blood vessels, including a prominent central artery, the nodal artery. Numerous nerve fibers can be seen peripherally.

The impulse generated by the SA node passes quickly to the AV node, stimulating atrial contraction in the process.

The long-standing belief that the impulse travels to the AV node by diffuse radiation along all atrial muscle fibers is probably inaccurate, as specific bundles of atrial muscle (internodal atrial muscle), which preferentially conduct the impulse, have been identified. Three such specific bundles – the anterior, middle and posterior internodal tracts – have so far been described. These are histologically indistinguishable from other atrial fibers.

The atrioventricular node is composed of specialized muscle fibers.

The AV node is located beneath the endocardium of the medial wall of the right atrium, just in front of the opening of the coronary sinus and immediately above the tricuspid valve ring. It is thus situated at the base of the interatrial septum, at the junction between atria and ventricles, and between the central fibrous body and endocardium.

Histologically the AV node is composed of a network of small muscle fibers identical to those of the SA node, but less haphazardly arranged. As in the SA node, the fibers of the AV node are embedded in a fibrocollagenous stroma and have rich blood and nerve supplies.

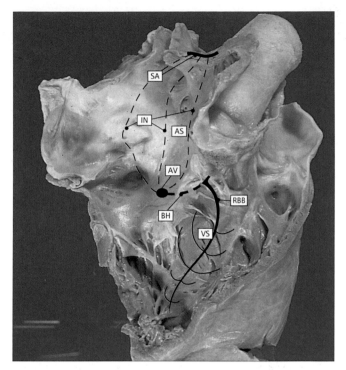

Fig. 9.21 Conducting system of the heart.
Photograph of opened right side of the heart trimmed to expose the septum between the two atria (AS) and the septum between the two ventricles (VS). The sinoatrial node (SA), internodal atrial muscle (IN), atrioventricular node (AV), bundle of His (BH) and right bundle branch (RBB), are indicated; the left bundle branch runs down on the left ventricular side of the interventricular septum.

Fig. 9.22 Sinoatrial node.
(a) Micrograph showing the sinoatrial (SA) node situated in the atrial wall close to the entrance of the superior vena cava (SVC). The node is highlighted in this pentachrome stain by the prominent blue-staining fibrocollagenous support tissue in which the cardiac pacemaker cells are embedded. Note the nodal artery (NA).
(b) Medium power micrograph showing the irregular whorled network of small nodal fibers (F) embedded in the bulky fibrocollagenous stroma (S). A small nodal artery (NA) is present.

The bundle of His, and the bundle branches arising from it, convey impulses to Purkinje fibers and the ventricles.

The small fibers at the anterior end of the AV node are more regularly arranged and eventually become a distinct bundle of parallel fibers that forms the main bundle conducting the impulse from the AV node to the ventricles. This conducting bundle, the **bundle of His**, penetrates the collagen of the central fibrous body, and then runs anteriorly for a short distance along the upper border of the muscle of the interventricular septum before dividing into right and left bundle branches.

The left bundle branch arises fan-like over a broad area as individual fibers, which leave the bundle of His; the remaining fibers form a distinct right bundle branch.

The left bundle branch fascicles run down beneath the endocardium of the left side of the interventricular septum

in two main groups, a posterior group and a smaller anterior group.

The right bundle branch runs down beneath the endocardium of the right side of the interventricular septum as a single bundle.

The right and left bundle branches connect with a complex network of specialized conduction fibers, the **Purkinje fibers**, which are large muscle fibers with vacuolated cytoplasm due to a high glycogen content, and scanty myofibrils. They lie in clusters of up to about six fibers (Fig. 9.23).

The heart has a rich vascular supply.

Because of its constant contractile activity the heart has enormous energy demands and therefore requires a substantial arterial supply. The left ventricle has the greatest oxygen demand and consequently the best arterial

Fig. 9.23 Purkinje fibers
(a) Micrograph showing the large pale-staining Purkinje fibers (P) lying just under the endocardium (E) lining the interventricular septum and separated from the myocardium (M) by a zone of loose fibrocollagenous tissue.

(b) The Purkinje fibers can be distinguished from normal cardiac muscle by a higher glycogen content as detected by a periodic acid-Schiff (PAS) stain and by high levels of the normal muscle protein αB-crystallin, as shown in this immunoperoxidase-stained preparation.

supply. Thus, any interruption in the cardiac arterial supply affects the structure and function of the left ventricle in particular (see Fig. 9.24).

The heart is supplied by two coronary arteries that arise as direct side branches of the aorta, just above two of the cusps of the aortic valve (see Fig. 9.17a). These are the left and right coronary arteries. Histologically the main coronary arteries are medium-sized muscular arteries (see Fig 9.5). They run in the epicardium and send branches into the myocardium, with a fine capillary bed running around the individual cardiac muscle cells. The least well-perfused part of the left ventricular muscle is the zone just below the endocardium.

Venous tributaries run with the major coronary arteries before draining into a large venous channel, the coronary sinus, which runs in the atrioventricular groove on the posterior aspect of the heart, before opening into the right atrium at the coronary sinus opening.

THE HEART

- has a central fibrous core and is made up of epicardial, myocardial and endocardial layers

- epicardium (pericardium) covers the outer surface of the heart, contains the main coronary artery branches and is covered externally by smooth mesothelium

- myocardium is the contractile component of the heart and is composed of cardiac muscle cells which are striated and linked by intercalated disks

- the endocardium lines the internal surface of heart chambers and is covered by flat endothelial cells which lie on a layer of fibroelastic tissue

- the conduction system is composed of muscle fibers modified for impulse conduction rather than contraction

- valves have a central fibrous core covered by fibroelastic tissue with endothelium on their surfaces

- atrial muscle cells secrete atrial natriuretic hormone

- the heart has a rich blood supply from two main coronary arteris (left and right) which arise as direct branches of the aorta just above the aortic valve ring

CORONARY ARTERY DISEASE

The most common and important disease of the heart is narrowing of the coronary arteries by atheroma. This impairs the function of the left ventricle because it reduces the blood flow and therefore oxygen supply to cardiac muscle. The coronary arteries are particularly prone to this common disease, with two main consequences.

ANGINA Slowly progressive reduction of coronary artery lumen by atheroma impairs oxygenation of the left ventricular muscle, leading to a characteristic pattern of chest pain (angina), which is usually brought on by exertion (i.e. when the left ventricular muscle is working harder).

MYOCARDIAL INFARCTION Complete obstruction of one of the coronary arteries or its branches (see Fig. 9.6) results in one area of the heart muscle being deprived of blood and therefore oxygen. Such affected heart muscle fibers die and are not replaced. This process is called myocardial infarction (see Fig. 9.24), colloquially known as a heart attack.

Fig. 9.24 Myocardial infarction.
Photograph showing a transverse slice across the left (L) and right (R) ventricles. The left ventricular myocardium is increased in thickness as a result of persistent high blood pressure (hypertension). Part of the left ventricular wall and septum shows reddish-black discoloration (arrow) due to infarction (i.e. death of tissue following sudden deprivation of oxygenated blood supply) resulting from occlusion of a coronary artery. Blood has seeped into the dead myocardium and rupture of the heart is imminent.

Fig. 9.25 Histology of the heart.

(a) Low power micrograph showing part of the wall of the left atrium (LAW) and left ventricle (LVW). Part of the mitral valve (MV), papillary muscles (PM) and chordae tendinae (CT) are also shown. Note that the left atrial wall has a relatively thick endocardium (E), whereas the thin endocardium of the left ventricle cannot be discerned at this magnification. Thick (Tk), thin (Tn) and medium (M) pericardium can all be seen on the outer surface of the heart.

(b) Medium power view of medium thickness pericardium from the area labelled M in (a). The outer layer (OL) is mesothelial-covered collagenous and elastic tissue, beneath which is a narrow adipose tissue layer (A) containing blood vessels (V).

Fig. 9.26 Small and large arteries.

(a) This photomicrograph shows a small muscular artery (A) cut in transverse section, together with some distended thin-walled small veins (V). With the H&E stain, the elastic lamina can be difficult to see; it is more clearly seen in a special stain for elastic tissue (see Fig. 9.5b and c).

(b) Micrograph showing the H&E appearance of a typical large elastic artery in the systemic circulation, in this case the aorta, at high magnification. The media is composed of alternate layers of relatively indistinct smooth muscle fibers and laminae of intensely eosinophilic, slightly refractile, elastic tissue.

Fig. 9.27 Small blood and lymphatic vessels.
ⓐ Micrograph of small vessels in adipose tissue, showing capillaries (C). One capillary is opening into a postcapillary venule (PCV), into which a direct metarteriole (M) is also opening.
ⓑ Micrograph of a large lymphatic vessel containing pink-staining lymph. Note that the muscle in the media merges into an indistinct adventitial layer. The nuclei of some of the endothelial cells are just visible.

Fig. 9.28 Anatomy of the heart.
ⓐ Photograph of opened right side of the heart. In the right atrium (RA), note the opening of the superior vena cava (SVC), the inferior vena cava (IVC), the coronary sinus (CS) and the thin atrial wall (AW). The arrow marks the site of the sinoatrial node.

In the right ventricle (RV), note the flaps of the right atrioventricular (tricuspid) valve (TV) separating the ventricle from the atrium, the pulmonary outflow tract (PT) with the pulmonary valve (PV) between it and the pulmonary artery trunk (PA).
ⓑ Photograph of opened left side of the heart. Blood enters the left atrium (LA) through the pulmonary veins (PV), and leaves through the left atrioventricular (mitral, bicuspid) valve (MV) into the left ventricle (LV).

In the left ventricle, note the thick muscular wall (VW), the papillary muscles (PM) and the chordae tendinae (CT), which link them to the leaflets of the mitral valve. Blood leaves the left ventricle through the aortic outflow tract and the aortic valve (AV) and enters the aorta (A).

1. IN THE HEART

(a) the main coronary arteries run in the epicardium
(b) myocardial cells have central nuclei and are striated
(c) the endocardium contains elastic tissue
(d) the valves are composed of dense collagenous tissue and lack an endocardial covering
(e) the percardial sac is lined by mesothelial cells

2. IN THE ARTERIAL SYSTEM

(a) large elastic arteries do not contain smooth muscle in their media
(b) muscular arteries have both an internal and external elastic lamina
(c) muscular arteries do not have an intimal layer
(d) the tone of smooth muscle is regulated by factors secreted by the endothelium as well as innervation by the autonomic nervous system
(e) vasa vasorum supply blood to the walls of large arteries

3. IN THE CARDIAC CONDUCTING SYSTEM

(a) cardiac contractions originate in the sinoatrial node
(b) internodal atrial muscle carries signals directly to the left and right bundle branches
(c) Purkinje fibers are indistinguishable from adjacent myocardial cells
(d) the atrioventricular node gives rise directly to the bundle of His
(e) the atrioventricular node is the only part of the conducting system composed of neuronal tissue

4. IN THE LYMPHATIC CIRCULATORY SYSTEM

(a) lymphatic capillaries take fluid from the extracellular space
(b) the term chyle is used to describe lipid-containing lymph draining from the intestines
(c) large lymphatic vessels have smooth muscle in their walls
(d) valves assist the flow of lymph
(e) lymph which goes to the lymph nodes returns to the venous system via a main lymphatic such as the thoracic duct

10. Respiratory System

INTRODUCTION

The respiratory system transfers oxygen from the air into the blood, and carbon dioxide from the blood into the air.

Blood oxygen is used for cellular respiratory processes which generate carbon dioxide as a by-product. The gaseous exchange occurs in the distal part of the respiratory tract where air-containing cavities (alveolar sacs) are in intimate contact with thin-walled blood vessels. The proximal part of the respiratory tract (upper respiratory tract) forms a series of transport passages by which air passes between the atmosphere and the gas exchange areas of the alveolar sacs (Fig. 10.1). On its way to the alveolar air sacs, the air is cleaned (by removal of particulate matter) and moistened, and its temperature is approximately equated to that in the farthest reaches of the lung.

In addition, the proximal part of the respiratory tract has specialized structures involved in the perception of smell and flavor (olfactory mucosa) and the production of sound (larynx).

UPPER RESPIRATORY TRACT

Ciliated, mucin-secreting epithelium lines the upper airways.

The architecture of the nasal cavity and paranasal sinuses provides a large surface area for warming and moistening inspired air, and for trapping particulate matter.

Air enters the respiratory system through the nostrils, which are openings to the exterior at the front of the nasal cavity.

The external aspect of the nostrils is covered by skin which extends for a short distance into the opening of the nostril (the vestibule), but then becomes a non-keratinizing squamous epithelium. Although occasional patches of stratified squamous epithelium persist, most of the nasal and paranasal sinus cavities are lined by a pseudostratified columnar epithelium, many of the columnar cells bearing numerous cilia. Scattered among these columnar cells are mucus-secreting (goblet) cells with microvilli on their luminal surface. This pattern, with minor variations, is seen throughout most of the air-conducting part of the respiratory tract, and is known as **respiratory-type epithelium** (Fig. 10.2).

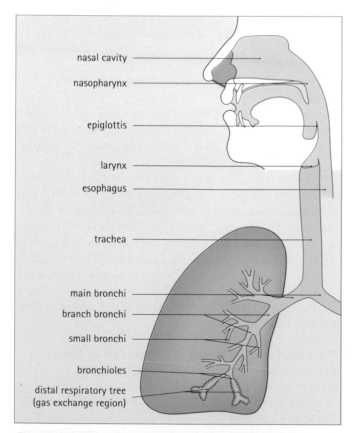

nasal cavity
nasopharynx
epiglottis
larynx
esophagus
trachea
main bronchi
branch bronchi
small bronchi
bronchioles
distal respiratory tree (gas exchange region)

Fig. 10.1 Upper respiratory tract transport passages.
Diagram to show the part of the respiratory tract that transports air from the atmosphere to the distal respiratory tract where gaseous exchange takes place.

G

Fig. 10.2 Nasal epithelium.
Micrograph showing the characteristic ciliated columnar epithelium lining the nasal cavity. There are occasional scattered mucus-secreting goblet cells (G).

The nasal and sinus submucosa is highly vascular and contains both mucous and serous glands.

Beneath the nasal epithelium, the lamina contains many glands (Fig. 10.3) equipped with basal myoepithelial cells (see page 75). Three main types of gland can be distinguished. Most are mucous glands, which secrete mucus to supplement that produced by the goblet cells in the lining epithelium. Some are serous cells containing basophilic granules (similar to those seen in the salivary glands, see page 76), which probably produce small amounts of amylase. Lastly, there are serous cells containing eosinophilic granules (similar to those seen in the lacrimal glands), which produce lysozyme.

Inspired air is moistened by the secretions of the serous components of the glands, while a sheet of mucus secreted by the goblet cells lies on the mucosal surface and traps any inhaled particulate contaminants. The mucus is then wafted backward by cilia toward the pharynx, where it is swallowed or expectorated.

The lamina propria also contains variable numbers of immune cells (see Chapter 8), which are mainly lymphocytes, plasma cells and macrophages, together with a few neutrophils and eosinophils. Eosinophils are particularly numerous in people who suffer from allergic rhinitis (hay fever).

A characteristic feature of the lamina propria is the presence of many blood vessels which form an interconnecting network, the vessels being surrounded by a supporting stroma in which smooth muscle is prominent. This highly vascular submucosa makes a major contribution to the warming of inhaled air.

The paranasal sinuses are cavernous spaces in the maxillary, ethmoid, sphenoid and frontal bones of the face.

Known as the **maxillary**, **ethmoid**, **sphenoid** and **frontal** sinuses respectively, each sinus communicates with the

Fig. 10.3 Nasal lamina propria.
Micrograph showing subepithelial tissue of the nose. Numerous seromucous glands (G) discharge their secretions onto the epithelial surface through wide ducts (D) .

main nasal cavity through a series of orifices (Fig. 10.4a), and is lined by epithelium similar to that of the main nasal cavity. In addition to providing an increased surface area for the moistening and warming of inhaled air, the sinus cavities play a role in the nature of the sounds produced in speech and song.

The nasopharynx is a posterior continuation of the nasal cavities and becomes the oropharynx at the level of the soft palate.

The nasopharynx is lined by columnar epithelium (like that of the nasal cavities) and stratified squamous epithelium, which becomes more prevalent as the oropharynx is approached; there are also areas of an intermediate epithelium resembling urothelium (see Chapter 15).

The stratified squamous epithelium is normally non-keratinizing and increases in amount with increasing age; keratinizing squamous epithelium is always abnormal and indicates disease. Beneath the nasopharyngeal epithelium, abundant mucosa-associated lymphoid tissue (MALT) forms Waldeyer's ring. The most important component of this is the nasopharyngeal tonsil (**adenoids**), which is sited where the posterior wall of the nasopharynx joins its roof. MALT samples inhaled antigenic material and prepares defense mechanisms against it (see Chapter 8). The Eustachian tubes from the middle ear open into the lateral walls of the nasopharynx (Fig. 10.4b).

Olfactory mucosa is located in the roof of the nasal cavity.

The olfactory mucosa, which senses smell and the more sophisticated aspects of taste, is located in the roof of the nasal cavity, and extends a short way down the septum and lateral wall (Fig. 10.4a).

Olfactory mucosa has a pseudostratified columnar epithelium composed of olfactory receptor cells, supporting (sustentacular) cells and basal cells. The disposition of these cells results in the pseudostratified appearance since the nuclei of each type occupy different levels (Fig. 10.5a & b). Beneath the olfactory epithelium are small serous glands (of Bowman) with short ducts which penetrate the olfactory epithelium. Their secretion may act as the solvent in which odorous substances dissolve.

The olfactory epithelium is composed of basal, sustentacular and olfactory receptor cells.

BASAL CELLS. The nuclei closest to the basement membrane of olfactory epithelium belong to the small basal cells. These cells are not in contact with the lumen and form the stem cells from which new olfactory cells can develop. Olfactory cells normally survive for about one month and regenerate after damage, the only neurons to do so.

SUSTENTACULAR CELLS. The nuclei closest to the lumen in olfactory epithelium belong to tall sustentacular cells, which have a narrow base in contact with the basement membrane, expanding to more bulky cytoplasm near the lumen. The oval nuclei of sustentacular cells lie close to the lumen, while the perinuclear cytoplasm contains a moderate amount of rough endoplasmic reticulum and numerous mitochondria, implying a synthetic function. There are small cytoplasmic accumulations of yellow-brown pigment and numerous microvilli on the luminal surface.

OLFACTORY RECEPTOR CELLS. The olfactory receptor cells are bipolar neurons insinuated between the sustentacular and basal cells. They have a central bulge containing the nucleus; from this area extend two cytoplasmic processes, the dendritic and proximal processes. The **dendritic process** extends to the surface of the epithelium where its tip is expanded into a club-shaped prominence, the **olfactory vesicle**. This bears cilia, some of which protrude into the nasal cavity, while other lateral cilia insinuate between the microvilli of the sustentacular cells. The cilia have the typical 9 + 2 arrangement (see Fig. 3.17) for some of their length, but there is a long distal portion which contains only the two central fibers. The cilia are inserted into basal bodies in the olfactory vesicle.The **proximal process** is very narrow and passes down

between the basal cells and basal portions of the sustentacular cells to penetrate the basement membrane. It then joins other non-myelinated processes to form the so-called **fila olfactoria**, which ultimately form synaptic connections in the **olfactory bulb** (the first cranial nerve, Fig. 10.5c). The proximal processes are therefore regarded as axons.

NASAL CAVITY AND SINUSES

- nose and sinuses are lined by pseudostratified, ciliated columnar epithelium with goblet cells
- main function is to filter, warm and moisten inhaled air
- sinus cavities and turbinate bones provide a large surface area
- mucosa-associated lymphoid tissue (MALT) is present in the nasopharyngeal tonsil (adenoid)
- nasopharynx communicates with the middle ear cavity through the auditory (Eustachian) tube
- roof of nasal cavity is the site of olfactory mucosa which includes bipolar olfactory neurons

Fig. 10.4 Nasal cavity and paranasal sinuses.
(a) Coronal section showing the relationship between the nasal cavity and ethmoid and maxillary sinuses. The frontal (anterior) and sphenoid (posterior) sinuses are not shown in this plane of section. The surface area of the respiratory mucosa is increased by long curved turbinate bones arising from the lateral walls of the nasal cavity, and by the paranasal sinus system. Note the olfactory epithelium and its proximity to the olfactory nerves and bulbs.
(b) Sagittal section showing the relationship between the nasal cavity, the anterior nares (nostrils), vestibule, nasopharynx and frontal and sphenoid sinuses. The opening of the frontal sinus is not shown in this plane of section. Note the openings beneath the two upper turbinates of the ethmoid and maxillary sinuses, and the opening in the nasopharyngeal fold of the Eustachian tube from the middle ear.

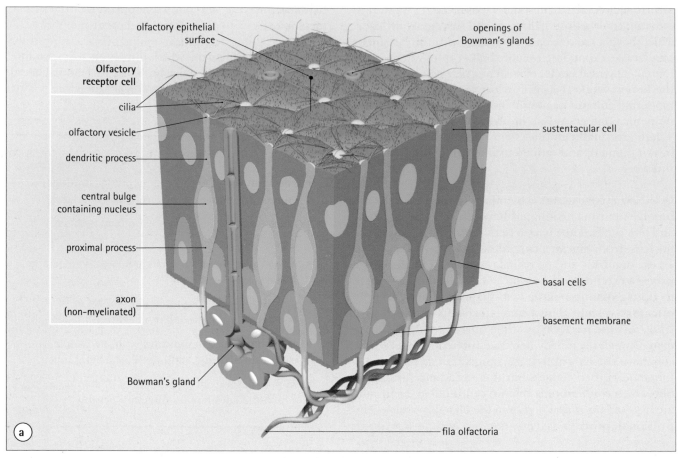

olfactory epithelial
surface

openings of
Bowman's glands

**Olfactory
receptor cell**

cilia

olfactory vesicle

dendritic process

central bulge
containing nucleus

proximal process

axon
(non-myelinated)

Bowman's gland

sustentacular cell

basal cells

basement membrane

fila olfactoria

a

b

c

Fig. 10.5 Olfactory mucosa.
(a) A three-dimensional drawing showing the components of the olfactory mucosa, Bowman's glands, and the nerves leaving the base of the olfactory epithelial cells on their way to the main olfactory nerve.
(b) Micrograph of a 0.5 μm acrylic resin section of human olfactory mucosa from an 18-week-old fetus before the associated bone plates have fully calcified. The nuclei of the basal (B), olfactory (O) and sustentacular (S) cells can be identified. The olfactory vesicles (V) on the luminal surface are just discernible. Compare with (a).
(c) Micrograph showing the nerve twigs (N) from the olfactory receptor cells (OC) fusing before passing upwards through the cribriform plate of the skull to join the olfactory nerve (ON), first cranial nerve, demonstrated using immunocytochemical method for neurofilament protein.

On its way to the trachea, air from the nasopharynx passes through the laryngeal region.

The laryngeal region has a complex architecture in order to:

- prevent inspired air entering the esophagus;
- prevent ingested food and fluid entering the trachea;
- permit the production of sound.

Laryngeal architecture is maintained by a series of cartilaginous plates (mainly the thyroid, cricoid and arytenoid cartilages). These are joined together by densely collagenous ligaments, and are mobilized by the action of small bands and sheets of striated muscle called the **intrinsic muscles of the larynx**.

The cartilages maintain the openness and shape of the airway, and move to prevent food inhalation during swallowing, which is also partly the responsibility of the epiglottis.

The epiglottis consists of a central sheet of elastic cartilage, covered by mucosa on both sides.

Movement of the epiglottis prevents ingested food and liquids passing into the trachea by covering the tracheal entrance during swallowing.

The anterior (lingual) surface is covered by stratified squamous epithelium continuous with that of the dorsal surface of the posterior part of the tongue.

The posterior surface, which faces the pharynx and larynx, is covered in its upper half by stratified squamous epithelium, and in its lower half by ciliated pseudostratified columnar epithelium. The lower half contains many seromucous glands, which penetrate deeply into the central elastic cartilage plate (Fig. 10.6.)

Fig. 10.6 Epiglottis.
Micrograph of epiglottis showing its central cartilaginous plate (CP) and seromucous glands (G), some of which split the cartilage, and the two types of epithelium (E) on its two faces.

The false and true vocal cords are folds of mucosa.

Below the epiglottis, the laryngeal mucosa is everted into the laryngeal lumen to form two pairs of folds, an upper pair of false vocal cords and a lower pair of true vocal cords.

Between these cords, an outpouching of laryngeal mucosa forms the **ventricle** (Fig. 10.7) and its upward extension, the **saccule**, on each side.

The areas where the ends of the true cords are attached to the anterior and posterior walls of the larynx are called the **anterior** and **posterior commissures**, respectively.

The **false cords** are covered by ciliated columnar epithelium (Fig. 10.7c), but islands of non-keratinizing stratified squamous epithelium are common in adults, becoming more extensive with increasing age.

Beneath the epithelium a loose fibrocollagenous supporting stroma contains numerous seromucinous glands and fibers of skeletal muscle from the thyroarytenoid muscle. Small islands of elastic cartilage and adipose tissue may also be found in adults, adipose tissue being most commonly seen in the elderly.

The **true cords** are covered by stratified squamous epithelium, which shows a rete ridge formation (see Chapter 18) on its free edge and inferior surface, although its upper surface is flat. The epithelium contains occasional melanocytes, but no significant melanin is formed. The immediate subepithelial support tissue (**Reinke's space**) contains loose fibrocollagenous tissue, which is virtually devoid of lymphatic vessels. This is an important factor in limiting or delaying the spread of cancers arising in the true vocal cords.

Beneath Reinke's space are the fibroelastic fibers of the vocal ligament, to which the skeletal muscle fibers of the vocalis part of the thyroarytenoid muscle are attached (Fig. 10.7c). There may be islands of elastic cartilage in the vocal ligament.

The **saccule and ventricle** are covered largely by respiratory-type ciliated columnar epithelium, and contain seromucous glands in their subepithelial tissue (Fig. 10.7d). In children, lymphoid aggregates are common, some with germinal centers.

The anterior and posterior commissures are covered with ciliated columnar epithelium, and their subepithelial zone consists of dense fibrocollagenous tissue containing seromucous glands. Lymphatics and blood vessels are common in both regions and are an important factor in the further spread of cancers of the vocal cords that invade locally to the commissures.

Fig. 10.7 Laryngeal region.

(a) Photograph of the laryngeal region opened in the midline posteriorly to show the epiglottis (E), the false cords (F), the true cords (T) and the openings of the ventricles (V) between them. This view also shows the anterior commissure (A).

(b) Photograph showing the vocal cords as seen from above when examined clinically with a laryngoscope. Note the epiglottis (E), false cords (F), true cords (T), the opening of the ventricles (V) and the anterior commissure (A) where the true vocal cords meet in the midline anteriorly.

(c) Low magnification micrograph showing the histology of the false (F) and true (T) cords. The false cord (F) is covered by ciliated columnar epithelium and contains seromucous glands. The true cord is covered by non-keratinizing stratified squamous epithelium and contains Reinke's space (R), fibres of the vocal ligament (VL) and the skeletal muscle fibres of the vocalis muscle (VM). (Inset) Micrograph showing the histology of the true and false cords at a higher magnification.

(d) Micrograph of the saccule, which is lined by ciliated columnar epithelium (CCE) and is rich in seromucous glands (G).

The trachea is lined with respiratory mucosa and is braced with cartilage.

Below the larynx, the airway continues as the trachea which runs down into the thoracic cavity, where it divides into two main bronchi, one to each lung.

The trachea is a tubular structure about 10 cm long and 2–3 cm in diameter which is rendered rigid and non-collapsible by a number – usually 15–20 – of incomplete circular rings of cartilage which occupy 70–80% of its circumference. Only a narrow strip of the posterior tracheal wall is deficient in cartilage; here the gap between the ends of each cartilage ring is bridged by a dense fibro-collagenous ligament rich in elastic fibers and bundles of smooth muscle (**trachealis** muscle) which permit some constriction of the tracheal lumen. The ligament linking the two cartilage ends prevents dilation (Fig. 10.8a).

The internal lining is a pseudostratified ciliated columnar epithelium containing scattered goblet cells. Subepithelial seromucous glands are particularly numerous in the posterior band devoid of cartilage (Fig. 10.8b).

The trachea bifurcates into two main bronchi, which are the tubes with the largest bore in the bronchial tree.

The **main bronchi** are extrapulmonary and enter each lung with the pulmonary arteries at the lung hilum. They then divide into **lobar bronchi**, one of which supplies each of the two lobes of the left lung (**left upper lobe bronchus** and **lower lobe bronchus**) and three lobes of the right lung (**right upper lobe bronchus**, **middle lobe bronchus** and **lower lobe bronchus**).

Each of the five lobar bronchi divides into a variable number of **segmental bronchi** delivering air to one of the bronchopulmonary segments, where the bronchi divide for a further variable number of generations, eventually terminating in **bronchioles**.

Throughout their course the bronchi have a similar structure to that of the trachea (Fig. 10.9), but there are variations. The basic structure comprises:
- a pseudostratified columnar ciliated epithelium;
- subepithelial fibrocollagenous tissue containing variable quantities of seromucous glands;
- variable amounts of smooth muscle, with elastic fibers arranged in longitudinal bands;
- variable amounts of partial cartilaginous ring.

Several cell types make up the epithelial lining of the bronchial tree.

The bronchial tree is lined by a ciliated columnar epithelium, which is pseudostratified in the larger bronchi and becomes less complex in smaller peripheral branches. The epithelium contains ciliated columnar cells, basal

Fig. 10.8 Trachea.
ⓐ Micrograph showing a child's trachea with an incomplete cartilage hoop (C), the free ends of the cartilage being joined by a band of muscle (M). The submucosa (S) contains numerous seromucous glands, particularly where the cartilage is deficient.

ⓑ Micrograph showing tracheal mucosa with ciliated respiratory epithelium (E) on its surface and seromucous glands (G) in the submucosa (S). The inner part of the tracheal cartilage ring (C) can be seen at the base of the micrograph.

cells, intermediate cells, mucus-secreting goblet cells and neuroendocrine cells (Fig. 10.10).

CILIATED CELLS are columnar in most of the bronchial tree, but are shorter and almost cuboidal in the most peripheral branches. They have a basal nucleus, and lysosomes and numerous mitochondria in their supranuclear cytoplasm. The luminal surface of each cell bears about 200 cilia and some microvilli, each cilium being about 6 μm long.

BASAL CELLS lie on the basement membrane and are small cells that are not in contact with the lumen. They form a stem cell population from which the other cell types develop.

INTERMEDIATE CELLS are probably stem cells transforming into either a ciliated columnar cell or a mucus-secreting goblet cell.

GOBLET CELLS are scattered between the ciliated cells and are most numerous in the main and lobar bronchi, becoming less common in the smaller branches. Their number increases in some chronic respiratory diseases.

NEUROENDOCRINE CELLS are small round cells with dark-staining nuclei and clear cytoplasm, similar to those seen in the alimentary tract (see Fig. 11.41), and are located on the basement membrane. They are scattered throughout the tracheobronchial tree, but are most numerous in the smaller bronchi. Neuroendocrine cells possess cytoplasmic processes and contain characteristic neuroendocrine granules. They secrete hormones and active peptides, including bombesin and serotonin, and are most numerous in the fetal lung; they may be scattered in the basal layer of the surface epithelium or congregate in small clumps (Fig. 10.11b).

Smooth muscle is present in the wall of bronchi.

The submucosa of the bronchial tree contains smooth muscle, seromucous glands and fibrocollagenous stroma with elastic fibers arranged in longitudinal bands.

In the main bronchi, the **smooth muscle** is largely confined posteriorly (as in the trachea), being attached to the ends of the incomplete cartilage rings, but in the intrapulmonary bronchi, the muscle is submucosal and arranged in an irregular spiral with two components, one spiraling to the left, the other to the right. It persists in the airway walls down to the smallest branches (bronchioles, see below), long after the cartilage component has disappeared.

Hypertrophy of the smooth muscle is an important component of some lung diseases (see Clinical Section, page 171).

The **submucosal bronchial glands** are seromucous glands which empty into the lumen through short ducts. Other deeper glands with longer ducts are located between and beneath the cartilaginous plates. The serous component is thought to secrete lysozyme and glycoprotein.

Fig. 10.9 Bronchial wall.
Medium-power micrograph showing a segment of the bronchial wall. Note the pseudostratified ciliated columnar epithelium (Ep), longitudinally running bands of elastin (El), bands of smooth muscle (SM), seromucous glands (G) and an isolated island of cartilage (C).

Fig. 10.10 Bronchial epithelium.
High-power micrograph of a thin acrylic resin section of the bronchial epithelium showing the various cell types present. Most of the cells are tall columnar ciliated cells (C) but scattered between them are occasional intermediate cells (I). Goblet cells are not seen in this section, but basal (B) and neuroendocrine (NE) cells are present on the basement membrane. Longitudinal elastic fibres (E) of the bronchial wall, here cut in transverse section, can also be seen.

Myoepithelial cells (see page 75) lie between the secretory and duct lining cells and their basement membrane, and some neuroendocrine cells are also present. The bronchial wall contains mucosa-associated lymphoid tissue (MALT).

Lymphocytes and IgA-secreting plasma cells are closely associated with the bronchial glands, and lymphoid aggregations are common, being most evident at bifurcations. The larger lymphoid aggregates occur in the proximal part of the bronchial tree and may have germinal centers.

Bronchi of all sizes contain some cartilage.

The main extrapulmonary bronchi have regular incomplete cartilage rings like the trachea, but the intrapulmonary bronchi have an irregular, roughly circumferential arrangement of cartilage plates connected by dense fibrocollagenous bands.

As the bronchi branch and get smaller and more peripheral, the cartilage plates decrease in size and number, and are mainly concentrated at bifurcations.

The bronchioles are the smallest part of the conducting airways.

Bronchioles are distal airways located between the cartilage-walled bronchi and the site where the ciliated epithelium ceases.

The bronchioles branch repeatedly, and as they do so reduce their luminal size. With the absence of cartilage, smooth muscle becomes a major component of their wall.

Bronchioles are lined by ciliated columnar epithelium without pseudostratification, and the cells become lower and near cuboidal in the small peripheral branches. Occasional goblet cells persist, as do small numbers of neuroendocrine cells (sometimes clustered to form so-called **neuroepithelial bodies** – see Fig. 10.11b – but there are no seromucous glands, and an additional cell type, the **Clara cell**, is found.

The Clara cell is neither ciliated nor apparently mucus-producing, and is most numerous in the terminal bronchioles. It contains numerous mitochondria and abundant smooth endoplasmic reticulum near the luminal surface, which bulges above the level of adjacent ciliated cells; small electron-dense granules are also seen in the apical cytoplasm.

The final bifurcations of the bronchiolar tree produce **terminal bronchioles** which are the smallest bronchioles, concerned solely with air conduction.

Fig. 10.11 Bronchiole.
(a) Micrograph of an H&E stained section showing a bronchiole (B) close to a pulmonary artery (PA) branch. The wall is composed only of muscle (M), and its epithelium (E) is similar to bronchial epithelium.
(b) Micrograph showing part of a bronchiole wall from a newborn stained by an immunoperoxidase method for bombesin, showing a so-called neuroepithelial body.

Clara cells

Contain:

- many large mitochondria, abundant smooth ER and some secretory granules – suggesting synthetic and secretory functions

- specific antiproteases and oxidases

Proposed functions include:

- protection against deleterious effects of inhaled toxins and carcinogens – a possible oxidase function

- protection against emphysema (see Clinical Section, page 171) – a possible antiprotease function

- some role in surfactant production or elimination

- possible stem cell, capable of producing other types of bronchiolar epithelial cells

Some words of caution: There is marked species variation in numbers and structure of Clara cells. Most of the research work has been carried out using rodents, in which the cells are numerous and distinct.

DISTAL RESPIRATORY TRACT

Gaseous exchange occurs in the distal respiratory tract.

The terminal bronchiole leads into the distal respiratory tree, which is concerned with gaseous exchange.

The first elements of this system are the respiratory bronchioles which are lined by cuboidal ciliated epithelium. This merges with the flattened epithelium lining ill-defined conduits outlined by a spiral of smooth muscle (alveolar ducts). The walls of these ducts are composed largely of the openings of laterally disposed air sacs (alveoli). Each alveolar duct terminates in two or three alveolar sacs formed from the confluence of the openings of several alveoli (Fig. 10.12a).

Alveoli are air sacs which are the main site of gaseous exchange.

Alveoli number 150–400 million in each normal healthy lung, and provide an enormous surface area (estimated at 70–80 m^2) for gaseous exchange.

Each alveolus is a polygonal air space about 250 μm in diameter when normally inflated, with a thin wall which contains pulmonary capillaries and forms the air–blood barrier.

Most alveoli open into an alveolar sac, or into an alveolar duct, but a few open directly into a respiratory bronchiole. Pores (of Kohn), which are 1–12 μm in diameter, permit communication between adjacent alveoli.

The cellular components of the alveoli are Type 1 and Type 2 pneumocytes, which lie on the alveolar basement membrane, and alveolar macrophages (Fig. 10.12b).

Type 1 pneumocytes are very thin cells which allow gaseous diffusion.

Type 1 pneumocytes represent about 40% of the alveolar cell population but form 90% of the surface lining of the alveolar sacs and alveoli.

Type 1 pneumocytes are attenuated flat cells with greatly flattened nuclei, and are joined together by tight junctions (see page 36). They contain scanty mitochondria and organelles, and their cytoplasm provides a very thin covering to the alveolar basement membrane, its thinness contributing to the efficiency of the air–blood barrier.

Type 2 pneumocytes secrete surfactant.

Type 2 pneumocytes represent 60% of the alveolar cell population numerically, but occupy only 5–10% of the alveolar surface area.

Unlike the thin, flat Type 1 cells, Type 2 pneumocytes are rounded cells which are commonly located in obtuse angles in the polygonal alveolus (Fig. 10.13a). Their nuclei are round and dark-staining, and their cytoplasm is rich in mitochondria and both rough and smooth endoplasmic reticulum. They also contain electron-dense

Fig. 10.12 Distal respiratory tree.
(a) Diagram showing the relationships between the terminal bronchiole, respiratory bronchiole, alveolar ducts, alveolar sacs and alveoli. The brown bands are smooth muscle.
(b) Low-power scanning electronmicrograph of an alveolar sac looking into two of the alveoli (A) that open into it. The two alveoli are separated by a wall, which is covered by Type 1 pneumocyte cytoplasm (T1). On the left is a pore of Kohn (PK), and a round Type 2 pneumocyte (T2) can be seen in the right alveolus.

vesicles and large spherical bodies of variably lamellated material, which is composed of phospholipid, protein and glycosaminoglycans, and forms the basis of pulmonary surfactant. Note that there is considerable species variation in the ultrastructure of the spherical surfactant-producing bodies, the classically described parallel multi-lamellation being best seen in dog and rat. In man, the lamellation is concentrically spherical. The granular surfactant material is extruded from the lamellar bodies through their microvillous luminal surfaces (Fig. 10.13).

When the alveolar epithelium is exposed to certain toxic agents, particularly if there is extensive destruction of the sensitive Type 1 pneumocytes, Type 2 pneumocytes increase in size and number; it is believed that some type 2 cells act as precursor stem cells for Type 1 pneumocytes.

Surfactant and the Type 2 pneumocyte

The main function of Type 2 pneumocytes is the production of pulmonary surfactant:

- surfactant is a complex mixture of phospholipids (mainly dipalmitoyl phosphatidylcholine), carbohydrates (glycosaminoglycans) and proteins (including SP-A, SP-B, SP-C and SP-D)

- when released from the Type 2 pneumocyte, surfactant produces a monolayer lining the internal alveolar surface, with a lower aqueous phase and a superficial lipid phase

- surfactant acts like a detergent by reducing alveolar surface tension, preventing collapse of alveoli during expiration, and facilitating expansion during inspiration

- Type 2 pneumocytes and surfactant are first detectable at about 28 weeks gestation, after which time premature babies are theoretically capable of respiratory survival

- between 28 weeks and term, amounts of surfactant may be inadequate or too rapidly spent, and articifical respiratory assistance may be needed

- surfactant failure leads to alveolar collapse, with Type 1 pnemocyte damage and so-called "infantile respiratory distress syndrome"

Fig. 10.13 Type 2 pneumocyte and surfactant.
(a) An H&E-stained thin acrylic resin section showing the confluence of the alveolar walls of three adjacent alveoli. In the angles are rounded cells with vacuolated cytoplasm; these are Type 2 pneumocytes (T2). The nucleus of a Type 1 pneumocyte (T1) is also seen.
(b) Electronmicrograph showing an active Type 2 pneumocyte. The cell is round and has a convex luminal face which is covered with microvilli. The most obvious intracytoplasmic organelles are large membrane-bound spherical bodies (B) containing lamellated lipoprotein material, which represents the surfactant substance. These can often be seen discharging their contents onto the luminal surface (arrows).
(c) Scanning electronmicrograph of two Type 2 pneumocytes, Note the microvilli (M), and small amounts of granular material (arrow) which is recently disgorged surfactant.

Alveolar macrophages phagocytose inhaled bacteria and particulate matter.

Normally alveolar macrophages lie on top of the alveolar lining cells and are also seen apparently free in the alveolar space, often containing phagocytosed material, particularly inhaled carbon particles.

Alveolar macrophages patrol the alveolar air spaces and the interalveolar septa (interstitium, Fig. 10.14), passing freely between the two. They phagocytose inhaled debris (e.g. fine dust, including carbon), and are an important defense mechanism against inhaled bacteria. They also remove superfluous surfactant, and secrete a large number of agents, including enzymes such as lysozyme, collagenases, elastases and acid hydrolases.

After phagocytosis, macrophages may enter the respiratory and terminal bronchioles, where they either pass into lymphatic vessels and hence become transported to regional lymph nodes, or they adhere to the ciliated

red cell

Type I pneumocyte

alveolar macrophage moving through alveolar pore of Kohn

interalveolar septum containing elastic and collagen fibers

fused basement membranes of capillary and Type 1 pneumocyte at areas of contact

alveolar capillaries

(a)

(b)

M

Tn

Tk

C

RBC

F

Fig. 10.14 Interalveolar septum and air–blood barrier.
ⓐ Diagram of the interalveolar septum showing the pulmonary capillaries coursing through the alveolar wall, sometimes in close contact with one wall, then the other.
ⓑ Transmission electronmicrograph through the alveolar wall. It is largely occupied by a capillary (C) containing a red blood cell (RBC) and a monocyte (M). The monocyte will leave the capillary and ultimately enter the alveolar lumen to become an alveolar macrophage. Note the thin (Tn) and the thick (Tk) parts of the alveolar wall.
Both sides of the alveolar wall are covered by a thin layer of Type 1 pneumocyte cytoplasm. In the thick part, between Type 1 pneumocyte cytoplasm and the capillary wall, there are collagen and elastic fibers (F).

mucus-coated epithelium, which is the first step on the mucus/cilia escalator. This eventually carries them up to the trachea and main bronchi, from which they are cleared in the mucus by coughing. Alternatively the macrophages may remain in the interstitium.

Elastic tissue is an important functional component of the alveolar wall.

Elastin has remarkable properties of stretch and recoil (see page 53) and has three important functions in the alveolar walls. Firstly, it allows the lungs to stretch to accommodate the inhaled air. Then, having thus stored energy, it allows air to be expelled from the alveoli by recoiling. Finally, it acts as a spring, tethering the soft-walled bronchioles, which contain no cartilage, to the lung parenchyma, and indirectly to the pleura, thus preventing bronchiolar and alveolar collapse during exhalation.

Gaseous exchange occurs across the air–blood barrier in the alveoli.

Oxygen diffuses from the alveolar cavity into the blood in the alveolar capillaries to become linked to red cell hemoglobin, and carbon dioxide diffuses from blood into the alveolar air. Each capillary is closely apposed to two alveolar cavities, and is therefore located in the interalveolar septum or interstitium. Where the capillary contacts the alveolar wall its basement membrane appears to fuse with that of the alveolar wall.

Parts of the interalveolar septum not occupied by the capillary contain fine collagen and elastic fibers together with some fibroblasts and macrophages.

Thus, in some places the capillary is in direct contact with the alveolar wall (thin part) but in others is separated from it by cells and fibers (thick part). The thin part is the site of gas exchange and thick part is where liquids can move between the air spaces and the interstitium. Macrophages move freely from alveolus to alveolus through the pores of Kohn. Both sides of the interalveolar septum are covered by a thin layer of Type 1 pneumocyte cytoplasm (Fig. 10.14).

INTERSTITIAL FIBROSIS

In some lung diseases, the fibroblasts in the interalveolar septa increase in number and secrete excess collagen and elastin. This results in fibrocollagenous thickening of the septa (interstitial fibrosis).

Interstitial fibrosis increases the rigidity of the lung and limits expansion, but most importantly impairs gaseous exchange because the presence of collagen fibers between the capillary and alveolar walls ruins their intimate contact.

CHRONIC OBSTRUCTIVE AIRWAYS DISEASE

The most common lung disease in the Western world is chronic obstructive airways disease, which is characterized by difficulty in getting air into and out of the distal respiratory tree.

There are three main disease processes causing chronic obstructive airways disease: asthma, chronic bronchitis and emphysema. These conditions may be present alone or in combination.

Asthma

Asthma is caused by a combination of bronchoconstriction and excessive production of particularly viscid mucus, both of which obstruct the airways.

Chronic bronchitis

In chronic bronchitis, the bronchial walls are thickened by a combination of muscle layer thickening, and increase in number and size of the mucous glands. This correlates with excessive mucus which is expectorated in this condition.

Emphysema

Emphysema is characterized by destruction of the walls of the alveolar ducts, sacs and alveoli with permanent dilatation of air spaces (Fig. 10.15). This leads to the loss of the elastic support for the bronchioles and results in their collapse, particularly during exhalation, and air trapping, as air is unable to pass the obstructed lumen.

Fig. 10.15 Emphysema.
Micrograph of lung from patient with severe emphysema, showing extensive destruction of the alveolar walls.

PULMONARY VASCULATURE

The lungs have a dual blood supply and venous drainage.

Blood to the lungs is provided by the pulmonary and bronchial arteries and veins.

The more important of the two systems physiologically is the pulmonary vascular system, since it is the capillary component of this system which is the site of gaseous exchange. The bronchial system provides oxygenated blood to the larger components of the bronchial tree (see page 165).

The pulmonary arteries supply the lung with relatively deoxygenated blood from the right side of the heart. Such blood has supplied the body's tissues with oxygen and collected carbon dioxide (see Fig. 9.1).

The pulmonary arteries enter each of the lungs at the hilum and closely follow the course of the adjacent bronchus and its branches, dividing more or less with the bronchi. The vessels culminate in the extensive intimate **pulmonary capillary** network in the interalveolar septa (see Fig. 10.14). The capillary network empties its reoxygenated blood into **pulmonary venules and veins**, which eventually convey the blood to the left side of the heart for distribution to other organs.

As the pulmonary arterial and venous system is a low-pressure system (i.e. pulmonary artery systolic pressure is 25 mm Hg, whereas systemic arterial systolic pressure is 110–135 mm Hg), the structure of its vessels differs considerably from those of the systemic circulation (see Chapter 9).

The proximal pulmonary artery branches are elastic arteries.

From their origin at the pulmonary valve ring to the intrapulmonary branches at the level where the bronchi lose their cartilage plates to become bronchioles, the pulmonary arteries are elastic arteries.

There are three main components (Fig. 10.16):

- a narrow intima composed of a single layer of endothelium lying on a narrow layer of scanty collagen fibers and myofibroblasts;
- a media composed of many layers of elastic fibers, which are irregular and fragmented in the pulmonary trunk and main pulmonary arteries, but more regular and intact in the peripheral branches. Between the elastic fibers are smooth muscle cells and some collagen;
- elastic laminae composed of longitudinally running fibers that form flat, interlinked strands of varying breadth. This particular orientation is probably an adaptation to counteract the stretching forces during lung expansion. In the aorta, which is exposed to circumferential stretch during systole, the elastic fibers are circumferential.

The distal pulmonary arteries are muscular arteries.

At about the bronchial/bronchiolar junction, the medial elastic laminae largely disappear and the arteries become muscular arteries.

These arteries continue to follow the bronchioles as far as the terminal and respiratory bronchioles, but also give off supernumerary arteries as side branches.

The media of the muscular pulmonary artery is composed largely of circularly orientated smooth muscle (Fig. 10.17a) and occasional collagen and elastic fibers. The organized laminated elastic tissue is confined to distinct internal elastic laminae (see Chapter 9)

Continuous branching of the muscular pulmonary arteries produces progressively smaller vessels with narrower bores and thinner walls, because of diminishing smooth muscle in the media (Fig. 10.17b). The muscle

Fig. 10.16 Elastic pulmonary artery.
Micrograph of an elastic pulmonary artery from a child. Note the endothelium (E), the scanty myofibroblasts (M) in the narrow intima (I), the thick media composed of fairly regularly organized alternating lamellae of elastic fibres (El) and intervening smooth muscle cells (SM) and collagen (C). The elastic is easily seen in this H&E section because the lamellae are so thick.

layer becomes discontinuous and finally disappears, the vessel then being called a pulmonary arteriole (Fig. 10.17c).

Arterioles are difficult to distinguish from venules. The alveolar capillaries are discussed in Fig. 10.14.

Pulmonary veins drain into the left atrium.

Oxygenated blood from the alveolar capillaries enters small venules, then large venules, small veins, large veins, and finally the main pulmonary veins which empty into the left atrium.

The small venules are composed of a thin intima lying on a narrow zone of collagen and elastic fibers. These small tributaries fuse to form larger venules, which run in the fibrocollagenous septa and are associated with increasing numbers of myofibroblasts and smooth muscle cells in the media (Fig. 10.18).

Larger veins have a distinct media with a variably continuous internal elastic lamina and irregularly arranged smooth muscle fibers.

The largest pulmonary veins have a media in which elastic fibers are irregularly interspersed with collagen and smooth muscle fibers, rather than confined to clearly defined elastic laminae.

Pulmonary vasculature varies considerably at the extremes of age.

Before birth the pulmonary vasculature is barely perfused because of the bypass through the patent foramen ovale and ductus arteriosus. Thus, the muscular pulmonary arteries have a small lumen, large endothelial cells and a thick media. In addition there are small bundles of longitudinally running smooth muscle fibers in the intima.

Fig. 10.17 Muscular pulmonary artery.
(a) Micrograph of muscular pulmonary artery stained with H&E. Note the media (M) and adventitia (A).
(b) Micrograph of a smaller muscular pulmonary artery stained by the elastic Van Gieson method to show the media (M) lying between two distinct dark-staining elastic laminae (EL). In addition to giving off a lateral supernumerary branch (S), this artery is bifurcating into two vessels with less well-formed arterial walls.
(c) Micrograph showing a small pulmonary arteriole. This is a thin-walled vessel resembling a small pulmonary artery from which the muscular media between the two elastic laminae has disappeared. Transitional vessels with only an occasional remnant of the spirally arranged muscular media can sometimes be identified.

These features change progressively to the adult pattern in the first few weeks of life, and new supernumerary arteries develop.

In old age, the veins and muscular pulmonary arteries thicken as a result of irregular fibrocollagenous thickening of the intima.

The bronchial arteries are direct lateral branches of the thoracic aorta.

The bronchial arteries provide a secondary blood supply which perfuses each lung at systemic arterial pressure to provide it with oxygenated blood.

The bronchial arteries follow the course of the bronchial tree and its branches to the level of the respiratory bronchioles, where they anastomose with the pulmonary artery branches. They also communicate with the pulmonary arterial system by capillary anastomoses in the bronchial submucosa.

In children, the bronchial arteries are histologically similar to other systemic muscular arteries (see Chapter 9). They have a muscular media and a distinct internal elastic lamina, but no cohesive external elastic lamina (Fig. 10.19a).

In adults, the bronchial arteries develop smooth muscle, arranged longitudinally in small bundles within the intima. These are particularly prominent in some forms of chronic lung disease, but are found from about 20 years of age in normal, healthy individuals (Fig. 10.19b).

The bronchial veins drain into the azygos and hemiazygos veins.

There are numerous anastomoses between the bronchial and pulmonary veins, the bronchial veins running, with the bronchial arteries, in the adventitia of the airways.

Fig. 10.19 Bronchial artery.
(a) Low-magnification micrograph of a bronchial artery from a two-year-old child stained by the elastic Van Gieson (EVG) method to show its muscular media (M) between the internal and external layers of elastic lamina (IEL) and (EEL). Elastic fibres appear black under the microscope. It is very similar to a normal systemic muscular artery and has a fibrocollagenous adventitial layer (A).
(b) High-magnification micrograph of a bronchial artery from a healthy 50-year-old man stained by the EVG method. It shows marked thickening of the intima (I) by longitudinal smooth muscle cells (yellow).

Fig. 10.18 Pulmonary vein.
Pulmonary veins (V) are thin-walled vessels which run in the fibrocollagenous septa with pulmonary lymphatics (L). Small venules resemble pulmonary arterioles, but the larger veins contain collagen and elastic fibres, as well as smooth muscle, outside the basement membrane.
The smooth muscle cells and elastic fibres are haphazardly arranged, but in large pulmonary veins the elastic fibres may form an interrupted or continuous elastic lamina. There are no valves in pulmonary veins of any size.

There are no lymphatic vessels from the alveolar air sacs and interalveolar septa.

Any fluid in the air spaces is absorbed into the thick part of the alveolar wall. This fluid diffuses proximally in the interstitium until it enters small lymphatics at about the level of the respiratory bronchioles. The small lymphatics merge to form larger vessels that follow the bronchial tree proximally as far as the lung hilum, draining into a series of peribronchial lymph nodes on the way.

Another system of lymphatics runs in the visceral pleura and fibrocollagenous septa that divide the lung parenchyma into discrete lobules; these peripheral pleural lymphatics drain directly into the pleural space.

PLEURA

The pleurae are the linings of the thoracic cavity.

The lungs are contained within the thoracic cavity, which is capable of increasing and decreasing in size by intercostal muscle relaxation and contraction. The internal lining of the thoracic cavity and the outer surface of the contained lungs are smooth, low-friction bathed with a small quantity of lubricating fluid. These surfaces are the pleurae. The outer surface of the lung is the visceral pleura, which is composed of five ill-defined layers:

- an outer layer of flat, mesothelial cells;
- a narrow zone of loose, fibrocollagenous tissue, with no identifiable basement membrane between it and the mesothelium;
- an irregular, external elastic layer;
- an interstitial layer of loose, fibrocollagenous stroma containing lymphatics, blood vessels and nerves, together with some smooth muscle fibres;
- an ill-defined internal elastic layer containing short lengths of elastic fiber, some of which merge with those of the interalveolar septa of the most peripheral alveolar groups.

These layers vary markedly from site to site (Fig. 10.20) but are particularly irregular in the region of a fibrocollagenous, interlobular septum, where the ill-defined elastic networks of the pleura often fuse into a single layer before extending part way into the septum.

Parietal pleura forms the internal lining of the thoracic cavity. Merging with the visceral pleura at the hilum of each lung, it has a similar structure, but is usually simpler with only one layer of elastic fibers.

Parietal pleura sits on a layer of adipose tissue, beneath which is a layer of dense fibrocollagenous tissue, which is, in turn, continuous with the periosteum of the ribs and the perimysium of the intercostal muscles.

Fig. 10.20 Visceral pleura.
Visceral pleura stained by the elastic Van Gieson method to show its elastic (black) and collagen (red) content. The flat mesothelial cells on the surface cannot be identified, but the irregular external elastic layer (E) and ill–defined fragmented internal elastic layer (I) can be seen, as can the outer (OC) and the interstitial (IC) collagenous layers, the latter containing blood vessels (BV).

Fig. 10.21 Lung architecture.
Low-power micrograph showing the general architecture of the lung of a child. Bronchi (B), bronchioles (B1), the alveolar network (A) and the outer covering of pleura (P) are indicated.

Fig. 10.22 Distal air passages.
Micrograph showing a terminal bronchiole (T) giving off a respiratory bronchiole (R), which has divided into three alveolar ducts (AD) with alveoli opening into them. They terminate in the alveolar sacs (AS) into which a number of alveoli open directly.

1. THE TRUE VOCAL CORDS OF THE LARYNX

   (a) are covered by ciliated, columnar
       epithelium
   (b) are rich in lymphatics
   (c) are rich in capillaries
   (d) contain fibers of the vocal ligament
   (e) contain fibers of the vocalis muscle

2. ARRANGE THE FOLLOWING COMPONENTS OF THE RESPIRATORY TRACT, MOVING DISTALLY

   (a) alveolar duct
   (b) terminal bronchiole
   (c) alveolus
   (d) respiratory bronchiole
   (e) alveolar sacs

3. TYPE 1 PNEUMOCYTES

   (a) are more numerous than Type 2
   (b) are joined to each other by tight junctions
   (c) are rich in mitochondria
   (d) have prominent surface microvilli
   (e) are very resistant to inhaled toxins

4. TYPE 2 PNEUMOCYTES

   (a) have surface microvilli
   (b) are flat attenuated cells
   (c) are stem cells which can produce new
       Type 1 and Type 2 pneumocytes
   (d) can become detached to act as
       intra-alveolar macrophages
   (e) contain multi-lamellate bodies in their
       cytoplasm

11. Alimentary Tract

INTRODUCTION

The alimentary tract is best considered as a muscular tube lined internally by an epithelium that varies in structure according to specialized functions required at particular sites along its length; with a few local variations, the structure of the musculature is similar throughout.

The function of the alimentary tract is to take in raw food material and to fragment it into small portions. These are then acted upon by a series of secretions, mainly enzymes, which convert the large molecules into smaller molecules, thus permitting their absorption into the blood and lymph circulation.

The small molecules are mainly amino acids, small peptides, carbohydrates, sugars and lipids, which are transported by the blood and lymph mainly to the liver, where they are used as the building blocks in the synthesis of essential proteins, carbohydrates and lipids.

The alimentary tract can be divided into three functional compartments with an auxiliary gland system (Fig. 11.1).

ORAL CAVITY AND ITS CONTENTS

The oral cavity is lined by stratified squamous epithelium throughout but contains many highly specialized structures.

The mouth is lined by stratified squamous epithelium, the underlying submucosa containing varying numbers of salivary glands, which can secrete both a serous and a mucus fluid. Skeletal muscle fibers are common in the deeper layers and are responsible for altering the size and shape of the cavity and for moving food; skeletal muscle fibers form the bulk of the tongue, and are also numerous and important in the cheeks.

In some areas the deep tissues of the oral cavity consist of bone, either simple plates of bone (as in the hard palate) or modified bone (teeth). The immovable hard palate produces a rigid structure against which the tongue can move, while the teeth, which are embedded in bony supports (the mandibles and maxillae), are the main tools for fragmenting ingested food.

The lips are covered by squamous epithelium and contain glands and underlying muscle.

The oral orifice is bounded by the lips, the external aspects of which are covered by hair-bearing skin, with sebaceous glands and eccrine sweat ducts. Between the hair-bearing outer surface and the moist, fluid-bathed inner surface there is a transitional zone known as the vermilion

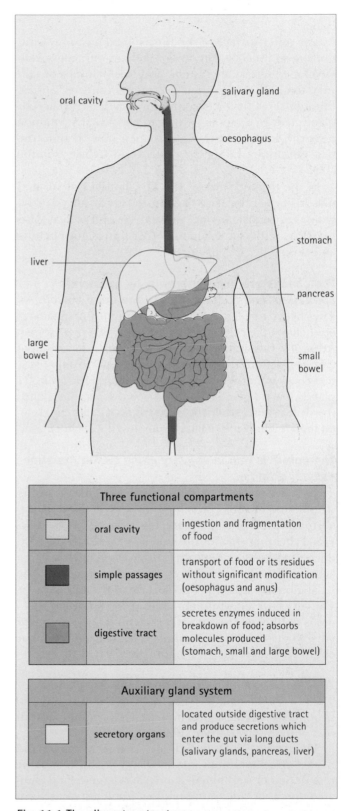

Three functional compartments		
☐	oral cavity	ingestion and fragmentation of food
■	simple passages	transport of food or its residues without significant modification (oesophagus and anus)
■	digestive tract	secretes enzymes induced in breakdown of food; absorbs molecules produced (stomach, small and large bowel)

Auxiliary gland system		
☐	secretory organs	located outside digestive tract and produce secretions which enter the gut via long ducts (salivary glands, pancreas, liver)

Fig. 11.1 The alimentary tract.

because of its pinkish-red appearance. Here the epithelium is non-keratinizing stratified squamous with a prominent rete ridge system (see Chapter 18) and the papillae between the epithelial downgrowths contain prominent blood vessels which are responsible for the pinkish-red color.

The inner surface of the lips is lined by a non-keratinizing stratified squamous epithelium with a less well-developed rete ridge system, and small clumps of salivary tissue disgorge their secretions onto its surface through short ducts. In addition, occasional sebaceous glands (Fordyce's spots), which are particularly common near the angles of the mouth, open directly onto the mucosal surface rather than into a hair follicle as in the skin.

In the deeper parts of the lips, bundles of striated muscle fibers (orbicularis oris muscle) are arranged mainly in a concentric manner around the oral orifice. This muscle is responsible, among other things, for opening and closing the oral orifice.

The cheeks are lined internally by squamous epithelium and contain glands and deep muscle.

The cheeks are lined by thick non-keratinizing squamous epithelium, the cells of which are often rich in glycogen. Areas of keratinization are common, usually as a result of chronic friction from ill-fitting dentures or from persistent cheek biting. The submucosa contains minor salivary glands (buccal glands) and occasional sebaceous glands (Fordyce's spots), while the deep tissues contain the skeletal muscle fibers of the cheek muscles (buccinator).

The palate is rich in salivary gland tissue (palatine salivary glands).

The surface epithelium of the palate is non-keratinizing stratified squamous epithelium with, in the hard palate, a prominent rete ridge pattern which reflects the frictional shearing stresses this area is subjected to by food during mastication. Beneath the salivary gland tissue, the submucosa is firmly tethered to the periosteum of the palatal bone plate. The oral surface of the soft palate is similarly covered with non-keratinizing stratified squamous epithelium which extends onto its free posterior edge where there is a transition to the ciliated columnar epithelium covering the nasal surface.

The floor of the mouth contains salivary glands.

The floor of the mouth is covered by thin non-keratinized stratified squamous epithelium which is continuous with that of the ventral surface of the tongue.

The floor of the mouth is also rich in salivary gland tissue, with many minor salivary glands in the floor of the mouth (minor sublingual glands) and larger glands situated on either side of the midline frenulum of the ventral surface of the tongue (major sublingual glands).

The tongue is muscular and covered in squamous epithelium.

The tongue is a highly muscular organ protruding upward and forward into the oral cavity from its floor. The ventral surface of the tongue is covered by thin non-keratinizing stratified squamous epithelium continuous with that of the floor of the mouth. In contrast, the dorsal surface, which is commonly in contact with the hard palate during feeding, talking and at rest, is covered with a thick keratinizing stratified squamous epithelium, which shows considerable specialization.

Fig. 11.2 Dorsal surface of the tongue.
The dorsal surface of the tongue can be divided into a posterior third (P) with smooth, dome-shaped elevations (E), and an anterior two-thirds (A) by a V-shaped line of circumvallate papillae (C). The surface of the anterior two-thirds is roughened by the presence of small filiform and fungiform papillae and by a surface keratin layer. In places the surface keratin may become thick and stained by food (coated tongue, arrow), particularly in the elderly (as here), and the coating may contain numerous bacterial colonies.

The upper surface of the tongue is divided into two main zones.

The dorsal surface of the tongue is divided into an anterior two-thirds and a posterior one-third. The two parts are separated by a V-shaped line of 6-10 dome-shaped protrusions, the circumvallate papillae (Fig. 11.2). Circumvallate papillae appear as flattened domes, the bases of which are depressed below the dorsal surface.

Each circumvallate papilla is surrounded by a narrow, moat-like channel, in the epithelium of which are numerous taste buds. These taste buds are thought to detect bitter taste. Small salivary glands discharge their secretions into the channels (Fig. 11.3).

The posterior third of the tongue is characterized by the presence of lymphoid tissue.

Low-smooth dome-shaped elevations of the covering epithelium of the posterior third of the tongue are due to lymphoid tissue (the lingual tonsillar tissue) in the submucosa (Fig. 11.4). This lymphoid tissue is part of the mucosa-associated lymphoid tissue system (MALT - see page 134) protecting (with the palatine tonsils and the pharyngeal adenoids) the oral portal of entry. Lymphocytes are numerous within the overlying non-keratinizing stratified squamous epithelium, which extends down into the lymphoid tissue as narrow clefts. Small salivary glands open into the bottom of the narrow clefts, becoming more prominent and numerous near the line of circumvallate papillae.

The surface epithelium of the anterior two-thirds of the tongue is raised in a series of elevations called papillae.

The three types of papillae in man are circumvallate (see opposite), filiform and fungiform.

FILIFORM PAPILLAE are the most numerous papillae and are found all over the dorsum of the anterior two-thirds of the tongue. They are tall, narrow and pointed (Fig. 11.5) and are keratinized, particularly at their tips. Filiform papillae contain no identifiable taste buds.

FUNGIFORM PAPILLAE (Fig. 11.5) are scattered apparently randomly among the filiform papillae on the dorsal surface of the tongue, and have a mushroom shape. Taste buds are present in their covering epithelium, those at the anterior tip of the tongue detecting sweet taste, and those just behind the tip and some way along the lateral borders detecting salty taste.

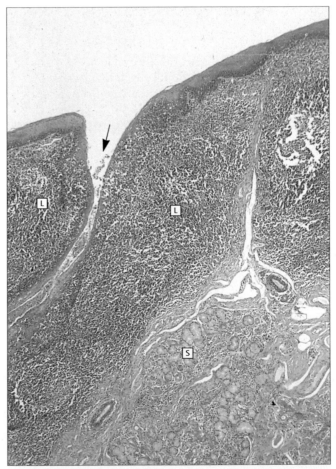

Fig. 11.4 Posterior one–third of tongue.
Posterior third of the tongue showing lymphoid tissue (L), cleft-like invaginations of the epithelium (**arrow**), and salivary glands (S) opening into the depths of the clefts.

Fig. 11.3 Circumvallate papilla.
The circumvallate papilla (P) is surrounded by a moat (M) into the bottom of which empty prominent salivary glands (S). Taste buds (TB) are particularly numerous in the walls of the moat.

Fig. 11.5 Fungiform and filiform papillae.
Photograph of part of the dorsal surface of the anterior two-thirds of the tongue showing the gross appearance of the mushroom-like fungiform papillae (**Fu**) and the smaller filiform papillae (**Fi**).

Taste buds are specialized sensory organs located in the epithelium of the tongue.

Each taste bud occupies the full thickness of the epithelium and comprises pale staining spindle-shaped cells in an oval cluster (Fig 11.6). The luminal surfaces of the cells open into a small defect in the epithelium, the taste pore, and each cell bears a number of microvilli. Ultrastructurally, some of the spindle-shaped cells have synaptic vesicles and are associated with small afferent nerve fibers; these are the taste receptor cells. Other cells with more electron-dense cytoplasm and scanty secretory granules near the luminal surface are thought to act mainly as supporting sustentacular cells, but may also secrete glycosaminoglycans into the taste pore.

Fig. 11.6 Taste buds in circumvallate papilla.
(a) This thin acrylic resin section, stained with H&E, is from a circumvallate papilla of a surgically removed human tongue from an elderly man. It shows the oval taste buds (TB) which occupy the full thickness of the epithelium. The luminal aspect of the spindle-shaped cells opens onto the surface at the taste pore, the beginning of which is shown here (P).
(b) An epoxy-resin section (0.5 μm thick) of a single taste bud, stained with Toluidine Blue stain to show the taste receptor cells with a mixture of spherical and spindle-shaped nuclei. A small bead of dark-staining glycosaminoglycan material is present in the taste pore.

There are also cells resembling the taste receptor cells but lacking the synaptic vesicles and afferent nerve connections. The turnover of these cells is rapid, (every 10–14 days), so there is a population of small rounded stem cells at the base of each taste bud from which the other cell types derive.

The taste buds of the dorsal tongue detect only acid, sweet, bitter, and salty, and provide early warning that food may be unpalatable. Appreciation of more subtle flavors depends on the smell receptors in the nose (see page 162).

Skeletal muscle in the tongue is arranged in many directions.

The musculature of the tongue comprises a complex pattern of skeletal muscle fibers. These fibers run in bands longitudinally, vertically, transversely and obliquely, with a variable amount of adipose tissue in between (Fig. 11.7).

This arrangement gives the tongue great mobility to manipulate food around the mouth for efficient fragmentation, and for moving fragmented food backward prior to swallowing; it also provides the fine control of tongue movement that is essential for speech.

Abundant islands of salivary tissue are present in the submucosa between the muscular core of the tongue and the surface epithelium in the region of the junction between the posterior one-third and anterior two-thirds. Some of the deeper salivary gland collections extend down into the superficial parts of the muscular zone.

ANTERIOR TWO-THIRDS OF TONGUE

- Covered by stratified squamous epithelium, thin on ventral surface, thick and papilliform on dorsal surface

- Filiform, fungiform and circumvallate papillae on anterior two-thirds; latter demarcate anterior and posterior parts of tongue

- Taste buds present on circumvallate and fungiform papillae

- Bulk is striated muscle with small amount of adipose tissue

- Salivary tissue in submucosa, mainly near circumvallate papillae

POSTERIOR THIRD OF TONGUE

- Covered by smooth, non-papillate stratified squamous epithelium

- Submucosa contains lymphoid aggregates (MALT), forming part of Waldeyer's ring

- Bulk is muscle and adipose tissue, with some salivary tissue in submucosa and muscle, mainly near circumvallate papillae

Fig. 11.7 Musculature of tongue.
ⓐ In the anterior two-thirds of the tongue the striated muscle bundles (M) are tightly packed with relatively little intervening adipose tissue (A). Note that the muscle bundles run in many directions. In the bulkier, less mobile posterior third of the tongue the adipose tissue is more abundant.

ⓑ Collections of salivary glands (S) are numerous in the submucosa and muscular core of the posterior tongue, particularly close to the junction between the posterior one-third and anterior two-thirds.

TEETH

INTRODUCTION

The main task of the oral cavity, the fragmentation of large food masses, is performed by the teeth, which are hard, heavily mineralized structures embedded in the raised alveolar ridges of the maxilla and mandible.

Teeth are arranged so that the free surface of those embedded in the mandible (lower teeth) oppose and contact those in the maxilla (upper teeth), allowing food material to be trapped between them.

The anterior teeth (incisor and canine teeth) have narrow, chisel-shaped or pointed free edges for chopping food into medium-sized pieces, while the posterior teeth (premolars and molars) have broader, flatter, free surfaces for grinding medium-sized food pieces into smaller fragments.

The mandible is joined to the body of the skull by the temporomandibular joint, which permits the mandible to slide backward and forward, and from side to side, thus aiding the grinding of food between the broad surfaces of the opposing molar teeth.

Each tooth can be divided into two anatomic components, the crown and the root.

The tooth is divided into two structural regions:
- the crown protrudes into the oral cavity;
- the root is embedded in the bone of the mandible or maxilla.

The junction between the crown and the root is called the neck. The mature tooth has five components: the central pulp cavity, dentine, enamel, cementum and periodontal ligament (Fig. 11.8).

The center of each tooth comprises the pulp which contains nutrient vessels and nerves.

The pulp cavity is the soft central core of the tooth and contains collagen and fibroblasts embedded in an acellular matrix. The cavity approximates in shape that of the tooth as a whole and its acellular matrix is composed of glycosaminoglycans.

Through the pulp cavity run the blood vessels that nourish the odontoblasts (see below) and the nerve twigs that provide dental sensation. These vessels and nerves enter and leave through a small **apical foramen** at the tip of the root.

The pulp cavity is narrow throughout most of the root (the **root canal**), but is expanded in the neck and crown (the **pulp chamber**). Its outer surface is lined by odontoblasts, which continually produce dentine. As dentine is progressively laid down, the pulp cavity diminishes in size.

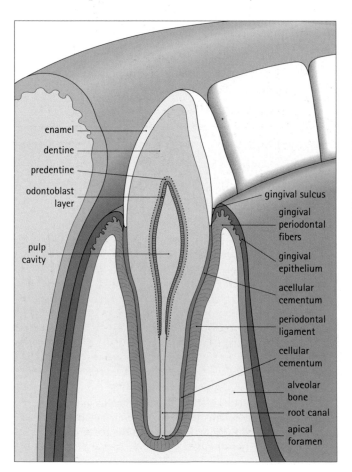

enamel

dentine

predentine

odontoblast layer

pulp cavity

gingival sulcus

gingival periodontal fibers

gingival epithelium

acellular cementum

periodontal ligament

cellular cementum

alveolar bone

root canal

apical foramen

Fig. 11.8 Mature incisor tooth.
The central pulp cavity, the outer layer of which contains cells (odontoblasts) that produce the specialized extracellular matrix components of the teeth, is surrounded by dentine, a relatively acellular mineralized material forming the bulk of each tooth.

The dentine of the crown of the tooth is covered by enamel, a heavily mineralized material forming a resistant outer coat. At the neck of the tooth, enamel is continuous with cementum. This is a bone-like material forming an outer coat to the dentine in the root. Cementum is linked to the alveolar bone of the mandible or maxilla by the periodontal ligament, which is composed of tightly packed collagen fibers embedded at one end into the cementum of the tooth and at the other end into the bone forming the tooth socket.

DENTINOGENESIS AND ODONTOBLASTS

The specialized mineralized matrix of the tooth is called dentine and is secreted by odontoblasts.

Dentine is composed of mineral salts and organic material. The mineral salts are calcium salts in the form of crystalline hydroxyapatite (about 70–80%) arranged as long, hollow parallel tubules, the **dentinal tubules**. Within these run the organic material in the form of fine cytoplasmic processes of the odontoblasts, and the Type 1 collagen fibers and glycosaminoglycans that they produce (about 20–30%).

Dentine is initially laid down by odontoblasts as a glycosaminoglycan matrix in which collagen fibers are linearly arranged. This non-mineralized predentine is synthesized by odontoblasts located at the outer limits of the pulp cavity (Fig. 11.9).

In man, the odontoblast cytoplasmic processes extend only 25–50% of the full length of the dentinal tubule, thus dentine close to the dentine–enamel border appears to contain empty tubules. In life these empty tubules may contain fluid which is lost during tissue processing.

As odontoblasts progressively synthesize new predentine at the inner surface of the pulp cavity (Figs 11.9 and 11.10), the cavity slowly decreases in size throughout life.

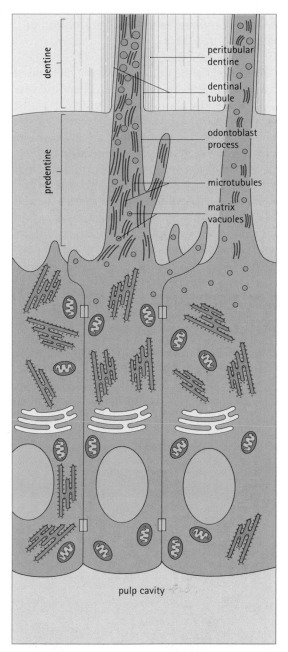

Fig. 11.10 Odontoblasts and dentinogenesis.
The functioning odontoblast is a tall, narrow cell, the base of which contacts cells and fibers of the pulp cavity (mainly fibroblasts and collagen). Its nucleus is basal and its cytoplasm is rich in mitochondria and rough endoplasmic reticulum. It has a large supranuclear Golgi complex. At the apex of the cell, the cytoplasm is drawn out into a long odontoblast process which runs through the predentine and dentine layers in the dentinal tubule, while small side branches penetrate the predentine. The cytoplasm of the odontoblast process and its branches contains numerous microtubules as well as small matrix vacuoles, which contain Ca^{++} and PO_4^- ions.

The matrix vacuoles play a key role in the mineralisation of the dentinal matrix. The mechanism is almost identical to that whereby matrix vesicles from osteoblasts produce mineralisation of osteoid matrix to produce bone mineralisation (see page 240).

Fig. 11.9 Dentine, predentine and odontoblasts.
Micrograph showing pulp cavity (P) lined externally by a layer of odontoblasts (O), external to which is a pale staining band of predentine (PD). The outer layer is mineralized dentine (D), in which the pattern of dentinal tubules can be seen.

Dentinogenesis commences with the formation of predentine by odontoblasts.

In predentine, randomly scattered collagen fibers (Type 1 collagen) produced by the odontoblasts are embedded in an extracellular matrix of phosphoprotein and glycosaminoglycans (mainly chondroitin-6-sulfate).

Mineralization is initiated by the discharge of the matrix vacuoles from the odontoblast process and its branches running through the predentine layer.

Some time after its formation, predentine becomes mineralized at its border with previously mineralized dentine; close to this predentine–dentine border the collagen fibers of predentine become more numerous and tightly packed. The dentine lining the dentinal tubules (peritubular dentine) is particularly compact and heavily mineralized (Fig. 11.11).

AMELOBLASTS AND ENAMEL FORMATION

Enamel is the hardest material in the body.

Enamel is composed almost entirely of the mineral hydroxyapatite $(Ca_{10}(PO_4)_6(OH)_2)$, which is arranged in tightly packed hexagonal enamel rods or prisms (Fig. 11.12) about $4\,\mu m$ in diameter, although some may measure up to $8\,\mu m$.

Each enamel rod extends through the full thickness of the enamel. The small interstices between adjacent rods are occupied by hydroxyapatite crystals. A small amount of organic matrix (protein and polysaccharide) represents the remnants of the matrix synthesized and excreted by the enamel-producing cells, the ameloblasts, prior to mineralization of the enamel.

Fig. 11.11 Dentinal tubules.
Scanning electron micrograph of dentine at a point well distant from the predentine layer. The mineral material contains regular empty dentinal tubules because the cytoplasmic processes of the odontoblasts extend only a short way into the tubules. Note the more compact dentine lining the tubules.

Fig. 11.12 Enamel.
ⓐ H&E-stained section of early forming enamel (E), being produced by a layer of ameloblasts (A). The enamel shows a distinctive pattern due to the arrangement of enamel prisms and abuts the dentine (D).
ⓑ Scanning electron micrograph showing the characteristic arrangement of tightly packed enamel prisms or rods.

Enamel is formed during tooth development by the ameloblasts.

Ameloblasts degenerate when the tooth erupts, after which time the enamel cannot be replaced by new synthesis. In the developing tooth (see Fig. 11.17), the functioning ameloblast is a tall, narrow cell, with its base attached to the cells of the stratum intermedium (Fig.

11.13). The nucleus is located basally and basal cytoplasm contains abundant mitochondria. The supranuclear cytoplasm contains a large, active Golgi complex and abundant rough endoplasmic reticulum, together with microtubules, which are predominantly longitudinally arranged, and secretory vacuoles which become larger and more numerous near the upper pole.

At the upper pole the cell elongates into a single large Tomes' process, and forms a fringe of smaller processes around its neck. The Tomes' process contains numerous microtubules and large numbers of secretory vacuoles.

The rough endoplasmic reticulum synthesizes various proteins and glycoproteins (including amelogenin and enamelin), which form the organic matrix of enamel (pre-enamel) and are packaged by the Golgi complex into secretory vacuoles. These then move into the Tomes' process and the small neck processes, discharging their contents onto the surface.

Mineralization of the matrix proteins by hydroxyapatite occurs almost instantaneously, producing small enamel crystallites, and, with progressive mineralization, the enamel rods or prisms.

The compact structured enamel prisms are probably derived from the surface of the main Tomes' process, while the small amount of less compact interprism enamel, which has a larger organic matrix component, is probably derived from the small neck processes.

Enamel covers the dentine only in the region of the exposed crown (Fig 11.14); in the root, the dentine is covered by cementum (see Figs 11.8 and 11.15).

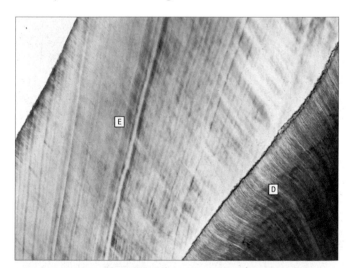

Fig. 11.13 Ameloblasts and enamel formation.
The functioning ameloblast is a tall, narrow cell, with its base attached to the cells of the stratum intermedium. The Tomes' process at the upper pole is rich in secretory vacuoles containing organic matrix proteins and numerous microtubules. Each Tomes' process has small associated cytoplasmic processes around it; these also produce some enamel but the main enamel prisms are produced by the Tomes' process.

Fig. 11.14 Formed enamel.
Unstained ground section of a mature human tooth showing the characteristic patterns of enamel (E) and dentine (D); the tightly packed dentinal tubules are clearly seen. The linearity of the compact parallel enamel prisms runs from the dentinal/enamel interface in straight lines to the surface. The coarse, slightly curved, oblique lines seen in this photomicrograph are an artefact produced by the grinding process used to make this section.

CEMENTUM AND PERIODONTAL LIGAMENT

Cementum is a bone-like tissue; it is calcified and contains collagen.

A thin layer of cementum covers the root of the tooth, being thin, compact and acellular (acellular cementum) over the upper region, but thicker and containing lacunae and cementocytes (cellular cementum) lower down (Fig. 11.15).

Cementocytes resemble osteocytes (see Chapter 13) and remain viable throughout life, being nourished through canaliculi which link the lacunae. They can become activated to produce new cementum when required.

In addition to the cementocytes, which are scattered throughout the cellular cementum, there is a layer of cells called cementoblasts, which are similar to the actively synthetic osteoblasts of bone (see Fig. 13.15).

Cementoblasts lie against the surface of the periodontal ligament and probably produce most new cementum by appositional deposition.

The periodontal ligament is a suspensory ligament tethering the tooth in the bony alveolar socket of the mandible or maxilla.

The periodontal ligament is composed of dense collagen and fibrocytes, with the fibers running across the gap between the cementum of the tooth and the bone of the alveolar socket (Fig. 11.16). As the collagen fibers are embedded in a ground substance, this ligament also acts as a shock-absorber, as well as permitting limited movement of the tooth within the bony socket.

At its cemental and alveolar limits, some of the collagen fibers are inserted into the cementum and bone. The alveolar bone at the inner margin of the socket is composed of woven bone rather than compact lamellar bone. Above the upper limit of the alveolar bone, the fibers of the periodontal ligament become the gingival periodontal fibers and blend with the submucosa of the gingivae.

TOOTH DEVELOPMENT

Teeth develop from both ectoderm and mesoderm.

Teeth develop from both ectoderm and from mesenchyme of mesodermal origin, the ectodermal component being the enamel derived from the enamel organ and the mesenchyme producing the rest of the tooth.

The enamel organ originates as a cellular downgrowth of the oral epithelium, initially in the form of a cap-shaped epithelial tooth bud connected to the overlying oral epithelium by the dental lamina. Beneath the epithelial tooth bud, a condensation of mesenchyme contributes to the rest of the tooth.

The stages in tooth formation are summarized in Figure 11.17.

Fig. 11.15 Cementum.
Micrograph showing the dentine (D), cementum and fibrous periodontal ligament (P) of the root of a tooth at the junction between the narrow compact acellular cementum (AC) and the broader cellular cementum (CC), in which osteocyte-like nuclei can be seen (O).

Fig. 11.16 Periodontal ligament.
H&E-stained section showing the relationship between the tooth (T), bony socket (B) and the fibrous periodontal ligament (PL) at the neck of the tooth.

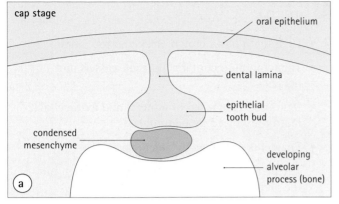

cap stage

oral epithelium

dental lamina

epithelial tooth bud

condensed mesenchyme

developing alveolar process (bone)

a

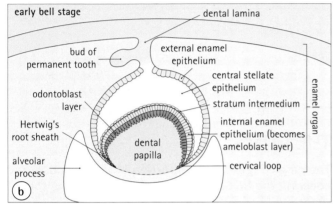

early bell stage

dental lamina

bud of permanent tooth

external enamel epithelium

central stellate epithelium

stratum intermedium

internal enamel epithelium (becomes ameloblast layer)

odontoblast layer

Hertwig's root sheath

dental papilla

alveolar process

cervical loop

enamel organ

b

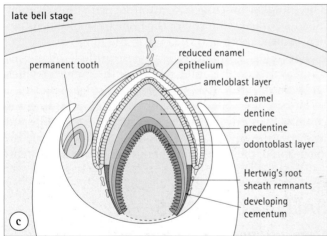

late bell stage

permanent tooth

reduced enamel epithelium

ameloblast layer

enamel

dentine

predentine

odontoblast layer

Hertwig's root sheath remnants

developing cementum

c

DL

A

E

DP

d

Fig. 11.17 Tooth development.

ⓐ Diagram showing early stage of tooth formation from both ectodermal (epithelial) and mesenchymal components.

ⓑ The cells of the epithelial tooth bud develop into the enamel organ, differentiating into a bell-shaped structure with a central core of loosely arranged stellate cells (stellate epithelium) and a peripheral layer of cuboidal or low columnar epithelium. The outer cell layer of the convex surface is the external enamel epithelium, and that of the concave surface the internal enamel epithelium.

The internal enamel epithelium differentiates into an outer layer of tall columnar ameloblasts (see Fig. 11.13) and a 2-3 cell thick inner layer called the stratum intermedium.

Where the external and internal enamel epithelium meet is called the cervical loop. An extension downward of cells of the external enamel epithelium forms the so-called Hertwig's root sheath which defines the final size of the tooth root, being later replaced by the cementum.

In the concavity of the enamel organ, the mesenchyme continues to condense to form the dental papilla, and a row of odontoblasts develops at its junction with the enamel organ, in contact with the ameloblast layer.

In deciduous teeth, like the incisor shown here, the permanent tooth arises from a side-growth from the dental lamina.

ⓒ Odontoblasts begin to produce predentine and this stimulates the production of enamel by the ameloblasts. Calcification of the predentine and pre-enamel begins almost immediately, and dentine and enamel continue to be laid down until the form of the tooth is complete. The dental papilla becomes enclosed by dentine to form the dental pulp.

The non-ameloblast components of the enamel organ become much reduced and eventually atrophy. When enamel formation is complete, the ameloblasts degenerate to form a thin layer of irregular cells which ultimately disappear when the tooth erupts.

The cells of Hertwig's root sheath begin to degenerate as the cementum is deposited by cementoblasts on the surface of the dentine of the tooth root. Partial development of the permanent tooth continues alongside the deciduous tooth in the same manner.

ⓓ Micrograph of a resin section of a developing tooth at the early bell stage, showing the enamel organ (E), including the ameloblast layer (A), the dental papilla (DP), and the degenerating dental lamina (DL).

DENTAL CARIES AND PERIODONTAL DISEASE

The most common disorders of teeth are:

- abnormal tooth eruption, leading to malalignment of teeth;
- dental caries;
- periodontal disease.

Dental caries results when bacterial plaque produces acid which dissolves the calcium hydroxyapatite of the enamel. Such focal decalcification may progress until the erosion involves the deeper dentine, from where the acids and bacteria can advance more rapidly down the dentinal tubules to the pulp cavity, causing tooth pain.

Continued bacterial damage can produce a tooth abscess in the soft pulp.

Destruction of the pulp cavity and its contained blood vessels leads to death of the odontoblast layer and eventual death of the tooth.

Periodontal disease is caused by the accumulation of bacterial plaque (calcified food and bacterial debris) in the gingival sulcus. This excites inflammation in the adjacent gum which gradually forces the gingiva away from the tooth, widening and damaging the gingival sulcus; deep periodontal pockets form in which food particles and bacteria become trapped. Bacterial proliferation then leads to further inflammation of the gum (gingivitis) and the periodontal ligament (periodontitis).

Persistent periodontitis destroys the periodontal ligament and the tooth becomes loose in its socket.

TEETH

- Each tooth has a crown, neck and root zone
- The tooth pulp contains nutrient vessels and nerves
- Dentine is composed of mineral and extracellular matrix produced by odontoblasts
- Enamel is produced by ameloblasts
- The periodontal ligament anchors the tooth into the alveolar socket of bone

THE GUMS

The gingiva (gum) is the portion of oral mucosa covering the alveolar bone ridge surrounding the tooth.

The gingival mucosa is continuous with the alveolar mucosa covering the rest of the bone. A small sulcus lies between the tooth and the bulk of the gingiva.

The sulcal epithelium is thin stratified squamous, whereas that on the outer surface of the gingiva is thick and keratinized with a prominent rete ridge pattern.

The submucosa in the region of the gingival sulcus is commonly infiltrated by chronic inflammatory cells and also contains gingival periodontal fibers which are an extension of the upper limit of the periodontal ligament.

SALIVARY GLANDS

There are three main salivary glands and many minor glands.

The mouth receives secretions from salivary gland tissue located both inside and outside the mouth. These glands may contain mucus-secreting cells, serous cells or a mixture of both. The serous glands secrete a watery solution containing enzymes (e.g. amylase, lysozyme), IgA secretory piece and lactoferrin, an iron-binding compound.

The largest salivary glands are located outside the mouth and transfer their secretions into the oral cavity by long ducts; smaller glands, sited mainly in the submucosa of the oral lining, are less well defined and empty their secretion into the mouth by short ducts.

The main salivary glands are the submandibular, the parotid and the large sublingual glands.

The submandibular salivary gland secretes a mixed serous/mucous product.

The submandibular glands are roughly ovoid in shape and are situated on either side of the neck just below the mandible. Their ducts open into the floor of the mouth, one on each side of the frenulum of the tongue.

The submandibular glands are typical mixed glands containing both serous and mucous elements, with serous elements predominating.

The secretory acini are composed mainly of epithelial cells, which are responsible for the serous secretion, and are plump cells filled with prominent, purplish-staining zymogen granules.

The mucus-secreting cells are pale-staining with abundant clear cytoplasm, and often form blind-ending tubules, the blind end bearing a demilune or crescent of zymogen-rich serous cells (Fig. 11.18).

The secretory acini empty into intercalated ducts which are lined by cuboidal or low columnar epithelium and merge to form intralobular ducts. These are characterized by tall columnar epithelium which stains pale pink and shows a characteristic striated pattern (see Fig. 3.23) of basal cytoplasm. Hence intralobular ducts are commonly called striated ducts.

Intralobular duct epithelium is biochemically active and modifies the concentration and content of the fluids produced by the secretory acini.

The intralobular striated ducts fuse to form larger interlobular ducts which are lined by a non-striated, often pseudostratified epithelium. Interlobular ducts then join to form the major ducts, some of which (particularly the main submandibular duct) may have a ciliated epithelium.

There is a network of myoepithelial cells between the epithelium and the basement membrane of the acini and much of the ductular system, contraction of the myoepithelial cells squeezing the secretion toward the major ducts.

The parotid salivary glands secrete a serous product.

The parotid glands are situated below and in front of the pinna on each side of the face. They are flat and well encapsulated and the facial nerve runs through them, dividing them into superficial and deep portions. Their long ducts open into the oral cavity opposite the second upper molar tooth on each side.

The parotids are composed entirely of serous glands rich in zymogen granules, with a variable amount of adipose tissue in the interstitium between parotid lobules (Fig. 11.19).

The sublingual glands secrete a mainly mucous product.

The large sublingual glands are located in the floor of the mouth, one on either side of the frenulum of the tongue. Their short ducts open into the mouth near to, or with, the submandibular ducts. These glands are composed predominantly of mucous cells.

Fig. 11.18 Submandibular salivary gland.
The submandibular salivary gland has both a mucous and a serous component. The serous component (S) contains numerous large zymogen granules, while the mucous component (M) is often arranged in duct-like structures, the ends of which are capped by the so-called serous demilunes (D). A striated duct (SD) shows the characteristic features of an ion exchange epithelium.

Fig. 11.19 Parotid salivary gland.
The parotid salivary gland is composed entirely of granular serous cells (S), with variable amounts of intervening adipose tissue. Note the cluster of small ducts (SD) and part of a major duct (MD).

There are numerous smaller groups of salivary gland tissue.

The oral cavity contains a large amount of salivary gland tissue scattered diffusely in the submucosa.

The most important are:

- lingual glands in the submucosa and muscle layers of the dorsal surface of the tongue (see Fig. 11.7b);
- minor sublingual glands close to the larger major sublingual glands (other tongue glands are found on the inferior surface of the tip of the tongue and on its lateral borders);
- labial glands on the inner surface of the lips;
- palatine glands in the submucosa of the soft and hard palates;
- tonsillar glands in the mucosa associated with the palatine and pharyngeal tonsils;
- buccal glands in the submucosa lining the cheeks.

The labial, sublingual, minor lingual and buccal glands are composed predominantly of mucous cells, but some serous cells may be present. The palatine and lateral lingual glands are entirely mucus-secreting.

TRANSPORT PASSAGES

The pharynx, esophagus and anal canal are comparatively simple transport tubes through which ingested food is transmitted by peristalsis without undergoing significant metabolic change. They are muscular tubes lined internally by stratified squamous epithelium and some mucous glands which provide lubricating mucus.

The pharynx is divided into oropharynx and nasopharynx.

The pharynx is located at the back of the mouth and transfers partly fragmented food from the oral cavity into the upper end of the esophagus. It also connects the nasal system of air chambers and the upper end of the trachea. The opening of the mouth into the pharynx is the **oropharynx**, while the nasal opening is the **nasopharynx**. The Eustachian tube from the middle ear (see Chapter 19) opens into the pharynx on each side.

The oropharynx and pharynx proper are lined by largely non-keratinizing stratified squamous epithelium. The nasopharynx is lined partly by stratified squamous epithelium, which changes to a ciliated columnar epithelium as the nasal cavities are approached.

The submucosa of the pharynx is well endowed with lymphoid tissue.

There is a particularly prominent aggregation of lymphoid tissue in the nasopharynx forming the pharyngeal tonsil (adenoids). At the junction between the mouth and pharynx, in the oropharynx, are large lymphoid tonsillar masses in the gap between the glossopalatine and pharyngopalatine arches on each side. These are the palatine tonsils. The tonsils are discussed on page 134.

ESOPHAGUS

INTRODUCTION

The esophagus lies between the pharynx and the stomach. It transports food in an undigested but fragmented form to the stomach, where digestion begins. It is about 25 cm long, originating from the pharynx at the level of the cricoid cartilage, and extending down the posterior mediastinum in the midline to the level of the diaphragm; it penetrates the left crus before opening into the stomach at the esophagogastric junction.

The esophagus is lined by squamous epithelium which lies over a lamina propria and a muscularis mucosae

The esophageal mucosa is composed of non-keratinizing stratified squamous epithelium, lamina propria and muscularis mucosae (Fig. 11.20). The basal zone of the

Fig. 11.20 Esophageal mucosa and submucosa.
The esophagus is lined by non-keratinizing stratified squamous epithelium (E), beneath which is a thick lamina propria (LP) and muscularis mucosae (MM). The submucosa contains abundant vessels and nerves together with esophageal mucous glands (OMG) which are characteristically surrounded by lymphocytic infiltrate.

epithelium may be several cell layers thick and consists of cuboidal or rectangular cells with dark nuclei and purple-staining cytoplasm in which there is no glycogen. Scattered in this layer are occasional melanocytes and neuroendocrine cells.

Above the basal zone the epithelial cells are larger and may be rich in glycogen, gradually becoming more flattened as the lumen is approached (Fig. 11.21).

The average epithelial thickness is 500–800 μm, but this is difficult to measure accurately because the lower border is irregular, and tongues of lamina propria extend up toward the luminal surface, giving an appearance similar to the rete ridge arrangement in the epidermis of the skin (see Chapter 18).

The esophageal lamina propria consists of loosely arranged collagen fibers and fibroblasts embedded in an acellular glycosaminoglycans matrix, with a normal scattering of lymphocytes and eosinophils, as well as occasional mast cells and plasma cells.

The muscularis mucosae is of variable thickness, being particularly thick at the lower end where it approaches the esophagogastric junction. In the upper esophagus the fibers appear to be arranged haphazardly, but in the lower third there are continuous sheets of longitudinal and circular smooth muscle.

The submucosa of the esophagus contains mucous glands, lymphoid tissue, nerves and blood vessels.

The submucosa of the esophagus is broad and contains mucous glands (see Fig. 11.20) which secrete acid mucins. Each gland has 2–5 lobes, which drain into a short duct lined by stratified columnar epithelium, the duct penetrating the muscularis mucosae, lamina propria and epithelial layer to open into the lumen. Lymphocytes, plasma cells and eosinophils are particularly common around the glands and their ducts (see Fig. 11.20). Aggregations of lymphoid cells forming small follicles are common in the esophageal submucosa near the squamous/columnar epithelial junction.

Esophageal submucosa is also particularly rich in blood vessels, lymphatics, nerves and ganglion cells.

The muscle of the esophagus contains both striated and smooth types.

The muscularis proper of the esophagus varies along its length, although it is generally arranged in discrete circular and longitudinal layers. In the upper third of the esophagus the layers are composed almost entirely of striated muscle, but a gradual transition to smooth muscle occurs in the middle third where both striated and smooth muscle fibers are found together. The muscle lay-

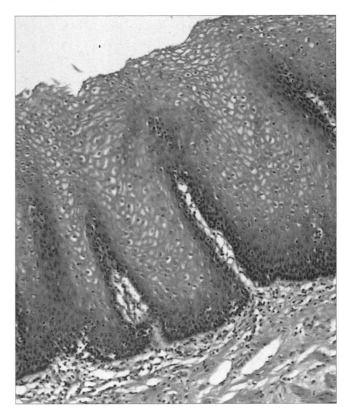

Fig. 11.21 Esophageal epithelium.
At high magnification, the esophageal squamous epithelium contains some pale-staining cells distended with glycogen; its lower border is irregular.

ers in the lower third are composed entirely of smooth muscle and are continuous with the smooth muscle layers of the stomach.

The esophagogastric junction is an important site of pathologic abnormality.

Unlike the rest of the esophagus, which is lined by stratified squamous epithelium, the short length (1–1.5 cm long) of esophagus below the diaphragm is lined by columnar epithelium similar to that of the cardiac region of the stomach; this is the esophagogastric (squamous/columnar) junction (Fig. 11.22). Disease results from exposure of the squamous epithelium of the lower esophagus to acid and digestive enzymes from the stomach.

Fig. 11.22 Esophagogastric junction.

(a) Macroscopic appearance of the junction between the esophagus and stomach. Most of the esophagus is lined by a stratified squamous epithelium (white), while the stomach epithelium appears brown.

(b) H&E section of the squamous/columnar junction in the region of the esophagogastric junction showing the abrupt transition between esophageal squamous epithelium (OE) and columnar gastric epithelium (GE). In the region of the junction, lymphoid aggregates (L) and esophageal mucous glands (OMG) are particularly prominent.

ESOPHAGEAL ULCERATION AND BARRETT'S ESOPHAGUS

The squamous epithelium of the esophagus is protected from exposure to gastric acid by:

- the anatomical arrangement of the esophagogastric junction;

- the small esophagogastric muscular sphincter, which in most cases prevents reflux of gastric contents into the lower esophagus.

However, the system is not foolproof, and reflux of acid gastric secretions may occur into the lower esophagus causing inflammation and pain. Under the constant irritating effect of reflux of acidic gastric secretions the epithelium in the lower esophagus changes its differentiation to a gastric-type of glandular epithelium. This condition is called Barrett's esophagus.

The islands of columnar epithelium in Barrett's esophagus are particularly prone to ulceration and inflammation (Fig. 11.23) and are also believed to predispose to development of one type of esophageal cancer

Fig. 11.23 Photograph showing the lower half of the esophagus (O) and the upper part of the stomach (S). Compare with Fig. 11.22a.
At the esophagogastric junction (OGJ) are four ulcers (U), which lie in inflamed columnar mucosa that extends up as far as the arrow. Above the arrow there is normal esophageal stratified squamous epithelium, which shows yellowish discoloration as a result of repeated vomiting.
Healing of such ulcers can lead to scarring of the lower end of the esophagus, and thereby narrowing of its lumen (i.e. an esophageal stricture), so that swallowing becomes almost impossible.

ESOPHAGUS

- Lined by non-keratinizing stratified squamous epithelium
- Submucosa contains mucous glands, lymphoid aggregates, and prominent blood vessels, particularly at lower end

- Muscle is striated type in upper third, smooth muscle in lower third, and both in middle third
- Lower esophagus is an important site of common diseases, particularly ulceration, stricture and cancer.

ANAL CANAL

The anal canal is a muscular conduit transporting feces for elimination.

The anal canal transports the residue of ingested food after it has been digested and most of its water content has been extracted (i.e. feces) from the rectum to the exterior in the process known as defecation.

Anatomically the anal canal is a tube 3–4 cm long (Fig. 11.24), the diameter of which is controlled by two sphincter systems.

The internal anal sphincter is composed of smooth muscle and is a localized thickening of the circular muscle of the lower rectum. It is under autonomic control and responds to distension of the rectal reservoir.

The external anal sphincter is composed of skeletal striated muscle and is continuous with the fascia and muscles of the pelvic floor. It is under voluntary control.

The anal canal is mainly lined by stratified squamous epithelium.

At its upper end the anal canal is lined by columnar epithelium identical to that of the rectum. This changes to a non-keratinizing stratified squamous type at the level of the pectinate (or dentate) line, which marks the site of the anal membrane of the fetus (i.e. the junction of gut endoderm and the ectodermal invagination of the proctodeal pit).

The pectinate line is a line of small crescentic valve-like mucosal extrusions, with small vertical folds, the anal columns, arising from their junctions.

Small branched tubular glands, the anal glands, open into the anal canal just above the pectinate line, while another set of glands, the prominent apocrine glands of the perianal skin (see Chapter 18), lie at the lower end of the anal canal (circumanal glands).

Two prominent venous plexuses are associated with the anal canal.

The internal hemorrhoidal plexus lies in the submucosa of the upper end of the canal above the level of the pectinate line.

The external hemorrhoidal plexus lies in the submucosa at the lower end in the region of the junction between anal canal and perianal skin.

Fig. 11.24 Anal canal.
Diagram of the anal canal showing the epithelial linings of the rectum (columnar), anal canal (non-keratinizing stratified squamous) and anal skin (keratinizing epidermis rich in hair follicles, eccrine and apocrine glands). There is a variable junctional zone of epithelium at the pectinate line.

The internal sphincter is a continuation of the circular smooth muscle layer of the rectum, and the external sphincter is composed of skeletal muscle under voluntary control.

The rectal longitudinal muscle loses its fibers at the level of the puborectalis muscle of the pelvic floor and continues as a fibroelastic septum between the internal and external sphincter.

Note the position of the internal and external hemorrhoidal plexuses; hemorrhoids (piles) result from enlargement of the internal hemorrhoidal plexus.

DIGESTIVE TRACT

The digestive tract is the site of several processes:
- major digestion of food material (some digestion begins in the mouth as a result of salivary secretion of diastase);
- absorption of the end products of digestion;
- absorption of ingested fluids and reabsorption of secreted fluids.

The digestive tract comprises the stomach, small intestine (i.e. duodenum, jejunum and ileum) and large intestine (i.e. caecum, appendix, colon and rectum). Its basic structure is shown in Fig. 11.25.

The digestive mucosa, composed of lining epithelium, lamina propria and muscularis mucosae, is the most variable component of the digestive tract and usually contains a mixture of epithelial cell types, both absorptive and secretory. The epithelium is supported by a variable layer, the lamina propria, which is composed of supporting cells and their products (including collagen). Within the lamina propria are small blood vessels, lymphatics, nerve fibers and cells belonging to the immune and defense systems (see Chapter 8), particularly macrophages and lymphocytes. The deep aspect of the lamina propria rests on a usually thin muscle layer, the muscularis mucosae.

The surface area of the digestive passages is increased by formation of folds and glands.

The efficiency of absorptive and secretory processes is improved by increasing the surface area of contact between the epithelial cells and the lumen. This is achieved by:
- intrusions or folding of the lining epithelium into the lumen (i.e. villi or plicae);
- inversions of the epithelium to form tubular structures, the lumina of which communicate with the main lumen;
- formation of complex glands within or exterior to the tract wall.

Examples of these structural modifications will be discussed in relation to specific areas of the digestive tract.

The submucosal layer contains vessels, nerves, and a specialized nerve plexus.

The submucosa lies between the mucosa and the main muscle layer of the digestive tract wall. It is composed of fibroblasts, collagen and acellular matrix, and contains

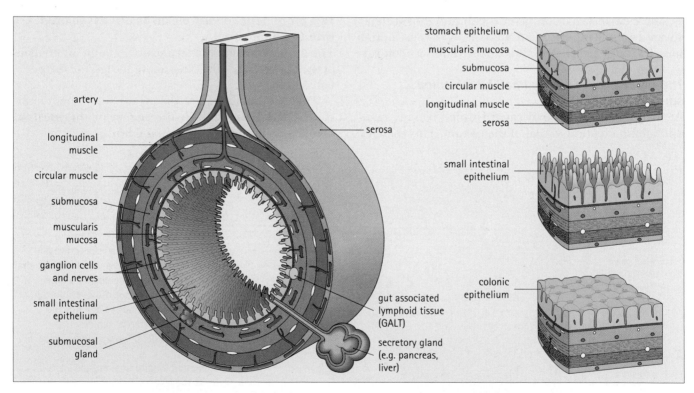

Fig. 11.25 Basic structure of the digestive tract.
The digestive tract is a muscular tube lined internally by specialized epithelium which for most of its length has a combined secretory and absorptive function. Three patterns of epithelial structure (stomach, small intestine and colon) are shown in this diagram.

Externally, the tract has an outer layer of flat mesothelium where it runs through the peritoneal cavity.

Various secretory organs, which are derived embryologically as outgrowths of the putative alimentary tract, lie partly or completely outside it. These organs (e.g. pancreas and liver) produce secretions which are vital for the tract to function normally; they are transferred to the digestive tract lumen by one or more ducts.

blood vessels, lymphatics and nerves which supply or drain their smaller equivalents in the lamina propria of the mucosa.

In addition the submucosa contains clumps of ganglion cells associated with the autonomic nerve supply of the tract, and in some areas contains lymphoid aggregates and follicles, which are part of the gut-associated lymphoid tissue (GALT) (see page 134).

The smooth muscle in the bowel wall is arranged in distinct layers which are each oriented in different directions.

The musculature of the alimentary tract is responsible for moving the luminal contents along the tract gradually from mouth to anus. It therefore extends beyond the digestive part of the tract into the transport passages (i.e. the oropharynx, esophagus and the anal canal). Movement is achieved by peristalsis, whereby a wave of contraction moves distally, forcing the luminal contents onward into the relaxed segment ahead.

There are two layers of smooth muscle throughout most of the digestive tract and a third layer in the stomach (see below). Traditionally identified as an outer longitudinal layer and an inner circular layer, they are in fact arranged spirally, with the inner circular layer being a compact spiral, and the outer longitudinal layer being a more elongated helix (i.e. a similar arrangement to that of the smooth muscle of the ureter, see Fig. 15.40).

Between the two main smooth muscle layers of the digestive tract are small blood and lymphatic vessels, together with the nerves and ganglion cells of the autonomic nervous system.

The basic pattern of two muscle layers that extend into the transport passages of the alimentary tract, proximally into the esophagus and distally into the anal canal, is modified by the presence of some skeletal muscle.

Localized thickenings of muscle in the bowel wall act as valves and are called sphincters.

In some areas, the basic muscle pattern is also modified by a localized increase in the circular muscle to act as a sphincter. Sphincter contraction occludes the lumen and thus prevents the passage of the luminal contents.

The pyloric sphincter is the most important sphincter and is located at the junction between the stomach and duodenum. By contracting, it delays stomach emptying, thereby permitting continued food breakdown in the stomach.

The esophagogastric sphincter is located between the lower esophagus and proximal stomach; it normally prevents reflux of gastric contents into the esophagus.

The ileocecal valve is situated between the terminal ileum and cecum; it delays discharge of ileal contents into the cecum.

The internal anal sphincter, sited at the upper end of the anal canal, retains fecal waste material in the rectum until controlled defecation.

The outer coat of the bowel wall is called the adventitia, being covered in some parts by peritoneum.

The adventitia is the outer coat of the digestive tract and surrounds the external layer of muscle. It is composed of loosely arranged fibroblasts and collagen embedded in matrix, with variable numbers of adipocytes.

The adventitia contains large blood and lymphatic vessels and nerves, the major arterial supply and venous drainage of the tract wall passing through it.

Some of the digestive tract is retroperitoneal but most is within the peritoneal cavity, and here the outer surface of the adventitia over much of its circumference is covered by a layer of flattened epithelium, the mesothelium (visceral peritoneum). This is identical to and continuous with the mesothelium lining the peritoneal cavity internally and covering the mesenteric attachment of the alimentary tract to the posterior abdominal wall (parietal peritoneum).

Adventitia covered by mesothelium (i.e. adventitia of stomach, most of small intestine and large intestine) is commonly called the **serosa**. Where adventitia is not covered by a mesothelium (i.e. adventitia of part of the duodenum and some of the colon), it merges with adjacent tissues.

Immunologic defense against antigens ingested in the digestive tract is provided by the gut-associated lymphoid tissue (GALT).

Throughout the digestive tract, the lamina propria contains cells of the immune system (see Chapter 8), including lymphocytes, plasma cells and macrophages. In addition to these cells there are individual intraepithelial lymphocytes (see below).

The lymphoid cells are commonly arranged as large follicles, often with germinal centers, and are partly located in the mucosa and partly in submucosa, thus splitting the muscularis mucosae. In the ileum, the follicles aggregate to form substantial nodules called Peyer's patches (see page 134).

Although lymphoid follicles and Peyer's patches contain both B and T lymphocytes, the diffuse, non-follicular infiltrate in the lamina propria is composed largely of T lymphocytes.

The mucosal epithelial cells that overlie the lymphoid follicles and Peyer's patches differ from the usual epithelial cells in both structure and function, and are called M cells (Fig. 11.26). They are cuboidal or flat rather than tall columnar, and have luminal microfolds rather than tall microvilli.

Fig. 11.26 Gut–associated lymphoid tissue (GALT).
Micrograph showing the typical arrangement of a nodule of
gut-associated lymphoid tissue (GALT) in the lamina propria.
The epithelial cells (M cells), closely associated with the
lymphoid aggregate, are cuboidal and show no cytoplasmic
specialization such as mucin droplet formation. Note the intraepithelial lymphocytes (IEL).

M cells are believed to take up antigenic macromolecules
from the intestinal lumen, incorporating them into endocytotic vesicles, and then transporting them to the lateral intercellular space in the region of an intra-epithelial
lymphocyte.

The gut has both intrinsic and extrinsic innervation.

The intrinsic innervation is collections of nerves and ganglion cells in the submucosa which form an interconnected network called submucosal (Meissner's) plexus
(Fig. 11.27a), while collections of nerves and ganglion
cells between the inner circular and outer longitudinal
components of the muscularis proper form a network
called myenteric (Auerbach's) plexus (Fig. 11.27b).

The extrinsic system comprises an autonomic input
from parasympathetic (stimulatory) and sympathetic
(inhibitory) abdominal plexuses which modulate the
activity of the intrinsic innervation of the gut. In addition sensory nerves derived from neurons in cranial and
spinal nuclei terminate in the bowel as tendril-like sensory endings.

The afferent autonomic impulses mediate visceral
reflexes and sensations such as hunger and rectal fullness.

The viscera are insensitive to pain, any painful sensations resulting from excessive contraction or distension
of the bowel muscle, or from the sensory nerves in the
peritoneum.

Fig. 11.27 Intrinsic innervation.
(a) High-power micrograph showing a cluster of ganglion cells (G) in the small bowel submucosa (Meissner's plexus).
(b) High-power micrograph showing clusters of ganglion cells (G) between the two muscle layers (M) of the muscularis proper (myenteric or Auerbach's plexus).

STOMACH

From the esophagus, food enters the stomach, which is a dilated portion of the digestive tract where fragmented food is retained while it is macerated and partially digested. At the lower end of the stomach, the pyloric sphincter (see page 195) prevents the passage of food until it is converted into a thick semi-liquid paste or pulp (chyme).

There are three layers of muscle in the stomach wall.

The muscular wall of the stomach differs from the standard digestive tract pattern by the presence of a third layer of oblique muscle fibers. These lie internal to the circular layer and assist in the complex churning action necessary to mix food thoroughly with the secretions of the gastric mucosa.

Fig. 11.28 Gastric mucous cells.
In this high-power micrograph, the gastric surface mucous cells have basal nuclei (N) and bulky luminal cytoplasm (C) filled with pale-staining mucus. As the neck region is approached (arrow) the cells (neck mucous cells) are smaller and contain less mucus. Note the prominent capillaries (Cap) and lymphoid cells (L) in the lamina propria.

The stomach muscle layers are thick. When contracted they decrease the stomach capacity and the mucosa is thrown up into longitudinal folds called rugae, which are most prominent on the convexity of the stomach (the greater curve). This is the state of the stomach when it is empty; when full the musculature relaxes and thins and the rugae stretch flat as the stomach distends.

The stomach is ideally equipped for its role as a reservoir by its distensibility, the presence of the pyloric sphincter, and the mechanisms preventing reflux at its upper end.

The gastric epithelium secretes hydrochloric acid, digestive enzymes and mucus. It also contains a population of hormone-secreting cells.

Food is converted into chyme by the secretions of the gastric mucosa into the lumen.

These are:

- a dilute solution of hydrochloric acid (approximately 0.16N);
- solutions of proteolytic enzymes, mainly pepsin;
- small amounts of other enzymes (e.g. rennin and gastric lipase);
- mucins, mainly in the form of neutral mucins.

The major functions of the gastric epithelium are the secretion of acid and digestive enzymes. It also secretes mucus to lubricate ingested food and to protect itself from the corrosive effects of the acid and enzymes. The surface area of the stomach epithelium is increased by downgrowths which form glands.

The secretions are produced by three main cell types. In addition there is a population of endocrine cells and population of stem cells from which the other cells types are derived. The cell types are:

- mucous cells,
- acid-producing cells (oxyntic or parietal cells);
- enzyme-producing cells (chief cells or peptic cells);
- stem cells;
- enteroendocrine cells.

Gastric mucous cells are of two types: surface mucous cells and neck mucous cells.

Surface mucous cells (Fig. 11.28) are tall and columnar with basal nuclei and clear-staining luminal cytoplasm distended by numerous small mucin vacuoles which are discharged into the stomach lumen by exocytosis. The cells also have prominent endoplasmic reticulum and the Golgi complex is located above the nucleus.

The luminal surface of surface mucous cells shows scanty short microvilli with a surface glycocalyx, and junctional complexes join adjacent cells near the luminal surface.

The lateral borders of the cells are often separated by a considerable intercellular gap, which is traversed by cytoplasmic protrusions of the lateral walls; this separation disappears as the apical surface is neared where the binding of adjacent cells is very tight. Surface mucous cells are also thought to produce blood group substances.

Neck mucous cells are smaller and less regular in shape than surface mucous cells, mainly because they are compressed and distorted by adjacent cells. They have a basal nucleus and finely granular cytoplasm due to the presence of small mucin vacuoles which are considerably smaller than those in the surface mucous cells.

The vacuoles are distributed throughout the cytoplasm and are not aggregated near the luminal surface as they are in the surface mucous cells. By light microscopy it is not always apparent that neck mucous cells contain mucin, and a PAS stain is often necessary to highlight it.

The acid-producing cells of the stomach are called parietal cells.

The acid-producing cells are large pyramidal cells with central nuclei and pale eosinophilic cytoplasm. The cytoplasm often appears vacuolated, particularly around the nucleus. The cell attachment to the basement membrane is broad, but their luminal aspect is narrow, being compressed between adjacent cells. Despite this these cells have a vast luminal surface area as a result of deep microvilli-lined invaginations producing so-called canaliculi (Fig. 11.29).

In the cytoplasm close to the canaliculi are clusters of round or oval vesicles which have clear centers and distinct membrane borders, and are thought to be involved in the transfer of substances from the cytoplasm to the lumen of the canalicular system. The rest of the cytoplasm is packed with round or oval mitochondria with closely packed cristae. This high concentration of mitochondria is responsible for the eosinophilia of the cell cytoplasm, particularly at the periphery. A small Golgi and some rough endoplasmic reticulum are also present.

Parietal cells also produce intrinsic factor, the glycoprotein that avidly binds to vitamin B12 to render it absorbable by the digestive tract.

ACID-PRODUCING CELLS

The acid-producing cells have abundant carbonic anhydrase, which is thought to play a vital role in generating H^+ ions for the production of hydrochloric acid (HCl).

Carbon dioxide diffuses across the basement membrane from blood capillaries into the cell, where it links with water molecules (a reaction catalyzed by carbonic anhydrase) to produce carbonic acid (H_2CO_3); this instantly dissociates into a H^+ ion and a HCO_3^- ion. The latter passes back into the blood, while the H^+ is pumped into the lumen of a canaliculus. Chloride ions (Cl^-) are actively transported across the cell into the canaliculus from the capillaries in the lamina propria.

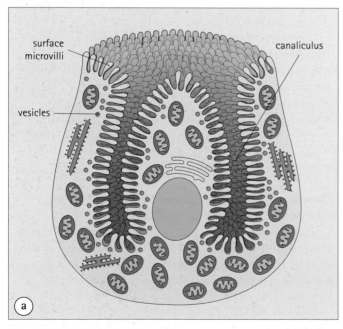

Fig. 11.29 Acid–producing cells.
(a) The acid-producing cell has an intricate system of invaginations (canaliculi) lined by microvilli, which produce the perinuclear vacuolated appearance seen on light microscopy. The rest of the cytoplasm is packed with mitochondria, particularly at the cell periphery. A small Golgi and some rough endoplasmic reticulum are also present, with vesicles close to the canaliculi.

(b) Electron micrograph showing the intricate canalicular system (C) of an acid-producing cell; the cytoplasm is largely occupied by tightly packed mitochondria (M).

Chief cells secrete the enzyme pepsin.

The enzyme-producing cells of the stomach are also known as chief or peptic cells They have large basal nuclei and contain eosinophilic refractile cytoplasmic granules and a rich rough endoplasmic reticulum (Fig. 11.30 and 11.31); they therefore resemble the exocrine cells of the pancreas (see page 207).

The granules contain the inactive enzyme precursor, pepsinogen, which is disgorged into the gastric lumen where it is converted by gastric acid into the active proteolytic enzyme, pepsin.

Pepsin is a potent enzyme, breaking down large protein molecules into small peptides, and converting almost all of the structural proteins into soluble small molecular weight substances; it is largely responsible for the conversion of solid food particles to fluid chyme.

STEM CELLS
The epithelial cells of the gastric mucosa are formed from stem cells

Stem cells are the precursor cells of all epithelial cells of the gastric mucosa. They are small cells with oval basal nuclei and show no cytoplasmic specialization when completely undifferentiated, but are capable of differentiating into mucous, acid-producing, enzyme-producing or endocrine cells.

Normally present in very small numbers in humans, they increase in number and activity when the gastric epithelium is continually damaged, for example in chronic irritation of the gastric mucosa (i.e. chronic gastritis). A surge of stem cell activity enables an ulcerated area of the stomach to be rapidly re-epithelialized. Such regeneration is an important final step in the healing of a stomach ulcer.

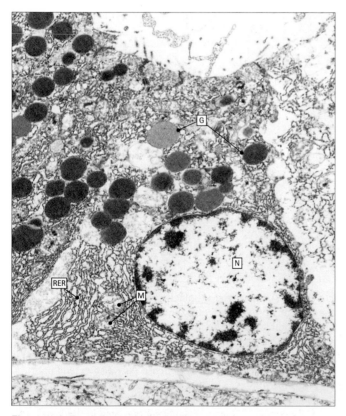

Fig. 11.30 Enzyme-producing cells.
Electron micrograph of an enzyme-producing cell showing its large basal nucleus (N), abundant mitochondria (M), abundant rough endoplasmic reticulum (RER), and the gray-staining spherical granules (G), which contain pepsinogen and are responsible for the eosinophilic granular appearance of these cells in H&E stained sections (see Fig. 11.31).

Fig. 11.31 H&E appearance of an acid-producing cell (A) from the body of the stomach. Note the enzyme-producing cells (E, see Fig. 11.30).

Endocrine cells in the gastric mucosa secrete a variety of hormones.

Enteroendocrine cells (see Chapter 14) of the stomach are small and round and are sited on the epithelial basement membrane. In H&E paraffin sections they have a round, central dark-staining nucleus and a rim of clear cytoplasm (Fig. 11.32a).

Ultrastructurally the cytoplasm contains membrane-bound neurosecretory granules, the shape, size, number and electron density varying according to the substance secreted.

Immunocytochemical methods demonstrate that:

- endocrine cells storing and secreting serotonin, somatostatin (Fig. 11.32b) and a vasointestinal polypeptide-like (VIP) substance are present in the cardiac, body and antral regions;
- cells secreting gastrin and a bombesin-like peptide are concentrated in the pyloric mucosa, where gastrin-secreting cells are concentrated mainly in the neck region, with rare scattered cells in the depths of the glands.

Fig. 11.32 Gastric endocrine cells.
ⓐ Micrograph of the base of glands in the body of the stomach showing the H&E appearance of gastric enteroendocrine cells (END). They are small with pale cytoplasm and a small, dark-staining central nucleus. Acid-producing (A) and enzyme-producing (E) cells are also evident.
ⓑ Micrograph of an immunoperoxidase stained section of stomach showing the distribution of somatostatin-secreting endocrine cells in the pyloric gastric mucosa. The cells are numerous in the neck region, with a few scattered cells in the deep glands.

The gastric mucosa can be divided into three histologic zones: a superficial zone, a neck zone and a deep zone.

There are three zonal divisions of the gastric mucosa. The superficial zone is composed of a layer of surface mucous cells with downgrowths which are variously called foveolae, pits or crypts.

The mucous cells lining the pits are not so tall and columnar as those on the surface; in addition they contain less mucin.

The superficial zone is roughly constant in its content and structure throughout the stomach.

The neck zone between the superficial and deep zones is narrow and composed largely of immature stem cells mixed with some neck mucous cells. The immature stem cells proliferate and migrate upward to replenish the predominantly mucous cells of the superficial zone, and downward to replenish the cell types in the glands of the deep zone.

The deep zone is composed of glands, the bases of which lie close to or in the muscularis mucosae, while the upper ends open into the bases of the superficial zone pits.

The structure of the deep zone varies, there being three main histologic patterns which delineate three main areas of the stomach: the cardia, the body and the pylorus (Figs 11.33 and 11.34).

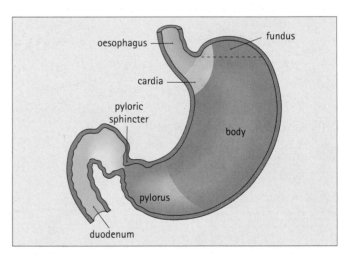

Fig. 11.33 Areas of the stomach.
Diagram of stomach showing the three histologically distinguishable areas. The cardia extends from the squamous/columnar junction at the lower end of the esophagus for a variable distance into the upper stomach, usually 2–3 cm down the lesser curve; cardiac mucosa may also extend part way into the fundus, which is an anatomic rather than a histologic feature.

Pyloric mucosa lines a roughly conical area in the lower third of the stomach, starting about halfway down the lesser curve. The area is very variable and tends to begin higher on the lesser curve in women.

Body mucosa occupies the rest of the stomach, including most of the anatomic fundus. The transition between the various mucosal patterns is commonly gradual, with a narrow junctional zone showing features of both.

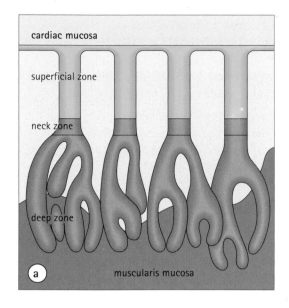

cardiac mucosa

superficial zone

neck zone

deep zone

a

muscularis mucosa

body mucosa

superficial zone

neck zone

deep zone

b

muscularis mucosa

S

N

D

c

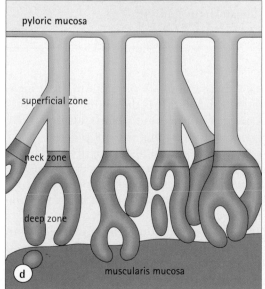

pyloric mucosa

superficial zone

neck zone

deep zone

d

muscularis mucosa

S

N

D

e

Fig. 11.34 Gastric mucosa.

ⓐ **Cardiac mucosa.** The superficial and deep zones of the cardiac mucosa are of about equal thickness. The surface and crypt epithelium is composed of mucous cells, while the deep zone is composed of tubular and branched glands lined by mucous cells, with scattered endocrine and acid-producing cells becoming more numerous near the junction with the body mucosa. Some of the more complex glands are coiled.

The muscularis mucosae is thick and irregular, and often sends bundles of fibers toward the surface, interdigitating with the glands. The histologic appearance of cardiac mucosa is shown in Figs 11.22b and 11.49.

ⓑ **Body mucosa.** The superficial zone of the body mucosa accounts for only 25% or less of the mucosa thickness. Most pits open directly and singly onto the surface, but some fuse before opening, to form a wider crevice.

The deep zone is composed of tightly packed long straight tubular glands that end blindly at the muscularis mucosae. At their upper ends the glands open into the bases of the crypts through a variably constricted neck region. The glands may open into single or larger fused crypts.

The superficial zone is covered by surface mucous cells, with neck mucous cells covering the deeper parts of the pits. At the neck region, neck mucosa cells are mixed with stem cells. The glands are composed of acid-producing cells, enzyme-producing cells, neck mucous cells and scattered endocrine cells.

ⓒ **Body mucosa.** H&E section of body mucosa showing the superficial zone (S) composed of mucus-secreting cells, a narrow neck zone (N) containing mainly stem cells and neck mucous cells, and the deep zone (D), largely composed of acid-producing and enzyme-producing cells.

ⓓ **Pyloric mucosa.** The superficial zone of the pyloric region occupies slightly more than 50% of the mucosal thickness, and the crypts are often branched.

The deep zone is composed of tortuous single or branched glands extending down to the muscularis mucosae.

The cell content of the superficial and neck zones is the same as in the cardiac and body mucosa. The glands are lined by mucous cells, but scattered acid-producing cells and numerous endocrine cells are also present. Acid-producing cells become more numerous close to the pyloric sphincter.

ⓔ **Pyloric mucosa.** H&E section of pyloric mucosa showing the superficial zone (S) occupying about 50% of the mucosal thickness. The narrow neck (N) and substantial deep (D) zones are composed of mucous cells which form branching glands in the deep zone.

GASTRIC ULCER

The stomach normally contains an acid solution, but is protected from the damaging effects of the acid by various mechanisms, including the presence of a thin layer of mucus over the surface of the epithelial cells.

In some circumstances, particularly in association with *Helicobacter pylori* infection, these protective mechanisms break down and the acidic gastric contents damage the mucosa. The resulting death of epithelial cells and lamina propria leads to the formation of a shallow ulcer. Continued exposure of such an unprotected area leads to the formation of a deep ulcer (chronic gastric ulcer), which can extend through the submucosa and the muscle layers (Fig. 11.35), and takes a long time to heal.

If an ulcer penetrates the full thickness of the stomach wall, the wall may perforate and the gastric contents can then pour into the peritoneal cavity, causing peritonitis and often death.

Treatment of gastric ulcer is based on removing or decreasing the levels of gastric acid either by neutralizing them (e.g. with oral alkalis) or by decreasing the amount of gastric acid produced by blocking its secretion by the acid-producing cells (e.g. using H_2 antagonists and proton pump inhibition.

Since gastric acid also enters the first part of the duodenum, this area may also be subject to ulceration (duodenal ulcer), as may the lower esophagus if reflux of gastric acid occurs (see Fig. 11.23).

Fig. 11.35 Chronic gastric ulcer.
Micrograph of an H&E section through a chronic gastric ulcer which has extended through the mucosa (M), submucosa (SM) and muscularis propria (MP).

STOMACH

- There are three layers of smooth muscle in the wall

- Mucosa is divided into cardia, body, and pyloric regions

- Parietal cells are specialized to produce acid and also secrete intrinsic factor

- Chief cells secrete the enzyme pepsin as an inactive precursor, pepsinogen

- Endocrine cells in the mucosa secrete gastrin, bombesin, somatostatin, and VIP

SMALL INTESTINE

INTRODUCTION
When the pyloric sphincter (see page 195) opens, partially digested food (chyme) empties from the stomach into the small intestine, which is the main site for the absorption of amino acids, sugars, fats, and some larger molecules produced by digestion of food. The small intestine also secretes enzymes to complete the digestive processes begun in the stomach. It begins at the pylorus, the distal limit of the stomach, and ends at the ileocecal valve, the proximal limit of the large intestine. At autopsy, when the longitudinal muscle is relaxed, the small intestine usually measures about 6 m, but in life it measures only about 3 m long. It is divided into three sections (duodenum, jejunum, and ileum), although the transitions from one to the other are not precise.

Duodenum is the proximal 20–25 cm of small intestine and is entirely retroperitoneal. It has the shape of a letter C, with the head of the pancreas fitting into its concave edge. The bile and pancreatic ducts open into the duodenum in this concavity.

Jejunum begins where the duodenum emerges from behind the peritoneum and extends to an ill-defined junction with the ileum.

Ileum extends from the jejunum to the ileocecal valve.

The small bowel has several modifications to increase its surface area.

As the major absorptive site, the small intestine shows architectural modifications to its mucosa and submucosa to increase its surface area.

The mucosa and submucosa are thrown up into a large number of folds or plicae arranged circularly around the lumen. These are most prominent in the jejunum (Fig. 11.36a) and are absent from the distal end of the small intestine.

The surface of the plicae is further arranged into villi which protrude into the intestinal lumen (Figs. 11.36 b & c and 11.37). Tubular glands or crypts extend down from the base of the villi to the muscularis mucosae. The small intestine has the standard arrangement of musculature (i.e. an external layer of longitudinal muscle and an inner circular layer) and a substantial submucosa in which GALT (see page 134) is particularly prominent.

Fig. 11.36 Small intestine – general architecture.

(a) Macroscopic view of small intestinal mucosal surface showing tightly packed circumferential mucosal folds or plicae.

(b) Low-power micrograph of the plicae (P) showing their complex mucosal surface, which is composed of large villi (V).

(c) Micrograph showing the villi (V) protruding into the small intestinal lumen; note the crypts (C) between their bases.

Fig. 11.37 In two dimensions, the villi appear to have the same structure, but in three dimensions their structure can be seen to correspond to one of three main patterns; they are either finger-like (F), leaf-like (L), or ridge-like (R), as shown in this scanning electron micrograph. There are also occasional intermediate forms. The proportions of these patterns vary from site to site and also with age. In babies and young children the villi of the duodenum and proximal jejunum are almost entirely leaf or ridge-like, finger-like villi appearing with age. The adult pattern is present by 10–15 years.

GLUTEN ENTEROPATHY (CELIAC DISEASE)

The absorptive function of the jejunum depends on the integrity of the villi. If enough villi are damaged, food material can not be absorbed, leading to weight loss, diarrhea, etc.

One important cause of extensive loss of villi is celiac disease, due to allergy to the wheat protein, gluten. The resulting immune-mediated inflammation leads to flattening of the jejunal surface with extensive loss of villi (Fig. 11.38).

Gluten enteropathy commonly presents in babies and young children with failure to thrive and to gain normal height and weight for their age.

The villi usually assume their normal structure when wheat and its products are excluded from the diet (i.e. a gluten-free diet), and the malabsorptive state subsequently improves.

Fig. 11.38 Gluten enteropathy (celiac disease). Micrograph of villous damage resulting from gluten sensitivity. The jejunal mucosal surface is flattened due to extensive loss of villi. Compare with Fig. 11.36c.

There are three functional zones of small intestinal epithelium.

The small intestinal epithelium can be divided into three functional zones. These are the villi, the crypts, and the neck zone where villi and crypts merge. The features of the villi are discussed with Fig. 11.39, and crypt structure is illustrated in Figures 11.40 and 11.41.

The cells of the epithelium are enterocytes, mucous cells, Paneth cells, endocrine cells and stem cells, and their numbers and distribution vary in the different zones of the epithelium.

Enterocytes are the main cell in the villi and are absorptive in function.

Enterocytes are tall columnar cells with round or oval nuclei in the lower third of the cell.

The luminal surface of enterocytes is highly specialized; each cell bears 2–3000 tightly packed, tall microvilli, which are coated by a glycoprotein, the glycocalyx (see Fig. 11.39c). This is composed of fine filamentous extensions of the microvillous cell membrane.

The glycocalyx contains a number of enzymes (brush border enzymes e.g. lactase, sucrase, peptidases, lipases and alkaline phosphatase), which are important in digestion and transport (see Fig. 11.39e).

Beneath the microvillous surface, the enterocyte cytoplasm contains lysosomes and smooth endoplasmic reticulum and paired centrioles in the terminal web region (see Fig. 3.15). Nearer the nucleus the cell is rich in rough endoplasmic reticulum and mitochondria and there is a prominent Golgi. Between the nucleus and the basement membrane are mitochondria and many ribosomes and polyribosomes. The lateral walls of enterocytes show complex interdigitations, and are the sites of Na^+ and K^+ ATPase activity. The lateral walls are separated from the microvillous surface by desmosomes and tight junctions (see Fig. 3.7).

The ultrastructural features of the enterocyte are linked to its absorptive function, and therefore many of the features and mechanisms are common to other active absorptive cells, such as those of the proximal convoluted tubule cell of the kidney. These absorptive mechanisms are illustrated and discussed in Chapter 15.

Fig. 11.39 Small intestine villus.
(a) Thin acrylic resin stained with H&E, showing a single villus which is covered by tall enterocytes (E) bearing a prominent microvillous brush border (MV). Scattered among the enterocytes are occasional mucous cells (M) and intra-epithelial lymphocytes (L). The stromal core contains small capillaries and lymphatics (not shown) and a number of lymphocytes, plasma cells and macrophages.
(b) Electron micrograph of a row of enterocytes. Note the microvillous border (MV), part of a mucous cell (M) and the endocrine cell with basal granules (E).
(c) Electron micrograph of microvillous brush border (MV) at high magnification. The glycocalyx (G) can be seen as a faint grayish haze on the surface of the microvilli.
(d) Scanning electron micrograph of part of the villus surface. Note the tightly packed enterocytes, the microvilli of which are partly obscured by the layer of glycocalyx. Mucous cells discharging their mucus (M) are clearly seen.
(e) Histochemical preparation of small intestine showing the distribution of the enzyme lactase (blue staining), which is localized to the luminal surface of the enterocytes. Like many other cell-bound enzymes responsible for food breakdown in the small intestine, the enzyme molecules reside in the glycocalyx.

Mucous (goblet) cells are mainly found in the upper two-thirds of the crypts.

Occasional mucous cells are scattered among the enterocytes of the villi (see Figs. 11.39a and c).

Mucous cells contain globules of mucin in their luminal cytoplasm, the mucin being discharged onto the surface when the cytoplasm is fully expanded by mucin granules. The scanty basal cytoplasm is rich in rough endoplasmic reticulum.

Mucous cells are least frequent in the duodenum, and increase in number in the jejunum and ileum, being most numerous in the terminal ileum close to the cecum.

Paneth cells are found in the lower third of the crypts.

Paneth cells have basal nuclei and prominent large eosinophilic granules in their luminal cytoplasm (Fig. 11.40). Ultrastructurally these granules are spherical and electron-dense, the remaining cytoplasm being rich in rough endoplasmic reticulum; these are features of a protein-secreting cell (see Fig. 3.20).

Paneth cells contain substances called defensins which are secreted and protect against infection.

Endocrine cells are located mainly in the lower third of the crypts, but are also seen higher up in the villi.

Endocrine cells in the small bowel resemble those seen in the stomach (see Fig. 11.32), being roughly triangular in shape, the broad base being in contact with the basement membrane, the narrow apex reaching the lumen. Their nuclei are spherical and their cytoplasm pale staining (Fig. 11.41).

Ultrastructurally, the cytoplasm contains neuroendocrine granules, and the luminal surface bears microvilli.

Small intestinal endocrine cells secrete a number of hormones and peptides, including serotonin (5HT), enteroglucagon, somatostatin, secretin, gastrin, motilin and vasoactive intestinal peptide (VIP).

Stem cells are found in the lower third of the crypts.

The replication of stem cells replenishes the stock of the other cells, including the Paneth and endocrine cells. Most replication is to replace the mucous cells and enterocytes of the villi since these cells have a rapid turnover, being shed from the tips of the villi about 5 days after production.

Before developing into the mature form of the two cell types, the stem cells differentiate into intermediate cells, which show some features of both mucous cells and enterocytes. These cells occupy much of the upper two-thirds of the crypts.

Stem cells and intermediate cells are particularly numerous when there is increased cell loss from the villi, which is a common feature of many diseases affecting the small intestine; the crypts increase in length and show increased numbers of cells in mitosis (i.e. crypt or gland hyperplasia).

The lamina propria of the small intestine is most clearly seen in the core of the villi, but also surrounds and supports the gland crypts.

The lamina propria of the small bowel is composed of collagen, reticulin fibers, fibroblasts and glycosaminoglycan matrix, through which run blood capillaries, lymphatics and nerves. It contains some smooth muscle fibers.

Fig. 11.40 Paneth cells.
Micrograph of the base of a small intestinal crypt from a paraffin section showing numerous Paneth cells (P) containing large numbers of bright red granules. A small endocrine cell (E) with ill-defined fine basal eosinophilic granules can also be seen.

Fig. 11.41 Endocrine cell.
Micrograph of the base of a small intestinal crypt showing a typical pale-staining entero-endocrine cell (E). In this thin acrylic resin section the Paneth cell (P) granules are difficult to see.

The blood vessels and lymphatics are particularly prominent in the villi, a central lymphatic (lacteal) running vertically down the centre of the core of each villus.

The lamina propria also contains lymphocytes, plasma cells, eosinophils, macrophages and mast cells.

The **lymphocytes** are largely T lymphocytes (approximately 70% T-helper and 30% T-suppressor, see Chapter 8); most of the **plasma cells** are IgA-producers. Lymphocytes are also present in the villous epithelium, usually in a basal position between the lateral intercellular spaces and, like those in the lamina propria, they are also T lymphocytes, but the subset pattern is different, about 80% being T-suppressor, the rest being T-helper types.

Eosinophils are common in the lamina propria throughout the digestive tract.

Macrophages are found mainly beneath the basement membrane in the upper reaches of the villi. They are thought to engulf particulate antigens and to ingest soluble antigens before presenting them to T lymphocytes.

Mast cells are seen mainly in the crypt region.

The submucosa of the small bowel contains vessels, lymphoid tissue and nerves.

The small intestinal submucosa contains lymphatics, blood vessels and the submucosal plexus of nerves and ganglion cells. In addition it contains part of the larger lymphoid aggregates of the gut-associated lymphoid tissue, which cross the muscularis mucosae.

In the first part of the duodenum the submucosa contains mucus-secreting Brunner's glands.

The small intestine has regional specializations in duodenum, jejunum and ileum.

The duodenum differs from the rest of the small intestine as follows:

- it is entirely retroperitoneal;
- its villous pattern contains a high proportion of leaf and ridge forms (see Fig. 11.37);
- it contains prominent mucus-secreting submucosal glands (Brunner's glands, Fig. 11.42); which penetrate and split the muscularis mucosae so that some acini are located within the lamina propria of the mucosa;
- it receives secretions of glands located outside the digestive tract through long ducts; these glands are the liver (see Chapter 12) and the exocrine component of the pancreas (see page 207).

Brunner's glands are similar to the submucosal glands of the pyloric region of the stomach, being composed of mucous cells lining short ducts which open into the bases or sides of the crypts of the mucosa. Brunner's glands secrete an alkaline mucoid material (pH 8.0–9.5) which may protect the duodenal mucosa from the acid chyme, bringing its pH toward the level at which the pancreatic enzymes are most effective.

Brunner's glands are also thought to secrete urogastrone, a peptide that inhibits acid secretion by the stomach. Endocrine cells can be demonstrated in these glands immunocytochemically.

The **jejunum** is the main absorptive site of the digestive tract, and shows not only the greatest development of plical folds (see Fig. 11.36a), but also the most complex villous system, with finger-like villi being predominant.

The **ileum** is characterized by the greatest development of GALT. The lymphoid cells aggregate into large nodules (Peyer's patches), which expand the lamina propria of the mucosa, split the muscularis mucosae and extend into the submucosa.

SMALL BOWEL

- Characterized by a mucosa raised into finger-like villi which contain abundant blood vessels and lymphatics

- Lined by columnar epithelium with goblet cells. Glycocalyx of surface epithelium has enzymes – for example, lactase and alkaline phosphatase

- Duodenum is associated with submucosal mucous glands (Brunner's glands)

- Contains mucosal endocrine cells which secrete gut hormones

- Has two layers of muscularis propria separated by a myenteric nerve plexus

Fig. 11.42 Brunner's glands. The first part of the duodenum is characterized by the presence of large, fluid-secreting mucous glands called Brunner's glands (B), which empty into the neck of the crypts (C). The Brunner's glands are partly located in the lower mucosa, but pass through the muscularis mucosae (MM) into the submucosa.

EXOCRINE PANCREAS

The exocrine pancreas is a glandular organ which secretes into the gut via a main duct system.

The pancreas is a long thin tapering structure extending from its head, which occupies the space formed by the concavity of the duodenum, to its tail, which is situated in the left hypochondrium near the hilum of the spleen.

The main pancreatic duct joins the distal end of the bile duct to open into the lumen of the duodenum at a small raised mound, the **ampulla of Vater**.

The pancreas has a thin, ill-defined fibrocollagenous capsule from which narrow irregular septae penetrate it, dividing it into lobules. Each lobule is composed of roughly spherical clusters (acini) of secretory exocrine cells (Fig. 11.43). Each acinus has an individual intra-acinar duct, which drains into progressively larger ducts.

Pancreatic exocrine cells are protein-secreting cells.

The acini are composed of protein-secreting cells (pancreatic acinar cells) which have a broad base and narrow apical surface covered by a few short microvilli.

The cells are rich in rough endoplasmic reticulum, which is concentrated mainly in the lower half of the cell, and is responsible for their cytoplasmic basophilia. The

upper half of the cell, close to the lumen, contains variable numbers of eosinophilic zymogen granules, which contain the pre-enzymes synthesized by the cell (Fig. 11.43a). Some cells contain large numbers of these granules, while others, which contain few or none, are thought to have recently disgorged their granules by exocytosis into the acinar lumen. It is thought that the pre-enzymes are synthesized by the rough endoplasmic reticulum and then transferred to the Golgi, which packages them into granules.

The pancreatic acinar cells produce and secrete the precursors of a wide range of enzymes.

The secretions of pancreatic exocrine cells are involved in the breakdown of food in the lumen of the duodenum, and include proteolytic enzymes (particularly trypsinogen, chymotrypsinogen, procarboxypeptidases A and B and proelastase) and lipolytic enzymes (prophospholipase and prolipase). The pancreas also secretes amylase, cholesterol esterase and ribonucleases.

Activation of the proenzymes occurs only in the duodenal cavity, with the conversion of trypsinogen to active trypsin by an enterokinase located in the duodenal brush border triggering a cascade of reactions in which the inactive precursors are converted to active enzymes.

Pancreatic secretion is alkaline due to the selective secretion of bicarbonate ions, which is thought to be performed by the ductular system rather than by the acinar cells.

The control of pancreatic secretions is mainly mediated through hormones, the most important being secretin and cholecystokinin (pancreozymin).

Secretin stimulates the formation of the bicarbonate rich fluid. Cholecystokinin is thought to stimulate the acinar cells to release their enzymes. Secretin and cholecystokinin are produced by the endocrine cells of the digestive tract mucosa, in response to the entry of acidic gastric contents into the duodenum.

Pancreatic secretions run in a ramified ductal system which merges into a main pancreatic duct.

The pancreatic ductal system begins in the acinus. Pale-staining centro-acinar cells represent the intra-acinar component of the intercalated duct, are lined by a simple monolayer of cuboidal epithelium, and form a complex network (Fig. 11.43b).

The intercalated ducts from individual acini fuse to form larger interlobular ducts, which run in the fibrocollagenous septa between the ill-defined pancreatic lobules and are lined by columnar epithelium.

Interlobular ducts join the main pancreatic ducts, which run longitudinally from the tail of the pancreas to its head and empty into the duodenal lumen at the ampulla of Vater. The main pancreatic ducts are lined by tall columnar epithelium containing a number of mucin-secreting goblet cells.

Fig. 11.43 Exocrine pancreas (a) Acini with acinar cells (PA) and eosinophilic zymogen granules (ZG) close to the lumen. (b) Part of the ductular system with centro-acinar cells (C) arising from the acini (A) as the intra-acinar component of the intercalated duct (D).

LARGE INTESTINE

The large intestine modifies the fluid content of feces as it passes for elimination.

The large intestine comprises the:

- cecum;
- ascending, transverse and descending colon;
- sigmoid colon;
- rectum.

The structure of the large intestine is fairly constant throughout, although there are regional variations, particularly between the cecum and the rectum.

The main function of the large intestine is to convert the liquid small intestinal contents to solid indigestible waste material, feces. This is achieved by extensive reabsorption of water and soluble salts from the bowel content, until it is semi-solid. With increasing solidity, mucin is required to lubricate its passage along the bowel. The **appendix** is a small appendage arising from the cecum.

The large intestinal epithelium is specialized for mucous secretion, salt and water absorption.

The epithelial component of the mucosa of the large bowel is a mixture of absorptive cells and mucous cells. These are arranged as simple, straight, non-branching tubular downgrowths extending from the surface to the muscularis mucosae. The cell types present are columnar cells, mucous cells, stem cells and endocrine cells (see Fig. 11.44).

Fig. 11.44 Large intestine.
(a) Micrograph showing large intestine mucosa. The surface is flat and simple straight tubular glands (TG) extend down to the muscularis mucosae (MM).
(b) The glands are lined by two populations of cells, the most numerous but less obvious being compressed tall columnar cells (C). The more easily seen cells are the mucous cells (mucus-secreting goblet cells, G), here stained blue by alcian blue.

(c) High-power micrograph showing both columnar cells (C) and goblet cells (G) in the upper part of the tubular gland, while the surface cells (S) are mainly columnar and contain little mucin.
(d) At the bases of the glands the cell population is a combination of uncommitted stem cells (S), goblet cells (G), columnar cells (C) and occasional small pale-staining endocrine cells (E).

Other epithelial cells are found adjacent to the lymphoid aggregates in the lamina propria and are tightly packed cuboidal or columnar epithelial cells which have relatively high nucleus to cytoplasm ratio and do not contain mucin. These cells are similar to the M cells associated with the lymphoid tissue in the small intestine.

Columnar cells are the most numerous type of epithelial cell in the large intestine. They are narrow slender cells and appear to be in a minority because they are compressed between the much larger mucous (goblet) cells. Their luminal surfaces have a microvillous brush border and there is evidence that they can produce and secrete a neutral polysaccharide, possibly glycocalyx material.

Columnar cells are thought to carry out the salt and water absorptive function of the colon. They lack brush border enzymes and so play no part in digestive breakdown, but have prominent lateral intercellular spaces, which suggests active fluid transport. Furthermore they are well equipped with Na^+ and K^+ ATPases in the lateral cell membranes.

Mucous cells possess large numbers of mucin granules, which produce the bulging rounded cytoplasm responsible for their synonym **goblet cells**. The mucin vacuoles are larger in the sigmoid colon and rectum than in the cecum and ascending colon, and there appears to be a difference in the type of mucin secreted. Mucin from the colon and rectum is highly sulfated; that from the cecum and ascending colon is less sulfated, and contains sialic acid radicals.

As the goblet cells approach the surface of the large intestine, they begin to discharge their mucus and continue to migrate upwards to form part of the surface epithelium, which is mainly composed of columnar cells.

Stem cells are the precursors of other cell types.

Stem cells form all of the specialized cells of the large bowel mucosa. They are located at the bases of the tubular down-growths and can develop into either mucous or columnar cells or into large intestinal endocrine cells.

Endocrine cells are comparatively few in number in the large bowel and are scattered among the other cells.

In the large bowel, endocrine cells are mainly in the lower half of each tubular downgrowth and have a broad base, narrowing to a small luminal surface covered with microvilli. Their neuroendocrine granules are situated basal to the nucleus and can sometimes be seen as small eosinophilic dots in H&E paraffin sections.

Immunocytochemical methods have shown that these cells contain a number of substances related to their endocrine function including chromogranin, substance P, somatostatin, and glucagon.

The large intestinal lamina propria consists of collagen, reticulin, and fibroblasts embedded in a glycosaminoglycan matrix.

There is a layer of compact collagen immediately beneath the basement membrane of the surface epithelium.

The cell content of the lamina propria includes lymphocytes and scattered eosinophils, the lymphocytes being mainly T cells. Also present are small lymphoid follicles (part of the GALT, see page 195), the larger of which breach the muscularis mucosae and extend into the submucosa. Cells containing PAS-positive granules, known as **muciphages**, are a common finding, particularly in the rectum.

The muscularis mucosae consists of a two-layered smooth muscle arrangement.

The muscularis mucosae of the large bowel has an inner circular and an outer longitudinal layer, but this distinction is usually only clear in abnormally thickened muscle layers. Elastic fibers are also present.

The muscularis mucosae is penetrated by fine nerve twigs from the submucosal plexus, the fine nerves continuing vertically into the lamina propria. The innervation of the colon is particularly important in the diagnosis of Hirschsprung's disease (see Fig. 11.47).

The muscularis propria is responsible for the main propulsive forces in the bowel wall.

The muscularis propria of the large intestine consists of an inner circular muscle layer and an outer longitudinal layer which is not continuous, being concentrated into three bands, the **taeniae coli**. These muscle layers are responsible for propulsion of the gut contents by peristalsis.

LARGE BOWEL

- Mucosa specialized for water and salt absorption and mucus secretion

- Mucosa characterized by long straight tubular glands of columnar epithelium containing goblet cells and absorptive cells

- Two layers to muscularis propria with intervening myenteric nerve plexus. Outer longitudinal muscle arranged as narrow bands (taeniae coli)

APPENDIX

The appendix has the same basic structure as the large bowel.

The appendix is a small, blind-ending tubular diverticulum arising from the cecum. It is normally 5–10 cm long and about 0.8 cm in diameter. Both measurements vary from person to person, but its diameter decreases with increasing age, being at its greatest at 7–20 years of age.

The wall of the appendix is composed of a muscularis propria, which has an outer longitudinal and an inner circular component like the rest of the digestive tract. The submucosa contains blood vessels, nerves and variable amounts of lymphoid tissue.

In children, the lamina propria and the submucosa contain abundant lymphoid tissue with prominent follicle formation (Fig. 11.45a). This is not present at birth, but progressively populates the appendix over the first 10 years of life, thereafter progressively disappearing, so that the normal adult appendix shows only traces of this tissue (Fig. 11.45b).

As the lymphoid tissue atrophies in the adult, the submucosa becomes progressively more collagenous, and in the elderly the mucosa itself may become more fibrotic, particularly near the tip.

The mucosal epithelium of the appendix is colonic in nature.

The mucosa of the appendix is composed of straight tubular glands containing tall columnar absorptive cells, mucin-secreting goblet cells and some enteroendocrine cells, which are mainly found in the bases of the glands. Enteroendocrine cells are also found in the submucosa, closely related to nerves and ganglion cells, particularly near the closed tip of the appendix.

Fig. 11.45 Appendix.
(a) Transverse section of appendix from a 10-year-old child. It is lined by large bowel type mucosa (M) in which there are large lymphoid follicles (F) extending into the submucosa (SM).

(b) Transverse section of appendix from a 36-year-old man at the same magnification as in (a). Note the relative reduction in size and the virtual disappearance of the lymphoid follicles (F).

DISORDERS OF THE LARGE BOWEL

The colon and rectum are subject to a number of disorders, many of which are transient, and the result of dietary indiscretion for example, following the ingestion of large quantities of beer! The three most important diseases of long duration in adults are:

- **cancer** of the large bowel epithelium

- **diverticular disease**, in which increased pressure in the bowel lumen forces mucosa through the muscle layers

- **ulcerative colitis**, which is a severe ulcerating disease of the colonic mucosa.

Ulcerative colitis

The cause of ulcerative colitis is not known, but large bowel mucosa is lost over an extensive area, with ulceration and destruction of the absorptive epithelium (Fig. 11.46).

This mucosal damage impairs water resorption from the colonic contents, and thus the normal solid feces are replaced by large quantities of watery diarrhea, which is similar in content and texture to the contents of the ileum. Destruction of the mucosa also leads to bleeding, so the watery diarrhea is often mixed with blood.

Hirschsprung's disease

In infants and children the most important disease of the large bowel is **Hirschsprung's disease**, in which defecation is not possible because a segment of the lower rectum is completely devoid of ganglion cells in the submucosa and muscularis layers. Normal innervation has been described on page 196 and illustrated in Fig. 11.27.

The affected segment of bowel is narrowed and the child's abdomen distends with unpassed feces, fatal perforation occurring if it is not treated.

Although the abnormality primarily affects the lower rectum, the aganglionic segment may be extensive, involving much of the distal colon.

Diagnosis is confirmed by rectal biopsy establishing that submucosal ganglion cells are absent. A characteristic feature is hypertrophy of preganglionic nerve twigs in the muscularis mucosae, submucosa and lamina propria (Fig. 11.47).

Fig. 11.46 Ulcerative colitis.
Micrograph of wall of sigmoid colon from a patient with ulcerative colitis. Note the complete destruction of the mucosa and some submucosa (SM); only a few scattered remnants of absorptive and mucus-secreting epithelium remain (arrow).

Fig. 11.47 Hirschsprung's disease.
Micrograph showing prominent nerve twigs in the lamina propria (LP), muscularis mucosae (MM) and submucosa (SM). This rectal biopsy from a child with Hirschsprung's disease has been stained by the cholinesterase enzyme histochemical technique.

Fig. 11.48 Esophagus.
This low-power micrograph shows the squamous epithelium (SE) of the lower third of the esophagus and the submucosa (SM), containing esophageal mucous glands (MG) surrounded by a prominent lymphocytic infiltrate. At this level of the esophagus the muscle layers (M) are composed entirely of smooth muscle. Higher in the esophagus there is a moderate amount of striated muscle. The outer adventitial layer (A) contains adipose tissue and a number of nerves and blood vessels.

Fig. 11.49 Esophagogastric junction.
This micrograph shows the junction between the squamous epithelium (SE) of the lower esophagus and the glandular epithelium (GE) of the stomach.

Two patterns of gastric mucosa can be seen, that closest to the esophageal squamous epithelium being cardiac-type (C, see Fig. 11.34a), which in this case forms a narrow zone before gastric mucosa of body-type (B, see Figs 11.34b and 11.34c).

In this region, the submucosa (SM) is highly vascular, as is the adventitial layer (A). The distinction of the muscle layers (M) into circular and longitudinal layers becomes indistinct in the esophagogastric area.

Fig. 11.50 Stomach wall.
Micrograph showing the stomach wall in the body region. The body mucosa is thick and composed largely of glands (G, see Figs 11.22 and 11.34). The distinct muscularis mucosae (MM) can be seen separating the epithelium from a loose textured submucosa (SM). The three muscle layers frequently seen in the stomach are evident. There is an inner oblique (OM) layer, a middle circular (CM) layer and an outer longitudinal (LM) layer. The stomach lies within the peritoneal cavity and its outer coat is therefore a serosal (S) layer covered by mesothelial cells.

Fig. 11.51 Small intestine.

This low-power micrograph from the first part of the jejunum shows the characteristic structure of the small intestinal wall.

The mucosal layer is thrown up into high folds (plicae P, see also Fig. 11.36a), the surfaces of which are modified to form numerous villi (V, see Fig. 11.37). This modification enormously increases the surface area of epithelium exposed to small intestinal contents in the lumen (L).

The submucosa (SM) is highly vascular and the double muscle layer (M) can be seen. The outer surface is covered by serosa (S).

The pattern of extensive plication becomes progressively less marked in the lower reaches of the small intestine.

Fig. 11.52 Colon.

Micrograph showing the colon with its flat surfaced mucosa (M) composed of simple tubular glands (G, see Fig. 11.44). There is a distinct muscularis mucosae (MM), which in this micrograph is breached in one area by a lymphoid aggregate (L) that lies partly in the mucosa and partly in the submucosa. This lymphoid aggregate is part of the GALT.

The submucosa (SM) is loose and fibrocollagenous, allowing movement of the mucosa on the muscle layer.

The muscle layer is composed mainly of circular muscle (CM), but there is a narrow discontinuous longitudinal muscle forming the taeniae coli (TC). There is a prominent collection of ganglia and nerves between the two muscle layers (arrows, see Fig. 11.27).

1. IN THE ORAL CAVITY

(a) the surface of the anterior two-thirds of the tongue is raised in a series of elevations called papillae

(b) taste buds are found around the base of circumvallate papillae and in fungiform papillae

(c) the tongue muscle is composed of complex interlaced pattern of non-striated smooth muscle fibers

(d) the periodontal ligaments tether the teeth in the alveolar sockets of the mandible or maxilla

(e) the floor of the mouth is lined by non-keratinized stratified squamous epithelium

2. SALIVARY GLANDS

(a) secrete a watery solution which contains amylase and lysozyme.

(b) the submandibular glands have a mixed population of serous and mucous cells.

(c) the parotid glands are composed of mucous-secreting cells.

(d) contain striated ducts which are lined by ion-pumping cells.

(e) are found on the inner surface of the lips and in the submucosa of the dorsal tongue

3. IN THE STOMACH

(a) acid is produced by chief (peptic) cells

(b) enzyme-producing cells secrete pepsinogen

(c) the mucosa in the body is characterized by long, straight, tubular glands containing acid-producing, enzyme-producing, mucin-producing and neuroendocrine cells

(d) the mucosa in the pylorus has relatively few acid-producing cells compared to the body region

(e) enteroendocrine cells secreting gastrin are concentrated in the cardiac region

4. IN THE SMALL BOWEL

(a) villi are seen macroscopically as large folds arranged circularly around the lumen

(b) enterocytes have a well-developed microvillous surface which forms the brush border

(c) Paneth cells are seen as large, vacuolated, pale-staining cells and are found mainly in the neck region of intestinal crypts

(d) Brunner's glands are serous in type and are found in the duodenum

(e) all mucosal epithelial cells are derived from common specialized stem cells located in the crypts

12. Liver

INTRODUCTION

The liver acts as a vast chemical factory, synthesizing large complex molecules from low molecular weight substances brought to it in the blood, particularly substances recently absorbed by the intestine and transported by a portal blood system. The liver also breaks down toxic substances brought to it by the hepatic artery, and synthesizes bile, which is transferred by a system of ducts (the biliary system) to the duodenum.

All of the biochemical functions of the liver are carried out by the epithelial parenchymal cell of the liver, the hepatocyte, and are dependent on complex interrelationships between:

- the vasculature (hepatic artery and portal vein branches, sinusoids and central veins);
- the hepatocytes;
- the bile drainage systems (the canaliculi and intrahepatic bile ducts, Fig. 12.1).

LIVER VASCULATURE

The liver receives blood from two vessels, the hepatic artery and the hepatic portal vein.

The hepatic artery perfuses the liver with oxygenated blood from the celiac axis branches of the aorta. On entering the liver it divides into increasingly smaller branches.

The hepatic portal vein carries blood from the digestive tract and spleen to the liver, the blood from the digestive tract being rich in amino acids, lipids and carbohydrates absorbed from the bowel, and that from the spleen being rich in hemoglobin breakdown products.

After entering the liver at the porta hepatis, the portal vein divides into smaller distributing veins, which then branch further, eventually forming terminal portal venules.

In the liver, the two input circulations (hepatic artery and hepatic portal vein) discharge their blood into a

Fig. 12.1 Architecture of the liver.

Hepatocytes (liver cells) are arranged as interconnecting flat plates between which are sinusoids containing blood supplied by small side branches of the hepatic artery and portal vein. Sinusoidal blood drains into a central terminal hepatic venule, each of which empties into an intercalated (sublobular) vein. Bile produced by hepatocytes enters narrow canaliculi which drain into small bile ducts running with the hepatic artery and portal vein branches.

common system of small vascular channels, the sinusoids (Fig. 12.2), which are in intimate contact with the hepatocytes.

The hepatic artery branches supply oxygenated blood containing metabolites for reprocessing and toxins for detoxification by hepatocytes.

The hepatic artery divides into successively smaller branches, the terminal elements running with the terminal branches of the hepatic portal vein before emptying into the hepatic sinusoids by short side branches (the arteriosinusoidal branches). A peribiliary plexus of small arterial branches supplies oxygenated blood into the large intrahepatic bile ducts before draining into the sinusoids.

The hepatic portal vein branches bring poorly oxygenated blood which contains material from the gut and spleen.

The blood is rich in carbohydrates, lipids and amino acids absorbed from the gut and hemoglobin breakdown products from the spleen. The main portal vein divides within the liver into progressively smaller branches (interlobar, segmental and interlobular branches), culminating in terminal portal venules which run with the terminal branches of the hepatic artery.

Lateral side branches (inlet venules) of the terminal portal venules empty blood into the sinusoids where it blends with blood from the terminal hepatic artery branches. The terminal parts of the hepatic portal and arterial systems run together in the portal tracts, which also contain bile ductules.

Hepatic sinusoids are the highly specialized liver capillary equivalents.

They are lined by a thin, discontinuous, highly fenestrated endothelium which does not rest on a basement membrane. Instead it is closely related externally to plates and cords of hepatocytes (Fig. 12.3), though separated from them by a space. This perisinusoidal space of Disse is the main site where material is transferred between the blood-filled sinusoids and hepatocytes in both directions.

The hepatic sinusoids are partly lined by a scattering of phagocytic cells (Kupffer cells), which are derived from circulating blood monocytes.

Sinusoids receive blood from the terminal portal venules and terminal branches of the hepatic artery and empty blood which has undergone considerable modification of its contents into terminal hepatic venules.

Blood leaving the sinusoids enters the central venules of the liver lobules.

Blood which has passed through the functioning liver parenchyma enters terminal hepatic venules (central veins of the lobules, see Fig. 12.7), which in turn unite to form intercalated veins; these then fuse to form larger hepatic vein branches. Hepatic veins are devoid of valves and open separately into the inferior vena cava as it passes through the liver on its way to the right atrium.

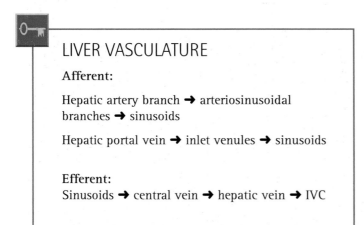

LIVER VASCULATURE

Afferent:

Hepatic artery branch ➜ arteriosinusoidal branches ➜ sinusoids

Hepatic portal vein ➜ inlet venules ➜ sinusoids

Efferent:
Sinusoids ➜ central vein ➜ hepatic vein ➜ IVC

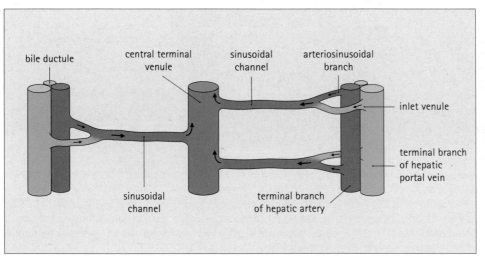

bile ductule   central terminal venule   sinusoidal channel   arteriosinusoidal branch

inlet venule

terminal branch of hepatic portal vein

sinusoidal channel   terminal branch of hepatic artery

Fig. 12.2 Hepatic microcirculation. Diagram of the hepatic microcirculation. Blood from the terminal branches of the hepatic artery and the portal vein enters the sinusoidal system via small side branches, the arteriosinusoidal branch and inlet venule, respectively. It then passes along the sinusoid lumina towards the terminal hepatic venule (central vein). The sinusoidal system is an interconnecting system of capillary-like channels in close contact with the functioning liver cells (hepatocytes); it is not a system of simple tubes as shown here.

HEPATOCYTES

The main functional cell of the liver is the hepatocyte.

Hepatocytes (liver cells), which are intimately associated with the network of blood vessels (sinusoids), are polarized polyhedral cells with three identifiable types of surface (see page 219). As would be expected in cells that are so metabolically active, their cytoplasm is packed with a wide range of organelles.

The nuclei are large, spherical and central, and contain scattered clumps of chromatin and prominent nucleoli. Many cells are binucleate, and nuclei are frequently polyploid; progressively more tetraploid nuclei develop with age.

The Golgi is large and active, or small and multiple, and is mainly seen near the nucleus, with an extension lying close to the canalicular surface.

The vesicles and tubules of the abundant smooth and rough endoplasmic reticulum are continuous with the Golgi. There are numerous free ribosomes in the cytosol, as well as large glycogen deposits and some lipid droplets, the glycogen often being closely related to the smooth endoplasmic reticulum.

Lysosomes (see page 21) of various sizes are numerous, some containing lipofuscin and lamellated lipoprotein. They are particularly large and numerous near the canalicular surface.

Peroxisomes (see page 22) usually number 200–300/cell.

Mitochondria are also abundant, numbering more than 1000/cell and are randomly scattered. This vast mitochondrial component gives the hepatocyte cytoplasm its eosinophilic granular appearance in H&E-stained paraffin sections.

Fig. 12.3 Hepatic sinusoids.
(a) High-power micrograph showing the relationship between the sinusoidal channels (S) and the cuboidal hepatocytes (H). Note the terminal hepatic venule, V.
(b) Micrograph of liver stained to demonstrate reticulin fibers (black), which run in the space of Disse between the hepatocyte surface and the endothelial cells lining the sinusoid (see Fig. 12.4

c & d). This method delineates the outline of the sinusoid (S) and the hepatocyte columns (H) and is used in the histologic diagnosis of liver disease on small cores of liver tissue obtained by needle biopsy (See Fig. 1.1).
(c) Immunoperoxidase preparation (showing lysozyme) identifying scattered phagocytic Kupffer's cells (K) in the sinusoid lining.

Fig. 12.4 Hepatocyte.

(a) Micrograph of a thin acrylic resin H&E-stained section of hepatocytes (H), which are roughly cuboidal and have a pale granular eosinophilic cytoplasm, much of the pallor being due to the presence of glycogen. The nuclei are central with a distinct nuclear membrane and prominent nucleoli.

Some of the hepatocyte surface lines the sinusoidal channel (i.e. sinusoidal surface, SS), while other surfaces are in contact with adjacent hepatocyte (i.e. intercellular surfaces, ICS), some of the adjacent hepatocyte surfaces having bile canaliculi (BC) running between them. Details of the canaliculi cannot be distinguished by light microscopy.

(b) Low-power electron micrograph showing some of the cytoplasm of two adjacent hepatocytes (H), joined by their canalicular surfaces (CS) in which a bile canaliculus (BC) can be seen. The other surfaces of the hepatocyte are the sinusoidal surfaces (SS)

bordering the sinusoid lumen (S). The space between the hepatocyte surface and the sinusoid is the space of Disse (SD).

(c) Medium-power electron micrograph showing the space of Disse (SD) between the sinusoidal surface of the hepatocyte (H) and the endothelial cell (E) lining the sinusoid. A number of irregular microvilli (MV) protrude into the space of Disse from the hepatocyte surface. The microvilli are much less regular in humans than in rodents. Some of the support fibers of the reticulin network (R) can be seen.

(d) Diagram showing the space of Disse lying between the hepatocyte and the discontinuous endothelium lining the sinusoid. The space contains microvillous processes from the hepatocyte surface and collagenous reticulin fibers, which form a supportive mesh.

Hepatocytes have three important surfaces.

The hepatocyte surfaces are important because they are involved in the transfer of substances between the hepatocyte, blood vessels and bile canaliculi.

The three types of surface are sinusoidal, canalicular and intercellular (Fig. 12.4).

Sinusoidal surfaces are separated from the sinusoidal vessel by the space of Disse.

They account for approximately 70% of the total hepatocyte surface. They are covered by short microvilli, which protrude into the space of Disse. Between the bases of the microvilli are coated pits (see Fig. 2.5), which are involved in endocytosis.

The sinusoidal surface is the site where material is transferred between the sinusoids and the hepatocyte.

Canalicular surfaces are the surfaces across which bile drains from the hepatocytes into the canaliculi.

They account for approximately 15% of the hepatocyte surface and are closely apposed except at the site of a canaliculus, which is a tube formed by the exact opposition of two shallow gutters on the surface of adjacent hepatocytes.

Canaliculi are about 0.5–2.5 μm in diameter, being smaller close to the terminal hepatic venule, and are lined by irregular microvilli arising from the canalicular surfaces of the hepatocytes.

Hepatocyte cytoplasm close to the canaliculi is rich in actin filaments, which are possibly capable of influencing the diameter of the canaliculus and thus the rate of flow.

The cell membrane around the canalicular lumen is rich in alkaline phosphatase and adenosine triphosphatase, and the canalicular lumen is isolated from the rest of the canalicular surface by junctional complexes (Fig. 12.5).

The intercellular surfaces are the surfaces between adjacent hepatocytes that are not in contact with sinusoids or canaliculi.

They account for about 15% of the hepatocyte surface.

These intercellular surfaces are comparatively simple, but specialized for cell attachment and cell-to-cell communication via communicating junctions (see Fig. 3.14).

Fig. 12.5 Bile canaliculi.
ⓐ Micrograph showing bile canaliculi highlighted by an immunoperoxidase method for CEA, which shows the canaliculi as brown lines or dots, depending on whether they have been sectioned longitudinally or transversely. The nuclei and outlines of hepatocytes (H) can be seen as can an occasional sinusoid (S).
ⓑ Electron micrograph of the canalicular surface of two apposed hepatocytes. Note the canaliculus (C) filled with microvilli and the junctional complexes (JC) separating the canalicular lumen from the rest of the apposed hepatocyte.

HEPATOCYTES

- Metabolically highly active so rich in cytoplasmic organelles

- High energy requirement so very many mitochondria

- Much of the cell surface is related to sinusoids where exchange of materials with blood takes place

- Part of the surface is in contact with bile canaliculi, where bile excreted from hepatocytes enters the biliary drainage system

INTRAHEPATIC BILIARY TREE

Bile produced by hepatocytes passes into bile canaliculi.

The bile canaliculi carry the bile back to the portal tracts (i.e. in the opposite direction to the blood).

As the canaliculi approach the bile ductules (Fig. 12.6a) in the portal tracts, they open into short passages lined by small cuboidal cells (the canals of Hering). From here, bile flows into the bile ductules in the portal tract.

Bile ductules anastomose freely, fuse and increase in size to form larger ducts, the trabecular ducts (Fig. 12.6b).

Many of these ducts fuse to form large intrahepatic ducts, which converge near the liver hilum into the main hepatic ducts (see page 223).

The basic functional unit of the liver is the lobule – (or is it?).

The components of the liver (i.e. the hepatocytes, terminal hepatic venules, portal triads and sinusoids) are arranged in a fairly constant pattern, which has been described as lobular, the classical lobule being composed of:

- a central terminal hepatic venule, into which drains a converging series of sinusoidal channels like the spokes of a cycle wheel;
- interconnecting plates of hepatocytes which surround each sinusoidal channel and run between the central terminal hepatic venule and the periphery of the lobule;

- peripherally arranged portal tracts, each containing terminal branches of the hepatic artery and portal vein and a small tributary of the bile duct.

Thus a ring of portal tracts forms the outer limit of each classical lobule.

The channels within each portal tract are surrounded by a small amount of fibrocollagenous tissue, and in some animals, particularly the pig, fibrocollagenous septa extend from one portal triad to another, clearly outlining the limits of each lobule. In humans, however, these fibrous septa are absent, and so the lobule is less clearly defined.

In the lobule, various zones of hepatocytes can be identified. These are the centrilobular, periportal and mid zones.

The centrilobular zone is composed of hepatocytes surrounding the central terminal hepatic venule, and is the zone most distant from the oxygenated arterial blood supply.

The periportal zone at the periphery of the lobule is closely related to the portal tracts. The outermost layer of periportal hepatocytes immediately adjacent to the portal tract is called the limiting plate; it is the first group of hepatocytes to be damaged in liver disorders that primarily involve the portal tracts.

As the cells of the limiting plate are exposed to hepatic artery and portal venous blood before other hepatocytes, they receive maximum exposure to any toxins in the systemic blood or absorbed by the digestive tract.

The mid zone is the zone of hepatocytes between the centrilobular and periportal zones.

Fig. 12.6 Intrahepatic bile ducts.

(a) Micrograph showing a small bile ductule (BD) in the portal tract. It has a simple structure with low cuboidal epithelium and a narrow surrounding zone of collagen (C) and some smooth muscle fibers. A terminal branch of the hepatic portal vein (HPV) and hepatic artery (HA) are also present in the tract.

(b) Micrograph of a transverse section of a trabecular duct (TD), which is larger than a bile ductule, with a larger lumen and a well-formed wall. It is surrounded by dense fibrocollagenous tissue of the trabecular septum (TS) in which it runs.

THE LOBULE CONCEPT

Lobule versus acinus concept and hepatocyte heterogeneity

The lobule concept has stood the test of time; however, it has recently been proposed that the structure of the liver should be considered in terms of another structural unit, the acinus (Fig. 12.7). The proposal is based on observations made on injection studies of the microcirculation of the liver; the acinus concept views the blood supply as the focal point, the periphery of one segment of the lobule being its short axis.

The architectural arrangement of the liver remains immutable. The lobular and acinar concepts are simply two different ways of looking at the structure. In man, neither lobules nor acini have a clearly visible outline, but most of the nomenclature used in the descriptions of disease processes (e.g. centrilobular necrosis, limiting plate inflammation) is based on the lobular concept.

In both concepts, one of the consequences is the realization that not all hepatocytes are equal ('hepatocyte heterogeneity'). Some of the differences consequent upon distance from the arterial supply have been mentioned above, but there are other functional and ultrastructural differences. For example, bile is mostly taken up in the periportal hepatocytes when the load is normal, the centrilobular hepatocytes only becoming involved in this function when there is a bile overload. Also, the centrilobular hepatocytes possess enzymes which enable them to be active in esterification reactions, whereas periportal hepatocytes are much less involved in this process but are rich in oxidative enzymes. There are probably many such differences in enzyme content, reflecting differences in function.

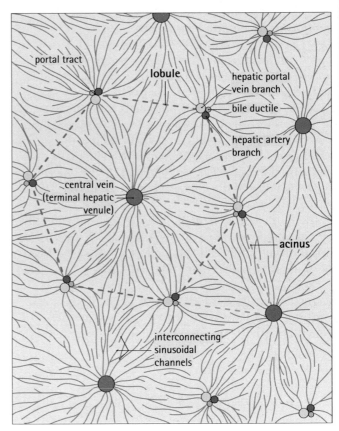

Fig. 12.7 Hepatic architecture - lobule and acinus. Diagram showing the architecture of the liver and the relationship between the vessels and ducts in the portal tract, the sinusoidal system and the central veins. The lobular and acinar concepts (see Fig. 12.12) are overdrawn.

LIVER FUNCTION

The liver has a wide range of functions which account for its complex structure.

BILE SYNTHESIS AND SECRETION. The liver produces bile, which in an alkaline secretion containing water, ions, phospholipids, bile pigments (mainly bilirubin glucuronide) and bile acids (glycocholic and taurocholic).

Bile is transported in the bile ducts from the liver to the gallbladder, where it is stored and concentrated prior to excretion into the duodenum via distal bile ducts.

Bile neutralizes the acid chyme, which enters the duodenum from the stomach, and bile acids in the bile emulsify fat globules in the chyme, thereby facilitating lipid digestion by lipases.

Most of the bile acids in the bile are reabsorbed in the ileum and recirculate to the liver, but about 10–15% is broken down in the intestine or lost in the feces. Liver cells synthesize replacement bile acids.

EXCRETION OF BILIRUBIN. Bilirubin is produced in the spleen from the breakdown of the heme component of hemoglobin. In the liver the bilirubin is conjugated with glucuronic acid, and the conjugate (bilirubin glucuronide) is excreted in the bile and thence the feces.

PROTEIN SYNTHESIS. The liver synthesizes many proteins, including albumen, and blood clotting factors such as fibrinogen and prothrombin.

GLUCONEOGENESIS. Lipids and amino acids are converted into glucose in the liver by gluconeogenesis.

STORAGE. Triglycerides, glycogen and some vitamins are stored in the liver.

DEAMINATION OF AMINO ACIDS. In the liver amino acids are deaminated to produce urea, which is excreted by the kidney.

CONJUGATION AND CHEMICAL BREAKDOWN OF TOXINS. The smooth endoplasmic reticulum of the liver possesses large numbers of enzymes that break down or conjugate toxic substances (e.g. alcohol, barbiturates, etc.) to convert them into other metabolites.

LIVER FAILURE

Liver disease can affect any of its functions, though when large numbers of hepatocytes are damaged, all of the functions tend to be disturbed.

Failure of synthetic functions.

The liver fails to produce important proteins such as albumen and the various protein clotting factors.

The reduced synthesis of albumen leads to a reduced oncotic pressure of the blood, which results in edema and accumulation of watery fluid in the peritoneal cavity (ascites).

Failure of clotting factor synthesis leads to spontaneous bleeding.

Failure of detoxification functions.

The liver fails to convert metabolic waste products into innocuous substances. Toxic substances therefore circulate in the blood and cause a number of symptoms including confusion, altered consciousness and eventually hepatic coma, which is rapidly fatal.

Failure of adequate bile secretion into the alimentary tract leads to retention of bile in the liver, with some of the components of the retained bile entering the blood and producing yellowing discoloration of the blood plasma and tissues (i.e. jaundice).

Chronic hepatic failure.

If hepatocyte damage is slowly progressive the abnormalities outlined above develop insidiously over a period of years. This is called chronic hepatic failure, and is most commonly associated with cirrhosis (see Fig. 12.8).

Acute hepatic failure.

If the liver disease is severe and of sudden onset, the metabolic abnormalities appear suddenly. This is acute hepatic failure, and is most commonly associated with some acute virus infections (e.g. hepatitis B virus infection) or exposure to liver toxins (e.g. paracetamol/acetamidophenol). In either case, acute hepatic failure results in the widespread death of liver cells.

CIRRHOSIS

Many slowly progressive diseases destroy hepatocytes and lead to distortion of liver architecture, particularly the relationships between the sinusoids, the portal venous system and the bile ducts.

Death of hepatocytes is followed by scarring, and, although hepatocytes can regenerate and produce a new population of cells, their connections with the portal system and the biliary drainage are destroyed. This pattern of liver disorder, known as cirrhosis (Fig. 12.8), is a common cause of chronic liver failure.

Cirrhosis is characterized by:
- continuing death of hepatocytes;
- collapse of normal architecture;
- increased production of fibrocollagenous tissue, leading to irregular scarring;
- attempted regeneration of surviving hepatocytes which form irregular nodules and have abnormal relationships with the microvasculature and bile drainage system. Regenerating hepatocytes are able to continue some synthetic functions, but eventually fail to keep pace with normal demands, and the symptoms of liver failure begin to manifest themselves.

Cirrhosis produces chronic liver failure and symptoms appear progressively over a period of some years, usually culminating fatally in coma or as a result of the complications of portal hypertension.

Portal hypertension.

In cirrhosis, the sinusoidal connections between the portal venous system and the draining central terminal hepatic venules and hepatic veins are destroyed.

Portal venous blood cannot therefore escape through its normal channels (i.e. through sinusoids into central terminal hepatic venules). Thus, the blood pressure in the portal venous system increases considerably and causes portal hypertension.

One escape route for portal venous blood is via anastomoses with the systemic venous system; these are normally closed when portal pressure is low, but open when portal pressure rises.

When these anastomotic channels are distended with blood, they are called varices.

One of the sites of such an anastomosis is at the lower end of the esophagus, which is unfortunate since the distended submucosal blood vessels (esophageal varices) bulge into the lumen of the esophagus and are easily eroded by gastric acid, resulting in torrential hemorrhage.

Bleeding from esophageal varices is a severe complication of portal hypertension and cirrhosis, and may be fatal.

Cirrhosis and portal hypertension most commonly follow persisting hepatocyte destruction due to alcohol toxicity, some forms of viral infection, and autoimmune liver disease.

Fig. 12.8 Cirrhosis.
Micrograph of cirrhotic liver. Compare with Fig. 12.12 and note the fibrous scarring (blue), which has distorted the normal architecture. There are nodules of regenerating liver cells but their connections with the vascular supply and bile drainage system are destroyed. Masson trichrome stain has been used here.

Bile formed in the liver is passed into the gut through the extrahepatic bile ducts.

The small tributaries of the intrahepatic biliary tree fuse to become increasingly larger channels, eventually fusing to become two large ducts, the right and left lobar bile ducts. These join at the hilum of the liver to form the common hepatic duct, which is the first part of the extrahepatic bile duct system (Fig. 12.9).

About 3–4 cm after leaving the liver, the common hepatic duct receives the cystic duct (a small duct from the gallbladder) and becomes the common bile duct.

The common bile duct is about 6–7 cm long and opens into the duodenum at the ampulla of Vater, having passed through the head of the pancreas and combined with the pancreatic duct.

GALLBLADDER

Introduction

The gallbladder is an ovoid sac with a muscular wall and is capable of moderate distention. It concentrates and stores bile, receiving dilute watery bile from the common hepatic duct, and emptying thick, concentrated, variably mucoid bile into the common bile duct.

Bile is transported in and out of the gallbladder through a short duct, the cystic duct. This duct contains a spirally arranged outgrowth of mucosa, which forms the spiral valve of Heister.

The gallbladder mucosa is covered by tall columnar epithelial cells specialized for absorption.

The lining cells have numerous microvilli on their luminal surfaces, and complex interdigitations of their lateral walls (Fig. 12.10). These differently specialized surfaces are separated by junctional complexes (see Fig. 3.13).

Gallbladder epithelial cells are adapted for salt and water absorption, and have abundant basal and apical mitochondria, and Na^+ and K^+ transport ATPases in their lateral walls.

Na^+ and Cl^- ions are actively pumped out of the cell cytoplasm into the lateral intercellular space to produce an osmotic gradient between it and the gall bladder lumen. Water is therefore drawn into the space from the lumen and then enters the abundant capillary network in the lamina propria.

This mechanism is similar to that employed by the proximal convoluted tubule epithelial cell in the kidney to absorb water and ions (see Chapter 15).

Gallbladder epithelium is thrown up into folds or plicae, which flatten when the gallbladder is distended.

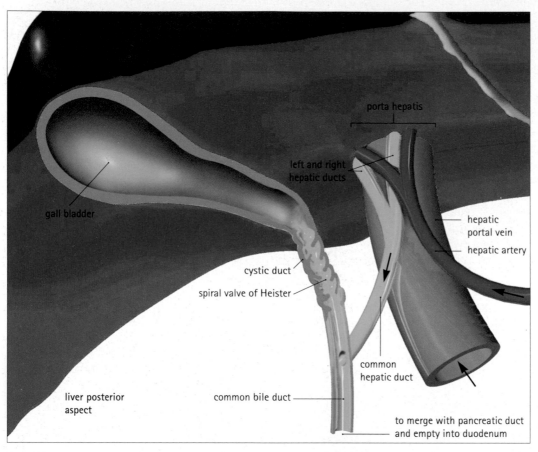

Fig. 12.9 Extrahepatic biliary tree.
Diagram of the drainage system whereby bile leaves the liver, is stored and concentrated in the gallbladder, and eventually enters the duodenum.
The right and left hepatic ducts emerge from the posterior aspect of the liver at the porta hepatis and join to form the common hepatic duct. A side branch of this duct (the cystic duct) conducts bile into and out of the gallbladder.
The common hepatic duct then continues as the common bile duct, passing through the head of the pancreas, where it merges with the pancreatic duct before entering the duodenum.

Fig. 12.10 Gallbladder.
ⓐLow-power micrograph of the gallbladder showing the mucosa (M) with its ridged mucosal folds, the submucosa (SM) and the muscular wall (MW).
ⓑHigh-power micrograph of gallbladder epithelium. The cells are tall and columnar with basal nuclei and a luminal surface bearing microvilli. The microvilli are discernible as a faint brush border (BB).

GALLSTONES

Gallstones (i.e. stones or calculi in the gallbladder or biliary tree) form when solid concretions of bile act as a nidus for calcium salt deposition. Small gallstones are asymptomatic; larger gallstones can cause obstructive jaundice or cholecystitis.

Obstructive jaundice.
Obstructive jaundice results from the blockage of a bile duct, for example by a gallstone that has passed out of the gallbladder and become impacted in the common bile duct on its way to the duodenum.

Blockage of the bile duct impedes the flow of bile into the duodenum. This results in:
- damming of bile in the proximal biliary tree, intrahepatic bile ducts and eventually bile canaliculi;
- passage of retained canalicular bile into the hepatic sinusoids and thence into the blood stream, producing jaundice;

- impaired intestinal breakdown of fat due to lack of the emulsifying bile acids normally present in bile;
- pale feces, normal fecal color being due to the presence of bile and its breakdown products.

Cholecystitis.
Gallstones may become impacted in the cystic duct (Fig. 12.11a) and obstruct the flow of bile at this point. This has the following consequences, which are the basic features of so-called chronic cholecystitis (Fig. 12.11b):
- the gallbladder contracts more strongly to try to overcome the obstruction, and consequently its musculature thickens;
- resulting high pressure within the gallbladder lumen pushes pouches of mucosa into the muscle layers (Rokitansky-Aschoff sinuses);
- stasis of bile within the gallbladder predisposes to infection and episodes of pain and fever are common.

Fig. 12.11 Obstructive biliary disease.
(a) Photograph of a greatly enlarged gallbladder with a gallstone (GS) impacted in its neck, close to the cystic duct. Obstruction of bile drainage has led to bile stasis and consequent infection, producing red inflamed mucosa (arrow).
(b) Micrograph of a chronically obstructed gallbladder. The muscle layer (M) is thickened by hypertrophy and a pouch of epithelium-lined mucosa (Rokitansky-Aschoff sinus, ARS) has bulged through it. Compare with Fig. 12.10a.

BILIARY SYSTEM

- Bile produced by hepatocytes from breakdown products of hemoglobin

- Bile passes from canalicular surface of hepatocytes → bile canaliculi → bile ductules in portal tracts → trabecular ducts → intrahepatic bile ducts → lobar ducts → common hepatic duct.

- Bile concentrated in gall bladder by extraction of water by absorptive epithelium, then stored

- Concentrated bile expelled from gall bladder by contraction of its smooth muscle wall into common bile duct, thence into duodenal lumen.

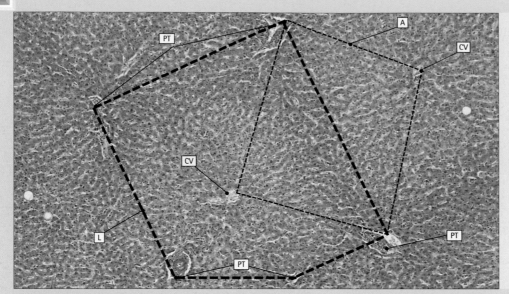

Fig. 12.12 Liver architecture.
Low-power micrograph showing the general liver architecture. Note the central terminal hepatic venules (CV), portal tracts (PT) and interconnecting cords of hepatocytes.
The concepts of the hepatic lobule (L) and hepatic acinus (A) are overdrawn (see Fig. 12.7).

Fig. 12.13 Liver sinusoids and hepatocytes.
Micrograph showing sinusoidal channels (S) passing between interconnecting columns of hepatocytes (H) on their way to the central terminal hepatic venule (CV).

Fig. 12.14 Portal tract.
Portal tracts contain a small bile ductule (BD), a terminal branch of the hepatic artery (HA), and a component of the distal part of the hepatic portal venous system (PV). All are contained within a fibrocollagenous supporting stroma.

1. THE BLOOD ENTERING THE LIVER THROUGH THE HEPATIC PORTAL VEIN

(a) is highly oxygenated
(b) contains material absorbed from food in the small ntestine
(c) contains hemoglobin breakdown products from the spleen
(d) enters the hepatic sinusoids
(e) contains formed bile for metabolic breakdown by hepatocytes

2. IN THE LOBULAR CONCEPT OF THE LIVER

(a) the terminal branch of the portal vein is at the centre of the lobule
(b) the portal tracts are located at the periphery of the lobule
(c) blood passes from the periphery to the center of the lobule
(d) bile passes from the hepatocytes to the center of the lobule
(e) the hepatocytes of the limiting plate are at the periphery of the lobule

3. BILE

(a) is a product of hemoglobin breakdown in the liver
(b) is stored and concentrated in the gall bladder
(c) accumulates in the liver and blood when the common bile duct is blocked
(d) passes into the duodenum at the duodenal papilla (ampulla of Vater)
(e) is acidic and augments the effects of gastric acid in digestion

4. HEPATOCYTES

(a) are rich in peroxisomes
(b) have a canalicular surface which is involved in bile secretion
(c) are separated from the sinusoid endothelium by the space of Disse
(d) contain glycogen
(e) rest on a reticulin scaffold

13. Musculoskeletal System

INTRODUCTION

The musculoskeletal system, which provides mechanical support and permits movement, is composed of skeletal muscle, tendons, bones, joints and ligaments.

Skeletal muscles act as contractile levers, and are connected to bone by **tendons**. **Bones** act as rigid levers, articulating with other bones through **joints**, which are kept in relationship by **ligaments**.

A special characteristic of muscle, tendons and joints is the possession of a rich sensory nerve supply, which detects position of the body and velocity of movement. The integration of this sensory information by the central nervous system is vital for the musculoskeletal system to function normally.

The main functional attribute of bone is its specialized extracellular matrix, which is hardened by the deposition of calcium enabling it to function as a rigid lever.

The rigid, hard character of bone belies its importance as a metabolic reservoir of mineral salts and the fact that it is in a constant state of dynamic remodeling.

Fig. 13.1 Development of skeletal muscle.
This photomicrograph shows elongated rhabdomyoblasts, with abundant pink-staining cytoplasm, developing in primitive mesenchyme in human embryonic tissue.

SKELETAL MUSCLE

Skeletal muscle is responsible for voluntary movement.

The histologic characteristics of skeletal muscle cells and the structural basis of muscle contraction are described on pages 65–69.

Individual muscle cells are arranged into large groups to form anatomically distinct muscles. These are characterized by:

- an orderly alignment of the constituent cells to generate a directional force following contraction;
- anchorage to other structures by highly organized fibrocollagenous support tissues;
- a rich blood supply reflecting high metabolic demands;
- innervation and control by specialized neurons (motor neurons) which terminate on muscle cells at specialized nerve endings (motor end plates);
- incorporation of specially adapted skeletal muscle cells into structures called spindles, to act as sensors of muscle stretch.

Embryologically, muscle fibers develop from mesenchymal tissues.

In embryogenesis, skeletal muscle develops from primitive mesenchymal tissues of the mesoderm. Small spindle-shaped or strap-shaped cells with a single nucleus and abundant pink-staining cytoplasm develop from primitive mesenchymal cells. These are skeletal muscle cell precursors, the rhabdomyoblasts (Fig 13.1). Numerous individual rhabdomyoblasts then fuse to form multinucleate muscle fibers, the cells enlarging in size when they become connected to the nervous system and receive motor stimulation.

Residual cells with the function of rhabdomyoblasts (i.e., capable of differentiating further into functional striated muscle cells) persist in adult skeletal muscle as **satellite cells**, (see Fig 13.6). Following muscle damage and loss of fibers, these cells proliferate and may produce new muscle cells.

A muscle is composed of many muscle fibers.

A mature muscle fiber is composed of large numbers of myofibrils bounded by a cell membrane termed the sarcolemma (see Figs. 5.2 and 13.2).

Each skeletal muscle cell is typically extremely long (up to 10 cm in length), and it is therefore more usual to use the term skeletal muscle fiber rather than cell.

Many muscle fibers are arranged together to form a muscle (Fig. 13.3). Although elongated, individual muscle cells do not extend the full length of a muscle, but are arranged in overlapping bundles, the force of contraction being transmitted through the arrangement of the support tissues.

(a)

(b)

Fig. 13.2 Skeletal muscle fibers.
(a) Micrograph of skeletal muscle fibers in a longitudinal section showing prominent cross striations. The dark bands are termed A bands (anisotropic, i.e. birefringent in polarized light), while the light bands are termed I bands (isotropic, i.e. no interference with polarized light). These bands correspond to the arrangement of thick and thin filaments in myofibrils (see Fig. 5.2). Nuclei (N) appear as elongated structures just beneath the cell membrane and each fiber contains many nuclei.
(b) Micrograph of skeletal muscle fibers in a transverse frozen section showing roughly hexagonal profiles with flattened sides

where they are compressed by adjacent fibers. Nuclei (N) appear as small circular profiles at the periphery of each fiber. Individual myofibrils are generally not identifiable by light microscopy.

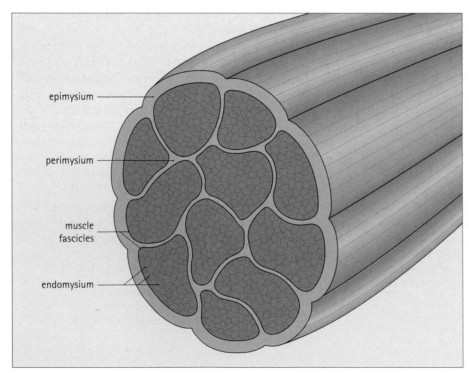

Fig. 13.3 Organization of muscle fibers into muscle.
Individual muscle fibers (see Fig. 5.1) are surrounded by endomysium, which is composed of sheets of external lamina identical to basement membrane (see page 56).

Endomysium secures the muscle fibers to each other and contains both capillary blood vessels and individual nerve axons (see Chapter 6).

Clusters of muscle fibers are held together by fine sheets of fibrocollagenous support tissue (perimysium) to form fascicles. Blood vessels, lymphatic vessels and nerves run in the endomysial support tissues.

An anatomically defined muscle is composed of many fascicles, which are surrounded externally by a thick layer of fibrocollagenous support tissue, the epimysium.

epimysium

perimysium

muscle fascicles

endomysium

Different muscles are characterized by different physiologic and metabolic properties.

The physiologic and metabolic properties of individual skeletal muscles are determined by differences in the structure of their constituent muscle fibers.

In both animals and man it has been possible to define several subtypes of muscle fiber by macroscopic, physiologic, biochemical and histochemical criteria, but there are marked inter-species variations.

Histochemical staining for specific enzymes delineates several types of fiber and is a useful method for analyzing muscle. Two main types of fiber are identified (types 1 and 2), and type 2 fibers can be subdivided into types 2A, 2B and 2C (Fig. 13.4). Type 2C fibres are thought to be a primitive form of type 2 fibre and, with appropriate innervation, are probably capable of developing into 2A or 2B fibres. Such histochemical staining is used routinely in the study of muscle pathology and allows the histologic diagnosis of certain muscle diseases.

Histochemical staining can also be correlated with other functional and biochemical attributes of muscle (Fig. 13.4c).

Not all muscles have the same proportions of type 1 and type 2 fibers. In general, muscles with a role in maintaining posture (e.g. calf muscles) have a high proportion of type 1 fibers, while muscles used for short bursts of power have abundant type 2 fibers.

Different individuals are genetically endowed with variable proportions of muscle fiber types in defined muscles, and this may limit athletic prowess at a particular sport; training does not affect the proportion of fibers in any given muscle, but does influence their size.

Fig. 13.4 Fiber types.
(a) Micrograph of a transverse frozen section of muscle stained by an enzyme histochemical method to demonstrate NADH transferase which indicates oxidative capacity. Two different subtypes of fiber are evident. Type 1 fibers (1) show a high level of activity and stain darkly while type 2 fibers (2) are paler because of their lower level of activity.
(b) Micrograph of muscle stained for one form of myofibrillar ATPase at pH 4.2. This technique also delineates two fiber types. Type 1 fibers stain darkly, having a high level of activity, while type 2 fibers have a low level of activity and stain lightly. Note that the type 1 and 2 fibers are arranged in a haphazard or checkerboard pattern.
(c) Table detailing the physiologic features of different fiber types.

Fiber type	metabolism	contractile behaviour
1	oxidative	slow twitch
2A	oxidative and glycolytic	fast twitch, fatigue resistant
2B	glycolytic	fast twitch, fatigue sensitive

DISEASES OF MUSCLE

Several diseases of muscle have been attributed to specific metabolic or structural abnormalities (Fig. 13.5a).

Duchenne muscular dystrophy is the most common inherited muscle disease and characteristically affects male children. Such individuals become unable to stand unaided in early childhood and develop progressive muscle weakness, becoming wheelchair-bound by their mid teens and typically dying in early adult life.

The abnormality in Duchenne muscular dystrophy is due to a defect in the gene coding for a protein termed dystrophin (Fig. 13.5b). This protein links the actin cytoskeleton of muscle to the external lamina, its absence leads to abnormal muscle fiber fragility.

Fig. 13.5 Diseases of muscle.
(a) Micrograph of frozen section of skeletal muscle from a child showing the typical appearance of dystrophy, which is a congenital primary disorder of muscle. There is marked variation in fiber size, with some large fibers (L) and some abnormally small fibers (S). Some fibers are dead (D) and are being removed by phagocytic cells.
(b) Micrograph of normal skeletal muscle stained by an immunocytochemical method for dystrophin (which stains brown), showing its localization in the sarcolemma. In Duchenne muscular dystrophy this protein is absent.

Muscle has a rich blood supply because of the high energy demands of contraction.

Large arteries penetrate the epimysium and divide into small branches, which run in the perimysial support tissues, forming perimysial arteries and veins. These branches terminate in a vast capillary network, which runs in the endomysium. Each muscle fiber is served by several capillary vessels.

Normal adult skeletal muscle cells do not undergo cell division.

Any increased demands placed on a muscle, for example by weight training, result in increased muscle size because the cells themselves increase in size (i.e. hypertrophy).

It is possible, however, for skeletal muscle cells to regrow because a pool of inactive stem cells in adult muscle called satellite cells can be stimulated to divide following damage. These cells are not discernible by light microscopy, but may be seen ultrastructurally (Fig. 13.6). They are infrequent and appear as small spindle-shaped cells lying just beneath the external lamina of a muscle fiber.

Fibers that have regenerated in adult life following damage to a muscle can be detected histologically because they commonly contain centrally placed nuclei rather than the peripheral nuclei typical of normal fibers.

Muscle contains stretch receptors.

Although there are no pain receptors in skeletal muscle, there are receptors sensitive to stretch, which function as part of a feedback system to maintain normal muscle tone (i.e. the spinal stretch reflex arc).

Sensory fibers that provide information on the tension of skeletal muscle arise from two sources:
* encapsulated nerve endings responding to stretch in the tendon associated with a muscle;

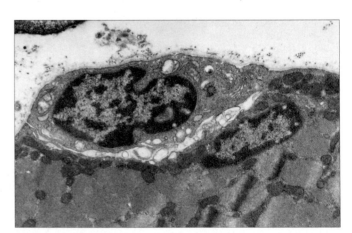

Fig. 13.6 Satellite cells.
Electron micrograph showing a satellite cell. These cells, small and spindle-shaped, are found immediately beneath the external lamina of a muscle fiber and act as stem cells in adult muscle.

- spiral nerve endings (sensory afferent fibers) sensing stretch and tension of specialized muscle fibers contained in a special sense organ in muscle called the muscle spindle (Fig. 13.7).

Fig. 13.7 Sensory innervation of skeletal muscle.
(a) Diagram illustrating the sensory innervation of muscle, which arises from two sources: encapsulated nerve endings in the tendons respond to stretch, and spiral nerve endings in muscle spindles sense stretch and tension.

The muscle spindle is composed of a fusiform capsule of fibrocollagenous tissue (continuous with the perimysium) surrounding a group of 8–15 thin muscle fibers. These fibers are termed intrafusal fibers to distinguish them from normal skeletal muscle fibers (extrafusal fibers).

Two types of intrafusal fiber can be distinguished; those with a fusiform shape and central aggregate of nuclei (nuclear bag fibers) and those of uniform width with dispersed nuclei (nuclear chain fibers).

Specialized motor nerve fibers (γ efferent fibers) innervate the intrafusal fibers and adjust their length according to the state of stretch of the muscle, which is detected by spiral nerve endings. The spiral nerve endings are wrapped around the intrafusal fibers and form special sensory afferent fibers running back to the spinal cord.
(b) Micrograph of frozen section from a child's muscle showing a muscle spindle, identified by its circular fibrocollagenous capsule (C) and its content of intrafusal muscle fibers (M).

The muscle spindle sensory mechanism maintains normal tone and muscle coordination.

Motor nerves to muscle terminate in motor end plates.

Large nerves, containing both motor and sensory axons, enter muscles by penetrating the epimysium and branch to form small nerves which run in the perimysium.

Perimysial nerves contain axons to fulfil both motor and sensory functions. The motor axons destined to innervate skeletal muscle (α efferent fibers) enter the endomysium as nerve twigs and branch to innervate several fibers.

At the end of each twig each axon becomes modified to form a motor end plate, and it is this which activates skeletal muscle contraction (Fig. 13.8).

Activation of the motor axon causes the release of acetylcholine from its storage granules by exocytosis. Acetylcholine then diffuses across the gap between the axon and muscle fiber and interacts with specific membrane receptors to cause depolarization of the muscle fiber which initiates contraction (see page 68).

The activity of secreted acetylcholine is rapidly curtailed by the activity of an enzyme called acetylcholinesterase, which is bound to the basement membrane investing the junctional folds.

In addition to nerve fibers controlling voluntary movement, specialized motor axons (γ efferent fibers) innervate fibers in the muscle spindle.

SKELETAL MUSCLES

- are composed of organized packets of striated muscle cells (see Chapter 5)

- most muscles contain a mixture of different muscle cell types, according to the function of the muscle as a whole

- muscle cell types are type 1 (slow twitch), type 2A (fast twitch, fatigue-resistant) and type 2B (fast twitch, fatigue-sensitive)

- individual muscle cells are incapable of regeneration by cell division, but a stem cell population of resting satellite cells is available partly to replenish muscles with functional contractile units after damage

- are dependent on nervous stimulation through motor end plates for contractile function and maintenance of structure

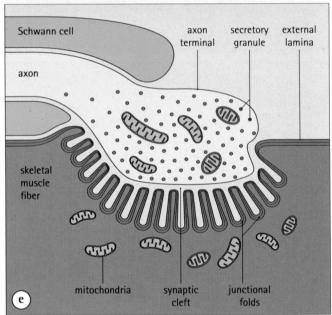

Fig. 13.8 Motor innervation of skeletal muscle.

(a) A thin resin section of skeletal muscle stained with toluidine blue showing a small perimysial nerve, which contains both motor (efferent) and sensory (afferent) fibers.

(b) A methylene blue-stained teased preparation of muscle showing several nerve twigs (T) branching from a single axon to innervate muscle fibers. There is a bulbous swelling (the motor end plate, MEP) at the end of each twig at the site of connection with the muscle. The group of fibers innervated by a single axon is a motor unit.

(c) Micrograph of a thin resin section of skeletal muscle stained with toluidine blue to show the motor end plate (MEP). The axon terminates in a dome-shaped swelling of the nerve terminal in direct apposition to the cell membrane of the muscle fiber, to form the MEP. This is invested by a layer of Schwann cell cytoplasm (S).

(d) Electron micrograph of a motor end plate showing the cell membrane of the muscle fiber thrown into a series of deep folds (junctional folds, JF) beneath which the sarcoplasm (S) contains numerous mitochondria (M). In the terminal swelling of the motor axon, neurosecretory granules (G), containing the transmitter substance acetylcholine, and mitochondria are abundant.

The terminal swelling of the axon is separated from the muscle cell membrane by a gap of 30—50 nm (the synaptic cleft, C), which includes the external lamina of the muscle.

(e) Diagram of motor end plate. The sarcoplasmic membrane in the region of the motor end plate contains specialized receptors which, when activated by acetylcholine, permit muscle cell membrane depolarization.

MYASTHENIA GRAVIS

Myasthenia gravis is a disease caused by the formation of antibodies to the acetylcholine receptor on the sarcolemma in the junctional folds of the motor end plates. The antibodies bind to the acetylcholine receptors and thereby prevent released acetylcholine from interacting with the receptors and causing depolarization.

Affected individuals develop tremendous muscle weakness manifest by fatiguability, inability to lift the arms, failure to maintain an upright posture of the head, and drooping of the eyelids.

Treatment is by the administration of drugs (anticholinesterases) which inhibit the action of the enzyme acetylcholinesterase. This potentiates the action of released acetylcholine and allows it to bind to receptors not blocked by antibody.

Myasthenia gravis is an autoimmune disease.

MUSCLE ATTACHMENTS

In order to transmit the force of contraction, the cell surface at the end of the muscle fibers is adapted for attachment to highly organized fibrocollagenous support tissues which anchor the muscle to other structures.

Such anchorage may be provided by:
- anatomically distinct tendons;
- broad areas of anchorage to a bony surface ;
- broad areas of anchorage to sheets of fibrocollagenous support tissue (fascia) which run between muscles.

Tendons attach some muscles to bone.

Tendons are long cylindrical structures of tightly packed longitudinally running collagen fibers, with the nuclei and scanty cytoplasm of fibrocytes compressed almost flat between them (Fig. 13.9). Tendons are therefore relatively acellular and have low oxygen and nutrient demands; in order to maximize their strength they are relatively avascular and contain only scanty capillaries. Because of this poor vascularity, tendons which have been partly or completely transected by trauma are extremely slow to heal, e.g. achilles tendon rupture.

Many tendons lie within fibrocollagenous tendon sheaths.

Where tendons run over bone they are encased in a sheath containing synovial fluid, which acts as a lubricant. The tendons of the fingers, for example, have a well-developed set of tendon sheaths.

The collagen fibers of tendons are firmly tethered to the muscle fibers in specialized areas called myotendinous insertions or junctions (Fig. 13.10), while at the bone end the collagen fibers of the tendon merge with the collagen of the periosteum.

The original tendon collagen is probably incorporated into bone when the periosteum makes new bone, as in bone growth during childhood (see page 246); such intraosseous tendon collagen fibers are called Sharpey's fibers.

Maintenance of the tendon at the site of bony attachment is the responsibility of the spindle cells of the periosteum, which also have the capacity to convert into chondroprogenitor cells (i.e. chondroblast precursors) or osteoprogenitor cells (i.e. osteoblast precursors, see Fig. 13.14). For this reason, the tendon close to its attachment to the bone may contain small islands of cartilage or bone.

Fig. 13.9 Tendon.
Micrograph of tendon showing highly organized regular bundles of collagen (C) with a few interspersed fibrocytes.

Fig. 13.10 Myotendinous junction.
At the point where skeletal muscle is attached to a tendon or fascia individual skeletal muscle fibers develop a complex interdigitating surface which is tightly anchored to the support tissues.

This micrograph of a myotendinous junction (MTJ) shows apparent splitting of the rounded contour of a muscle fiber to form several small rounded structures separated by fibrocollagenous tissue. Such splitting of the terminal portion of the fiber increases the surface area available for anchorage to support tissues and thus contributes to the mechanical strength of insertion.

BONE

INTRODUCTION

Bone is a highly specialized support tissue which is characterized by its rigidity and hardness. Its four main functions are: to provide **mechanical support** (e.g. ribs), to permit **locomotion** (e.g. long bones), to provide **protection** (e.g. skull) and to act as a **metabolic reservoir** of mineral salts.

Bone is composed of:

- support cells (osteoblasts and osteocytes);
- a non-mineral matrix of collagen and glycosaminoglycans (osteoid);
- inorganic mineral salts deposited within the matrix;
- remodeling cells (osteoclasts).

Bone contains a specialized extracellular matrix material called osteoid.

Osteoid is a collagenous support tissue of type 1 collagen embedded in a glycosaminoglycan gel containing specific glycoproteins (e.g. osteocalcin) which strongly bind calcium. Deposition of mineral salts in the osteoid gives bone its characteristic rigidity and functional strength.

Osteoblasts and osteocytes produce and nourish the osteoid, into which inorganic mineral salts are deposited to make it rigid and hard. Osteoclasts constantly reshape the deposited bone (i.e. the mineralized osteoid).

Bone is constantly being remodeled.

Bone is a dynamic tissue, being formed and destroyed continually under the control of hormonal and physical factors. This constant activity permits the process of modeling (i.e. modification of the bone architecture to meet physical stresses).

Bone turnover is normally low in adults, but in babies and children it is high to allow the growth and active remodeling required to cope with new demands, for example with the onset of walking.

In the adult, bone turnover can increase from its normal basal level to meet any increased demand, for example to repair a fracture (see below). In addition, increased bone turnover can be the result of pathological processes. It can lead to bone disease.

The two main patterns of bone are called woven and lamellar.

Two types of bone can be identified according to the pattern of collagen forming the osteoid:

- woven bone is characterized by haphazard organization of collagen fibers and is mechanically weak;
- lamellar bone is characterized by a regular parallel alignment of collagen into sheets (lamellae) and is mechanically strong (Fig. 13.11).

Woven bone is produced when osteoblasts produce osteoid rapidly; the collagen fibers are deposited in an irregular, loosely intertwined pattern. This occurs initially in all fetal bones (see Fig. 13.23), but in this case the resulting woven bone is gradually replaced by remodeling and the deposition of more resilient lamellar bone.

In adults, woven bone is created when there is very rapid new bone formation, as occurs in the repair of a fracture or in Paget's disease (see Fig. 13.22). Following a fracture woven bone is remodeled and lamellar bone is deposited, but in Paget's disease the woven bone persists and leads to mechanical weakness and bone deformity. Virtually all bone in the healthy adult is lamellar.

Osteoid and Bone Matrix

- bone matrix is 90% osteoid collagen, which is mainly type 1 collagen

- osteoid collagen is a triple-stranded polymer of three polypeptide alpha chains

- defective osteoid collagen may be a cause of inherited disease characterized by bone fragility (e.g. osteogenesis imperfecta)

- additional bone proteins include osteocalcin, osteonectin, osteopontin, and various other proteins combined with carbohydrate molecules. The precise function of these proteins is not known, but some readily bind calcium and other mineral ions, and may therefore have a role in mineralization

Fig. 13.11 Woven and lamellar bone.
Polarizing micrograph of repairing bone showing both recently formed woven bone (W) at the centre and original lamellar bone (L) on either side. Note the haphazard arrangement of the collagen fibers in the woven bone and the regular parallel arrangement in the lamellar bone.

OSTEOID

- is a specialized form of type 1 collagen embedded in a glycosaminoglycan gel

- the supporting gel contains specific proteins, e.g. osteocalcin, which have affinity for calcium

- is synthesized and secreted by osteoblasts, which also orchestrate deposition of mineral salts

- may be deposited by osteoblasts in regular parallel sheets (lamellar) or haphazardly (woven)

- healthy bone formed from lamellar osteoid is strong and efficient

- bone formed from woven osteoid is comparatively weak, bulky and inefficient, and is usually pathological, resulting from fracture or Paget's disease

Bones have a dense outer cortex and an inner trabecular region.

Most bones have a basic architecture composed of:
- an outer cortical or compact zone;
- an inner trabecular or spongy zone.

Cortical bone forms a rigid outer shell, which resists deformation, while the inner trabecular meshwork provides strength by acting as a complex system of internal struts. The spaces between the trabecular meshwork are occupied by bone marrow (see Chapter 7).

In bones with a substantial weight-bearing function, the trabecular pattern is arranged to provide maximum resistance to the physical stresses to which that bone is normally subjected.

The specialized support cells of the bone reside either on its surfaces or within small spaces in formed bone termed lacunae.

The details of normal bone architecture are shown in Figs 13.12 and 13.13.

Fig. 13.12 Bone architecture – cortical and trabecular bone.
(a) Low-power scanning electron micrograph showing the architecture of bone (cortical and trabecular) and its relationship to bone marrow (see Chapter 7). The cortical bone (C) is dense and forms a compact outer shell which is bridged by narrow, delicate plates of trabecular bone (T). The spaces between the trabecular bone are occupied by yellow marrow (adipose tissue) or hemopoietic red marrow. Here the marrow (M) has retracted from the bone during tissue preparation.
(b) Medium-power scanning electron micrograph showing more detail of cortical (C) and trabecular bone (T). The outlines of a number of Haversian systems (H) of various sizes, each with a central canal, can be seen.
(c) Polarizing micrograph of a single osteon (Haversian system). A central Haversian canal (H) is surrounded by concentric layers of lamellar bone, which contains a number of dark-black spaces marking the sites of osteocytes (O). Outside the Haversian system are less regularly arranged interstitial bone lamellae (I), which act as packing between adjacent Haversian systems.

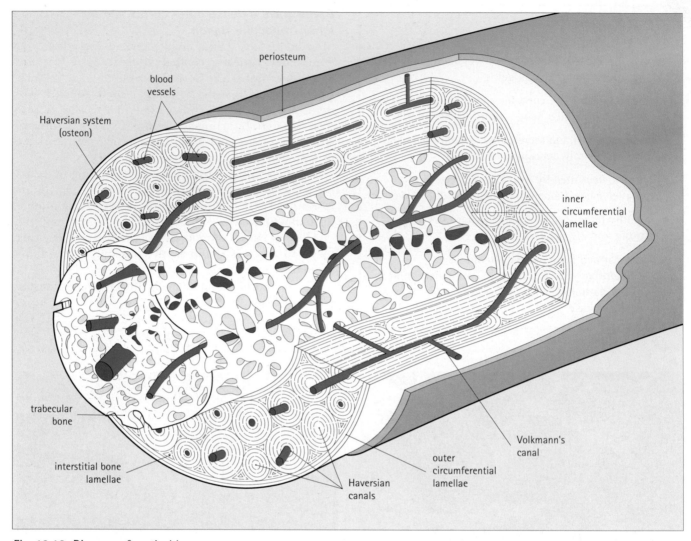

Fig. 13.13 Diagram of cortical bone.

There is a network of Haversian canals which are linked by transverse Volkmann's canals. The canals contain blood vessels and some nerves. Each Haversian canal is surrounded by concentric layers of lamellar bone. These layers contain concentrically arranged rings of osteocytes, each lying in its small lacuna and communicating with osteocytes in its own and adjacent layers through cytoplasmic processes lying in narrow canaliculi.

The Haversian canal and its concentric bone and osteocyte system is called a Haversian system or osteon. The interior of each Haversian canal is lined by flat osteoprogenitor cells or inactive osteoblasts, as are the inner surface of the cortical bone plate and the outer surfaces of the bone trabeculae. This layer, called the endosteum, provides a source of new osteoblasts necessary for new bone formation if remodeling is needed. Cortical remodeling in the Haversian canals is common.

The Haversian canal systems, interspersed with irregularly arranged interstitial bone lamellae which act as packing, occupy the bulk of the cortex; inner and outer circumferential bone lamellae separate the Haversian systems from the endosteum and the outer surface of the bone, the fibrocollagenous periosteum.

ABNORMALITIES OF BONE ARCHITECTURE

Abnormal bone architecture may result from:
- damage both to cortical and trabecular bone due to fracture;
- decreased cortical and trabecular bone due to osteoporosis;
- destruction of trabecular bone due to cancer;
- maldevelopment of bone.

Osteoporosis. In old age, both cortical and trabecular bone become thinned (osteoporosis, see Fig. 13.21) and are therefore more fragile and more prone to fracture. Fracture of the neck of femur is common in the elderly. Osteoporosis may also develop following disuse, for example in the leg bones of a wheelchair-bound person. There is some evidence that hormonal disturbances may induce osteoporosis in post -menopausal women.

Bone involvement in cancer. The bone marrow is a common site of spread of some forms of cancer, particularly cancers that originate in the breast (see Fig. 18.31), bronchus, thyroid and kidney. Proliferation of tumor cells frequently destroys the trabecular bone, and thus leads to an increased tendency to bone fracture (pathological fracture), an important complication of widespread cancer.

Maldevelopment. There are a number of diseases arising from impaired bone formation during embryological development. Many of these are incompatible with survival and such children commonly die *in utero* or shortly after birth. The most common maldevelopment of bone that is compatible with life is achondroplasia, resulting in a form of dwarfism characterized by a normal sized trunk but short limb bones.

BONE CELLS

Four main types of cell maintain bone.
Cells concerned with the production, maintenance and modeling of the osteoid are:
- osteoprogenitor cells;
- osteoblasts;
- osteocytes;
- osteoclasts.

Osteoprogenitor cells are the stem cells of bone and form osteoblasts.
Osteoprogenitor cells are derived from primitive mesenchymal cells. They form a population of stem cells that can differentiate into the more specialized bone-forming cells (i.e. osteoblasts and osteocytes).

In mature bone in which there is no active new bone formation or remodeling, the osteoprogenitor cells become flattened spindle cells closely applied to the bone surface, when they are sometimes called inactive osteoblasts.

In actively growing bone, however, for example in fetal bone or in a period of high turnover in adult bone, these cells are much larger and more numerous, containing plump oval nuclei and more abundant spindle-shaped cytoplasm (Fig. 13.14), converting into cuboidal active osteoblasts.

Fig. 13.14 Osteoprogenitor cells.
Micrograph of toluidine blue-stained epoxy resin section showing numerous plump spindle-shaped osteoprogenitor (Op) cells in the developing skull bone of a 15-week human fetus. Derived from primitive mesenchymal cells, they are transformed into osteoblasts (Ob), which are larger and more cuboidal. The osteoblasts have begun to deposit osteoid collagen (C).

Osteoblasts synthesize the organic component of the bone matrix (osteoid).

Osteoid consists of type 1 collagen, glycosaminoglycans and proteoglycans.

When fully active, osteoblasts are cuboidal or polygonal cells. They have basophilic cytoplasm, which reflects the abundance of rough endoplasmic reticulum in their cytoplasm, resulting from their role as active protein synthesizing and secreting cells. For details of osteoblast structure and function see Figs 13.15 and 13.18.

Fig. 13.15 Osteoblasts.

ⓐ Micrograph of an acrylic resin section of actively growing fetal bone stained by Goldner's method, which distinguishes mineralized bone (green) from unmineralized osteoid. Note the zone of unmineralized newly formed osteoid (OS) adjacent to the row of actively synthesizing osteoblasts (Ob) on one side of the trabeculum. On the other side, a layer of now flattened osteoblasts has entered an inactive resting phase (ROb) and its recently formed osteoid is now almost fully mineralized (arrow).

ⓑ Micrograph of a toluidine blue-stained thin epoxy resin section of actively growing bone, with a row of cuboidal osteoblasts (Ob) actively synthesizing and secreting organic matrix (osteoid, OS); the cells have bulky basophilic cytoplasm due to their protein-synthesizing rough endoplasmic reticulum. Some of the osteoid is lightly mineralized (mOS).

ⓒ Low-power electron micrograph showing an osteoblast (Ob) at the face of newly forming bone. Note the zone of unmineralized osteoid (OS), which has recently formed between the active osteoblast and the older mineralized bone (mB).

ⓓ High-power electron micrograph showing the characteristic cytoplasmic features of an active osteoblast. The cytoplasm is rich in rough endoplasmic reticulum (RER) and there are prominent mitochondria (M); the collagenic protein precursors and glycosaminoglycans are synthesized in the RER and then packaged in the Golgi prior to transfer to the cell surface in secretory vesicles.

The cell surface shows numerous cytoplasmic processes (CP), particularly on the face in contact with existing osteoid (OS). The secretory vesicles discharge their contents from this surface to form identifiable osteoid collagen fibers (OC) embedded in an electron-lucent matrix (Mx) of glycosaminoglycans and proteoglycans.

The formation and secretion of collagen is described on pages 50–52.

Osteocytes are inactive osteoblasts trapped in mineralized bone.

When osteoblasts have completed a burst of osteoid-producing activity, most return to an inactive state, becoming flattened and spindle-shaped and closely applied to the now inactive bone surface. Some osteoblasts however become surrounded by mineralizing bone matrix and lie within small cavities (lacunae) in the bone. When this happens the cell is called an osteocyte (Fig. 13.16).

Fig. 13.16 Osteocytes.
ⓐ Micrograph of a toluidine blue-stained acrylic resin section of bone showing osteocytes trapped within mineralized bone matrix. Note their fine cytoplasmic processes, which lie in narrow canalicular channels within the mineralized bone and link one osteocyte with another.
ⓑ Electron micrograph of a recently entrapped osteocyte. It shows some of the cytoplasmic rough endoplasmic reticulum (RER) and mitochondria (M) of the osteoblast from which it is derived. Note the origin of one of its cytoplasmic processes (CP), the rest being out of the plane of section.

Adjacent osteocytes can communicate with each other by long cytoplasmic processes which lie in narrow channels called canaliculi. Usually they are arranged haphazardly but in cortical bone they assume a regular pattern (see page 235–236).

The function of osteocytes is not known, but each osteocyte in its lacuna maintains a narrow zone of osteoid around it and retains the prominent Golgi and a fraction of the rough endoplasmic reticulum of its parent osteoblast. This suggests that it may be able to maintain the organic matrix.

Through their interconnecting cytoplasmic processes, osteocytes receive nutrients sufficient to survive. They may also resorb formed bone matrix to release calcium (a process called osteocytic osteolysis), though the evidence for this is poor.

TUMORS OF OSTEOBLASTS AND OSTEOCYTES

Osteosarcoma

The most important tumor derived from bone cells is osteosarcoma which is a malignant tumor of osteoblasts. It is most common in children and usually involves the bones around the knee joint, either the lower end of the femur or the upper end of the tibia.

The tumor cells resemble osteoblasts in structure and in function, in that they synthesize osteoid; however, the production of osteoid is scanty, haphazard and irregular, and it does not mineralize normally.

The malignant osteoblasts are largely primitive and more closely resemble immature osteoprogenitor cells than mature osteoblasts.

Osteosarcoma spreads extensively via the bloodstream, often producing secondary (metastatic) tumors in the lungs.

Osteoid osteoma

Benign tumors of osteoblasts occur as localized swellings in bone. Again the tumor cells produce osteoid but, in contrast to osteosarcoma, there is more osteoid formation and a greater degree of mineralization.

In one form of osteoma the cells produce large amounts of regular osteoid which becomes fully mineralized, producing a dense, hard bony nodule; this is ivory osteoma and may be derived from osteocytes.

Osteomas are benign and do not spread.

Osteoclasts erode mineralized bone.

Osteoclasts are large cells with multiple nuclei and abundant cytoplasm and are thought to be derived from blood monocytes. It is not known whether they form from fusion of a number of monocytes or from repeated monocyte nuclear division not associated with cytoplasmic splitting.

Osteoclasts are found attached to the bone surface at sites of active bone resorption, often in depressions where they have eroded into the bone. These depressions are called resorption bays or Howship's lacunae.

For details of osteoclast structure and function see Fig 13.17.

MINERALIZATION OF OSTEOID
Rigidity of bone is determined by deposition of minerals.

The hardness and rigidity of bone is due to the presence of mineral salt in the osteoid matrix. This salt is a crystalline complex of calcium and phosphate hydroxides called hydroxyapatite ($Ca_{10}(PO_4)_6(OH)_2$).

For mineralization to occur, the combined local concentrations of Ca^{++} ions and PO_4^- ions must be above a threshold value. A number of factors operate to bring this about:

- a glycoprotein (osteocalcin) in osteoid binds extracellular Ca^{++} ions, leading to a high local concentration;

Fig. 13.17 Osteoclast.

(a) Micrograph of a toluidine blue-stained epoxy resin section showing a single osteoclast (Oc), which has alighted on an irregular spur of bone prior to reabsorption. At a later stage the spur of bone will have been eroded and leveled as a result of osteoclast activity.

(b) Micrograph of Goldner-stained acrylic resin section of bone showing active resorption of bone on one face, with a multinucleate osteoclast (Oc) lying in a Howship's lacuna. There is active osteoblast deposition of new osteoid on the other face (arrow), in a bone which is undergoing active modeling (see Fig. 13.20).

(c) Electron micrograph of an osteoclast, demonstrating its richness in Golgi, lysosomes, secretory vesicles, and

mitochondria. At its interface with the bone, highly complex cytoplasmic protrusions from the osteoclast's surface appear as a ruffled border (R).

(d) High-power electron micrograph of the ruffled border region where numerous fine cytoplasmic processes (CP) extend from the surface of the osteoclast, some interdigitating with the collagenic fibers (C) of the osteoid. Fragments of mineralized osteoid (mOS) can be seen between the cytoplasmic processes.

(e) Micrograph of a frozen section of bone demonstrating abundant acid phosphatase activity (red) in an osteoclast (Oc) which is actively eroding the bone surface.

- the enzyme alkaline phosphatase, which is abundant in osteoblasts, increases local Ca^{++} and PO_4^- ion concentrations;
- osteoblasts produce matrix vesicles, which can accumulate Ca^{++} and PO_4^- ions, and are rich in the enzymes alkaline phosphatase and pyrophosphatase, both of which can cleave PO_4^- ions from larger molecules.

Matrix vesicles are round membrane-bound vesicles which are probably derived from the cell membrane. During osteoid formation they bud off from the osteoblast into the matrix and form the nidus for the initial precipitation of hydroxyapatite.

It is currently believed that osteoblast-derived matrix vesicles are the most important factor controlling the initial site of mineral deposition in osteoid, and that, once the first few crystals of hydroxyapatite have precipitated out, they grow rapidly by accretion until they join foci growing from other matrix vesicles. In this way, a wave of mineralization sweeps through new osteoid (Fig. 13.18).

Other cells that produce matrix vesicles are the ameloblasts and odontoblasts of the developing tooth (see page 185) and chondrocytes; hence the frequent mineralization of cartilage.

If the local concentrations of Ca^{++} and PO_4^- ions are normal, then mineralization occurs shortly after the new osteoid has been formed. However, when there is a state of high turnover, the osteoblasts produce large amounts of osteoid in a short time and mineralization lags behind, catching up only when the rate of new osteoid production falls.

During a lag phase, distinct layers of unmineralized osteoid can be seen between the layer of active osteoblasts and the previously mineralized bone. This is evident in the phases of rapid bone growth in fetal life, and also in adult life during periods of active remodeling of bone such as following fracture or as part of some disease processes.

Fig. 13.18 Mineralization of bone.
ⓐ Diagram of the events believed to occur in newly formed osteoid. Immediately adjacent to the irregular osteoblast surface is a zone (A) of freshly deposited osteoid collagen and glycosaminoglycan containing newly formed matrix vesicles.

Next is a zone (B), in which early crystals of hydroxyapatite are being deposited in slightly older matrix vesicles, and beyond it a zone (C) in which the foci of mineralization rapidly enlarge by accretion of mineral salts.

In zone D the individual foci of mineralization, each centered on a matrix vesicle remnant, have become almost completely confluent. In zone E mineralization is complete and the underlying osteoid collagen is obscured.

The junction between zones C and D is the so-called calcification front, but as this term is used inaccurately in an entirely different context in pathological studies of bone disease it is best avoided unless carefully defined.

ⓑ High-power electron micrograph showing early mineral deposition in a zone of recently formed osteoid from fetal bone. Note the early crystalline pattern of mineralization of a matrix vesicle (arrows) in zone B, enlargement of foci of mineralization in zone C, becoming confluent in zone D. Zones A and E are not shown.

OSTEOMALACIA (FAILURE OF MINERALIZATION)

Mineralization of osteoid can take place only if there are sufficient Ca^{++} and PO_4^- ions.

If the blood level of Ca^{++} ions is low (due, for example, to inadequate dietary intake by vegans or malabsorption resulting from small intestinal disease), or if PO_4^- ion levels are low (which is uncommon, and usually due to excessive PO_4^- ion loss in the urine), then mineralization is impaired. This leads to the disease known as osteomalacia (Fig. 13.19).

Patients with osteomalacia develop softening of the bone, which results in an increased tendency to bone fracture, either major fractures or a series of smaller microfractures producing bone pain.

Osteomalacia in the growing bones of children leads to the disease called rickets and produces permanent deformity of the soft, poorly mineralized bones.

Fig. 13.19 Osteomalacia.
Micrograph of iliac crest bone embedded in acrylic resin without prior decalcification from a patient with osteomalacia. Note the broad zone of unmineralized osteoid (red) and the central zone of mineralized bone (black) in this section stained by the von Kossa's silver technique.

BONE MODELING

Following initial deposition, the bone matrix and the struts forming trabecular bone are remodeled.
In rapid bone growth in fetal development and childhood, large quantities of bone are produced by osteoblastic synthesis of bone matrix, which is subsequently mineralized. The subsequent pattern of remodeling is determined by local mechanical stresses so that the bone matrix is aligned to resist local shearing and compressive stresses.

Modeling is achieved by a carefully balanced combination of:
- new bone deposition and mineralization by active osteoblasts (see Fig 13.18);
- selective resorption of formed bone by osteoclasts (Fig. 13.20).

Selective resorption of formed bone occurs where the osteoclast is in contact with the bone surface.
Resorption of bone is believed to proceed as follows:
- lysosomal enzymes are released from the osteoclast cytoplasm where it is in contact with the bone;
- the released enzymes hydrolyze the collagenous protein and glycosaminoglycans of the adjacent bone matrix;

- the disrupted bone matrix yields up its attached mineral salts;
- local acidic conditions, which possibly result from the secretion of organic acids such as carbonic, lactic and citric acids by the osteoclasts, break up the hydroxyapatite, thereby releasing soluble Ca^{++} and PO_4^- ions;
- some of the soluble breakdown products of demineralization and protein hydrolysis may be resorbed by the osteoclast by endocytosis.

Osteoclasts are highly mobile and resorb bone as they move along the bone surface.

In some bone diseases, the osteoclasts are stimulated into inappropriate resorptive activity, and at the same time appear to lose their mobility so that they remain localized to one area of the bone surface. In this situation they bore deeply into the bone at one site (tunneling resorption) instead of sweeping bone away from a large area.

Osteoclast resorption of bone can be stimulated by parathyroid hormone (parathormone).
Parathormone is secreted by the parathyroid glands, which maintain a constant level of Ca^{++} ions in the blood by increasing their output of parathormone in response to low serum Ca^{++} ion concentration (see page 262).

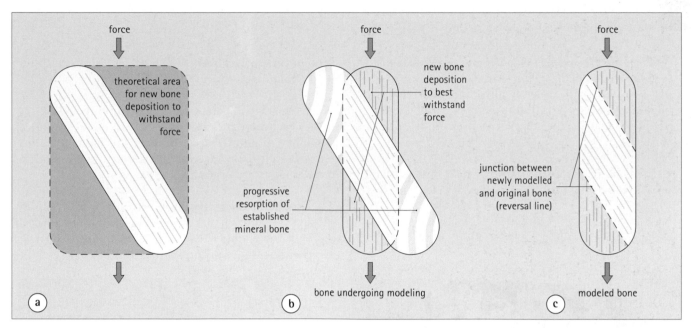

Fig. 13.20 Bone modeling.

(a) Diagram showing a piece of bone inappropriately orientated to best withstand the direction of the force to which it is exposed. The force could be resisted by deposition of new bone on the old in the area indicated, but this would produce a large heavy block of bone which, if repeated throughout the body as a whole, would result in such a bulky mass that movement would be impossible. A more efficient strength to weight ratio is achieved by modeling.

(b) Diagram to show how the bone can be modeled to become more efficient. The junctions between original bone and newly

modeled bone are not easily seen in histological sections of mineralized bone, but are evident when decalcified sections are examined, particularly if the section is examined in polarized light, which accentuates the different directions of the osteoid collagen fibers.

The junctions between different phases of bone deposition in different directions are called reversal lines, and are particularly numerous and haphazard when bone modeling has been random and uncontrolled, as in Paget's disease (see page 244).

(c) Diagram to show final modeled bone with reversal lines.

Parathormone increases the serum Ca^{++} ion level by stimulating osteoclastic activity, the increased resorption of bone resulting in the release of Ca^{++} ions into the blood. In addition, parathormone can increase blood Ca^{++} by reducing Ca^{++} ion loss by the kidney, and by increasing Ca^{++} absorption by the small intestine.

The effect of parathormone activity in the bone is not usually detectable histologically unless there is a prolonged and excessive parathormone secretion.

The elevation of blood Ca^{++} produced by osteoclast-driven bone resorption is not matched by a rise in serum PO_4^- because parathormone also stimulates PO_4^- excretion by the kidney.

Osteoclast activity and bone resorption is inhibited by calcitonin.

Calcitonin is a hormone produced by thyroid C cells (Fig. 14.19). It antagonizes parathormone and is secreted in response to a high serum Ca^{++} level. It has a direct effect on osteoclasts by inhibiting their activity in resorbing

bone, but also has an effect on the kidney where it increases the rate of excretion of both calcium and phosphate. The sum effect of calcitonin is to lower the levels of both calcium and phosphate ions in the blood. The ability of calcitonin to suppress the activity of osteoclasts in resorbing bone has been used in the treatment of Paget's disease (see page 244); treatment with salmon calcitonin sometimes reduces the level of activity of the disease.

There is normally a balance between osteoblast and osteoclast activity.

In normal healthy bone, osteoblast and osteoclast activity are well controlled so that the overall mass of bone remains constant and there is neither loss nor gain of bone once the mature bone mass has been achieved.

At the same time, both osteoblasts and osteoclasts are capable of increasing their activity in response either to an increased physiological demand, such as increased physical activity, or to bone fracture requiring repair and remodeling processes.

OSTEOPOROSIS AND PAGET'S DISEASE

Osteoporosis (Fig. 13.21) can occur as a result of disuse (e.g. prolonged bedrest, limb paralysis), and also in people who are otherwise healthy, particularly post-menopausal women. It results in an increased tendency to bone fracture, particularly compression fractures of vertebrae.

Paget's disease is of unknown cause, but probably results from uncontrolled osteoclast activity, leading to resorption of bone and osteoblastic attempts to fill in the remaining erosions (Fig. 13.22).

When the wave of osteoclastic resorption dies down or moves elsewhere, the osteoblasts continue to produce new bone in an attempt to repair the damage. Thus paradoxically the affected piece of bone usually ends up larger than it was originally.

The repaired bone is, however, less able to resist physical stress because the new bone deposition is haphazard and reparative, rather than organized and constructive; it is therefore more prone to fracture.

Fig. 13.21 Osteoporosis.
(a) Micrograph of a resin section of a bone biopsy from the iliac crest (see Fig. 1.1) showing normal cortical and trabecular bone, stained with a silver method, which makes calcified bone show up as black.
(b) Micrograph of bone from a patient with osteoporosis. When compared with (a), which shows bone mass of a healthy patient of the same age, it is clear that the cortical zone is narrower, and that the trabeculae are thinner and less numerous.

Fig. 13.22 Paget's disease.
Micrograph of a resin embedded, Goldner stained section from a patient with active Paget's disease. There is uncontrolled osteoclast (Oc) resorption of a bone, and osteoblasts (Ob) are attempting to fill in sites of recent osteoclast erosion in an adjacent site.

BONE CELLS

Osteoprogenitor cells

- are precursors of osteoblasts

Osteoblasts

- synthesize osteoid collagen, then mineralize it by depositing calcium and phosphate hydroxides (hydroxyapatite)

- produce matrix vesicles rich in Ca^{++} and PO_4^{++} ions and the enzymes alkaline phosphatase and pyrophosphatase, essential for mineralization.

- are only large, metabolically active cells when there is a requirement for new osteoid deposition; when inactive they are insignificant spindle cells lying on the bone surface (**bone lining cells**)

Osteocytes

- are inactive osteoblasts trapped within the bone they have made

Osteoclasts

- are multinucleate cells derived from blood monocytes

- are highly mobile cells capable of eroding mineralized bone by enzymic hydrolysis of osteoid collagen, with release of bone minerals

- Osteoclastic resorption of bone can be stimulated by parathyroid hormone in response to a low serum calcium level

In the fetus, new bone formation may be intramembranous or endochondral.

Bone develops in the fetus by two mechanisms:

- condensation from sheets of mesenchymal cells which act as bone-forming membranes (intramembranous ossification);
- transformation of previously deposited cartilage (endochondral ossification).

In intramembranous ossification, bone is formed between pre-existing membranes.

Intramembranous ossification results in the formation of flat bones such as those of the skull, and also contributes to some of the cortical bone shafts of long bones. In intramembranous ossification (Fig. 13.23), some of the primitive mesenchymal spindle cells of the mesenchymal membrane enlarge and develop abundant rough endoplasmic reticulum to become active osteoprogenitor cells and eventually osteoblasts.

The resulting osteoblasts begin to deposit bone in isolated islands, and remodeling begins instantly by combined osteoblast and osteoclast activity to form a network of trabecular bone.

Intervening residual mesenchymal tissue develops prominent blood vessels, and some mesenchymal cells eventually develop into hemopoietic bone marrow (see Chapter 7).

Further development is associated with increased bone formation on the outer and inner surfaces to form complete plates of bone (the outer and inner tables).

Fig. 13.23 Intramembranous ossification.

ⓐ Micrograph of an acrylic resin, Goldner-stained section from the skull of a developing fetus. Within the fibrocollagenous membrane, islands of primitive mesenchymal cells develop into clusters of osteoprogenitor cells (Op, see Fig. 13.14), which mature into osteoblasts. The osteoblasts then lay down osteoid (OS), which becomes mineralized (blue-green).

Although the initial bone islands are irregular in shape, remodeling by synchronized osteoblast and osteoclast activity produces flattened sheets of bone.

ⓑ Micrograph of fetal skull showing a slightly later stage in the same process. The bone is now roughly fashioned in the shape of a plate, with almost continuous outer and inner layers bridged by trabeculae (T). The spaces between the bone are occupied by primitive mesenchymal tissue, developing fibrocollagenous tissue, and a system of interconnecting vascular channels (V). Later still the bone plates thicken and hemopoietic marrow fills the spaces.

Endochondral ossification is the method whereby the fetus forms long and short bones using pre-formed cartilage models.

In this process, hyaline cartilage (see Fig. 4.15) is deposited in the shape of the required bone and is subsequently transformed into bone by osteoid deposition and mineralization.

Endochondral ossification permits elongation and thickening of the bone during fetal development and throughout childhood until bone growth ceases.

Hyaline cartilage develops from a mass of immature mesenchymal tissue, and assumes the approximate shape of the bone. In the case of a long bone this will include a shaft (diaphysis) with club-shaped expansions (the epiphyses) at either end (Fig. 13.24).

A layer of spindle-shaped mesenchymal cells, chondroblasts (see page 60) and some osteoprogenitor cells, surrounds the hyaline cartilage model and forms a perichondrium. Later, as osteoprogenitor cells outnumber chondroblast precursors, this layer is termed the periosteum.

At the mid-shaft of the diaphysis, osteoprogenitor cells transform into osteoblasts and lay down osteoid, which becomes mineralized to form a collar of bone around the diaphysis. Concurrently, the chondrocytes in the cartilage model multiply so that it increases in length and breadth; chondroblasts in the perichondrium/periosteum produce new cartilage. Calcium salts are then deposited in the cartilage matrix.

Once the bony collar has been formed, the diaphysis increases in diameter by bone deposition on the outer surface of the collar and resorption of bone on the inner surface.

Capillaries grow into the diaphysis of the model by penetrating the periosteum; they carry osteoprogenitor cells which then establish a primary ossification centre in the centre of the diaphysis.

The osteoprogenitor cells in the primary diaphyseal ossification centre transform into osteoblasts and begin to deposit osteoid, which progressively replaces the calcified cartilage of the original model.

Mineralization of the osteoid, followed by some remodeling, produces a network of trabecular bone

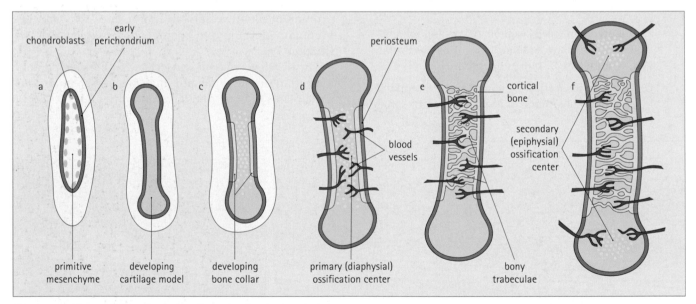

Fig. 13.24 Prenatal long bone development (endochondral ossification).

(a) Chondroblasts develop in primitive mesenchyme and form an early perichondrium and cartilage model.

(b) The developing cartilage model assumes the shape of the bone to be formed, and a surrounding perichondrium becomes identifiable.

(c) At the mid shaft of the diaphysis, the perichondrium becomes a periosteum through the development of osteoprogenitor cells and osteoblasts, the osteoblasts producing a collar of bone by intramembranous ossification. Calcium salts are deposited in the enlarging cartilage model.

(d) Blood vessels grow through the periosteum and bone collar, carrying osteoprogenitor cells within them. These establish a primary (or diaphyseal) ossification centre in the centre of the diaphysis.

(e) Bony trabeculae spread out from the primary ossification centre to occupy the entire diaphysis, linking up with the previously formed bone collar, which now forms the cortical bone of the diaphysis. At this stage the terminal club-shaped epiphyses are still composed of cartilage.

(f) At about term (the precise time varies between long bones),secondary or epiphyseal ossification centers are established in the centre of each epiphysis by the ingrowth along with blood vessels of mesenchymal cells which become osteoprogenitor cells and osteoblasts.

which progressively occupies the core of the diaphysis and merges with the denser compact bone of the peripheral bone collar.

At about the time of birth, blood vessels and osteoprogenitor cells grow into the cartilaginous club-shaped ends of the developing bone (epiphyses) at either end of the diaphyseal shaft and form secondary (or epiphyseal) ossification centers.

Long bones continue to grow throughout childhood and adolescence.

Increase in length is due to continued endochondral bone formation at each end of the long bones.

An actively proliferating plate of cartilage (the epiphyseal plate) remains across the junction between the epiphysis and diaphysis. This plate gives rise to apposition of new cartilage to the ends of the diaphysis, which is converted to trabecular bone, leading to a progressive increase in length (Fig. 13.25). Activity of the epiphyseal plate normally ceases after puberty.

New bone forms on the diaphyseal side of the epiphyseal plate as follows:

- cartilage on the epiphyseal face of the epiphyseal plate proliferates to produce columns of chondrocytes embedded in matrix;
- chondrocytes approaching the diaphyseal face of the epiphyseal plate become greatly enlarged and pale-staining, and begin to produce alkaline phosphatase, which facilitates calcification of the matrix;
- osteoblasts lay down osteoid on the calcified cartilaginous matrix as the first stage in the ossification of the calcified cartilaginous trabeculae;
- the deposited bone is remodeled as it is incorporated into the diaphysis.

The epiphyseal plate and the zone of ossifying cartilaginous matrix trabeculae form the metaphysis.

Increase in circumference of the diaphysis is achieved by formation of new bone on the outer surface of the cortical bone, which is subjected to slightly less active resorption on its inner aspect.

This not only increases the diameter of the diaphysis, but also the thickness of the cortical bone, which is necessary to cope with the increased physical demands resulting from increasing body weight and physical activity.

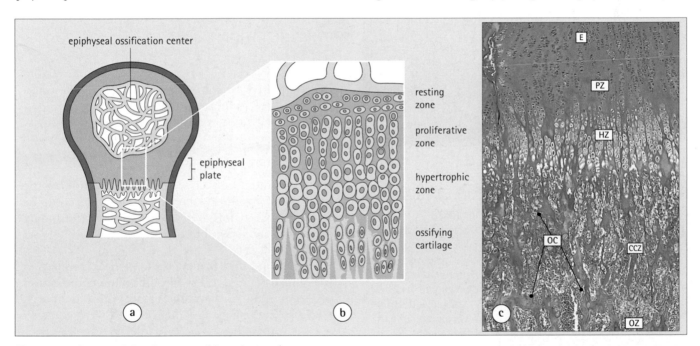

Fig. 13.25 Postnatal development of long bones (endochondral ossification).

(a) Diagram showing the initial enlargement of the secondary (epiphyseal) ossification centre within the epiphyseal cartilage, leaving an epiphyseal plate of cartilage and a surround of cartilage which will ultimately become the articular cartilage

(b) Diagram showing the fine detail of the epiphyseal plate between the secondary epiphyseal ossification centre on one side and the developing diaphyseal trabecular bone on the other. Chondrocytes in the epiphyseal plate proliferate in columns towards the diaphysis, becoming hypertrophied as they deposit cartilage matrix. The matrix becomes progressively mineralized before osteoblasts deposit osteoid on the calcified matrix model.

(c) Low-power micrograph of decalcified H&E-stained epiphyseal region from a long bone of a fetus, for comparison with b . Epiphyseal plate cartilage (E), the proliferative zone (PZ), the hypertrophic zone (HZ), the calcified cartilage zone (CCZ) and the beginning of the ossification zone (OZ) can be seen.

At this stage there is hemopoietic marrow in the spaces between the ossifying plates of cartilage (OC).

Secondary ossification centers develop in the epiphyseal cartilage at a later stage of development.

JOINTS

INTRODUCTION

Bones are connected to each other by joints, which permit varying degrees of movement between the joined bones.

Joints can be divided into two main groups:

- those that permit limited movement;
- those that permit free movement.

Some joints between bones are formed by fibrocollagenous or cartilaginous tissue.

In joints that permit only limited movement, the bones are connected by flexible fibrocollagenous or cartilaginous tissue. Such joints generally occur between bones subserving a primary supportive or protective role, for example between:

- the flat bones of the skull, which are joined by fibrous or ligamentous tissues (syndesmoses);
- the ribs and the sternum, which are joined by cartilage (synchondroses).

In old age, the support tissue forming both syndesmoses and synchondroses tends to be replaced by bone to form a rigid immobile joint (synostosis).

A clinically important group of joints of limited movement are those between vertebrae.

The bodies of the vertebrae are joined to each other to form the long uninterrupted column (vertebral column) by the intervertebral disks. These are thick rubbery pads which not only act as shock-absorbers but also permit some movement so that the column is flexible within limits.

Intervertebral disks are composed essentially of fibrocollagenous tissue containing some chondrocytes and cartilage matrix (fibrocartilage, see page 61). The two surfaces in contact with the vertebral bodies each consist of a thin layer of hyaline cartilage covering a concentrically lamellated rubbery structure of fibrocartilage (the annulus fibrosus). At the centre of the disk is a soft semi-fluid core of soft gelatinous matrix (the nuclear pulposus, Fig. 13.26).

Fig. 13.26
Intervertebral disk.
ⓐ Micrograph of an acrylic resin section of an intervertebral disk (I) between two vertebrae (V) stained with H&E.
ⓑ Micrograph of part of the same intervertebral disc at higher magnification, showing the annulus fibrosus (AF) forming a compact outer region adjacent to vertebral bone and the soft, semi-fluid at the centre nucleus pulposus (NP)

SCIATICA

Wear and tear on the intervertebral disks may lead to degeneration of the annulus fibrosus, with extension of the nucleus pulposus into it. This results in:

- impaired efficiency of the disk as a shock absorber;
- expansion of the annulus fibrosus, causing it to bulge.

If the annulus fibrosus bulges in the region of the spinal nerves as they emerge from the spinal cord, the nerves may be stretched and damaged, producing peripheral nerve symptoms.

Intervertebral disk degeneration is most common in the lumbar region of the vertebral column and causes pressure on the nerves, producing sciatica, pain travelling down the back and outer side of the leg.

Joints that allow free movement between adjacent bones are termed synovial joints.

The bone ends are held together by bands of collagenous tissue (ligaments) which may be external or internal to the joint cavity; external ligaments surround a fibrous capsule enclosing the heads of the bones, which are separated from each other by a lubricant fluid, synovial fluid.

Because the bone ends move against each other, they are coated with a smooth, friction-free layer of hyaline cartilage (articular cartilage), and the synovial fluid provides a thin lubricant film between the opposing articular cartilages.

The internal lining of the joint capsule is a specialized secretory epithelium, the synovium, which produces synovial fluid.

The synovium is composed of 1–4 layers of cells which merge on their deep surface with a zone of loosely arranged fibrocollagenous tissue containing adipocytes, fibroblasts, mast cells, and macrophages. This deep layer merges with the denser fibrocollagenous tissue of the joint capsule.

Synovial cells vary from flat, mesothelial-like cells through to spindle-shaped, polyhedral or cuboidal cells.

Two cell types have been defined in synovial membrane: type A cells are phagocytic and contain numerous lysosomes, while type B cells contain abundant rough endoplasmic reticulum and appear to be adapted for protein production. The synovial membrane has an abundant blood, lymphatic and nerve supply running in the loose fibrocollagenous tissue.

Ligaments, composed of dense collagenous tissue, stabilize joints.

Structures around the joint, which prevent excess movement, include collagenous external ligaments and tendinous muscle attachments (Fig. 13.27). External ligaments surround articular (synovial) joints, attaching one bone to the other over the outer surface of the joint capsule.

Ligaments are composed of tightly packed collagen fibers all running in the same direction, with compressed fibrocytes in between; thus they resemble tendon. They differ from tendon in that they contain elastic fibers. Ligaments strengthen the joint; they permit normal movement but prevent over-flexing or over-extension. The attachment of ligament to bone is similar to that of tendons.

In some complex joints there are internal ligaments (e.g. cruciate ligaments in the knee joints) to prevent overstretching or twisting, and fibrocartilaginous menisci (also in the knee) to stabilize and guide gliding movements.

Fig. 13.27 Synovial joint.
(a) Diagram of a simple synovial joint showing the two articulating bone ends separated from each other by synovial fluid and enclosed within a fibrocollagenous capsule. Surrounding ligaments and tendinous muscle attachments prevent excess movement.

(b) Low power micrograph of an interphalangeal joint of the finger. Note the ends of the articulating bone (B), the articular cartilages (AC) and the joint capsule enclosing the synovial cavity (SC), which contains synovial fluid. The synovial cavity is lined internally by synovium.

ARTHRITIS

Osteoarthritis

Some synovial joints, particularly the hip and finger joints, are exposed to persistent wear and tear over many years. This sometimes leads to degeneration of the articular cartilage, which loses its normal complement of hydrated glycosaminoglycans and so is unable to resist compressive forces. This leads to erosion of the cartilage and rubbing together of adjacent bone surfaces.

Eventually the surface bone becomes highly compacted and ivory-like; this is called eburnation.

The constant bone-to-bone trauma and excessive movement at the joint leads to a painful swollen joint with:
- thickening of the joint capsule;
- irregular protuberances of abnormal new bone at the edges of the articular surfaces (osteophytes);
- reduction in the synovial space.

These are the typical changes of osteoarthritis.

Rheumatoid arthritis

Another common form of arthritis is rheumatoid arthritis, an autoimmune disease causing immune-mediated damage to the synovial membrane and articular cartilage.

The synovial membrane becomes thick and extensively infiltrated by cells of the immune system (mainly lymphocytes and plasma cells), while the damaged articular cartilage is replaced by vascular fibrocollagenous tissue (pannus).

1. OSTEOBLASTS

(a) are derived from blood monocytes
(b) synthesize and secrete osteoid collagen
(c) produce matrix vesicles important in mineralization of bone matrix
(d) have abundant rough endoplasmic reticulum
(e) have a characteristic ruffled border on the surface closest to the bone

2. OSTEOCLASTS

(a) are derived from osteoprogenitor cells
(b) erode bone
(c) are stimulated by parathyroid hormone
(d) are stimulated by calcitonin
(e) are rich in alkaline phosphatase

3. SKELETAL MUSCLE

(a) develops from primitive rhabdomyoblasts
(b) contains type 1 fast-twitch fibers
(c) contains satellite cells which are phagocytic
(d) contains stretch receptors called muscle spindles
(e) contains motor nerve twigs which terminate in motor end plates

4. IN BONE DEVELOPMENT

(a) chondroblasts develop in primitive mesenchyme and form an early perichondrium and cartilage model
(b) the term diaphysis refers to the shaft region
(c) the term epiphysis refers to the club-shaped expansion at the end of long bones
(d) the epiphyseal plate can be divided into periosteum, bone collar and osteoprogenitor zones
(e) postnatal increase in length is due to endochondral bone formation near the end of long bones.

14. Endocrine System

INTRODUCTION

Cell communication is vital for any multicellular organism to function efficiently.

At a local level, cells communicate via cell surface molecules and gap junctions (see page 39), while remote communication is mediated by the secretion of chemical messengers which activate cells by interacting with specific receptors. Such secretion may be one of four types: autocrine, paracrine, endocrine or synaptic (Fig. 14.1).

Autocrine secretion occurs when a cell secretes a chemical messenger to act on its own receptors. This is particularly evident in the local control of cell growth by substances such as epidermal growth factor.

Paracrine secretion describes the secretion of chemical messengers to act on adjacent cells. This is also mainly concerned with the local control of cell growth and is also a mode of action of many of the cells of the diffuse neuroendocrine system (see page 269).

Endocrine secretion is the secretion of chemical messengers (hormones) into the blood stream to act on distant tissues.

Synaptic secretion refers to communication by direct structural targeting from one cell to another via synapses, and is confined to the nervous system.

The chemical messengers belong to four main molecular classes:

- amino acid derivatives (e.g. epinephrine/adrenalin, norepinephrine/noradrenalin, thyroxine);
- small peptides (e.g. encephalin, vasopressin, thyroid releasing hormone);
- proteins (e.g. nerve growth factor, epidermal growth factor, insulin, growth hormone, parathormone, thyroid stimulating hormone);
- steroids (e.g. cortisol, progesterone, estradiol, testosterone).

Most chemical messengers are water-soluble, hydrophilic molecules that diffuse freely and usually interact with a cell surface receptor protein. However, steroids and thyroxine are hydrophobic; after carriage to a cell by special proteins in the blood, they pass through its membrane to interact with receptor proteins inside.

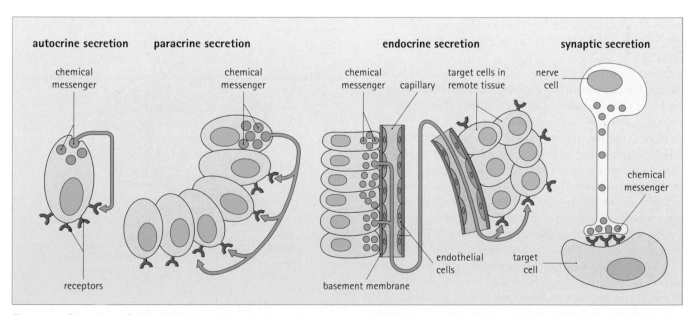

Fig. 14.1 Secretion of chemical messengers.
Diagram showing the four mechanisms of chemical messenger secretion.

ENDOCRINE CELL AND TISSUE SPECIALIZATION

Cells whose main role is to secrete messenger substances are termed endocrine cells.

Endocrine cells are found in three distinct anatomic distributions:

- gathered together in one specialized organ to form an endocrine gland (e.g. adrenal, pituitary and pineal glands);
- forming discrete clusters in another specialized organ (e.g. ovary, testis, pancreas);
- dispersed singly among other cells in epithelial tissues, particularly in the gut and respiratory tract, in which case they form part of what is referred to as the diffuse neuroendocrine system.

Endocrine cells and tissues have special characteristics related to their secretory function.

Certain cells termed neuroendocrine cells have membrane-bound vesicles, which are granules containing the chemical messenger. Secretion is achieved by exocytosis, in which the membrane of the vesicle fuses with the cell membrane, thereby discharging its contents outside the cell. Certain neuroendocrine cells transiently store the messenger as specific neuroendocrine granules, which can be identified in cells using immunohistochemical staining techniques.

Endocrine tissues are usually vascular to facilitate rapid dissemination of secreted products into the bloodstream. In contrast to other types of secretory cell, the secretory pole of endocrine cells is adjacent to the capillary vessel wall, while the nucleus is found at the opposite pole.

Autocrine and paracrine messengers act relatively slowly, having to diffuse into the bloodstream. They act on local cell receptors and are rapidly destroyed once secreted, thereby limiting their activity.

Endocrine messengers act relatively slowly, having to diffuse into the blood stream, circulate to a target organ, and then enter a target cell. Many neuroendocrine cells secrete amines or peptides and have common metabolic features involving the uptake of amines which then undergo decarboxylation in the process of hormone synthesis. This has led to the term APUD cells (amine precursor uptake and decarboxylation).

Cells containing neuroendocrine granules and of neuroendocrine lineage have a restricted set of specific metabolic isoenzymes and structural proteins which can be detected histochemically. γγ-Enolase is an isoenzyme in the glycolytic pathway that is present in high concentration in neuroendocrine cells together with PGP 9.5 (ubiquitin-C-terminal hydrolase). In the neuroendocrine granules, chromogranin is a component of the core protein and synaptophysin is a glycoprotein in their membrane. Histochemical detection of these substances enables their use as markers of neuroendocrine differentiation.

PITUITARY

The pituitary is a multi-functional endocrine gland.

The pituitary gland secretes a large number of hormones to activate many peripheral endocrine cells, for example those in the adrenal glands, thyroid, testes and ovaries.

The pituitary is a bean-shaped gland approximately $12 \times 10 \times 9$ mm in size and weighing 0.4–0.9 g in the adult. It is sited beneath the brain, to which it is linked by the pituitary stalk, and is surrounded by the bone of the base of the skull in a depression of the sphenoid bone termed the sella turcica (Fig. 14.2).

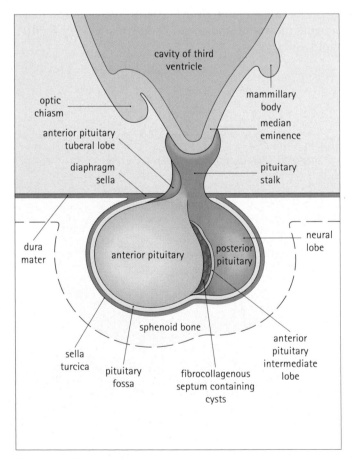

Fig. 14.2 Pituitary gland.
Diagram showing the pituitary gland and its relationship to surrounding structures.

Anatomically the pituitary is divided into two parts.

The anterior pituitary (adenohypophysis) is an epithelial-derived tissue with three distinct components: the distal lobe (pars distalis) forming the major portion of the gland; the intermediate lobe (pars intermedia), which is a rudimentary zone in man but prominent in other mammals; and the tuberal lobe (pars tuberalis), which is a layer of cells running up the pituitary stalk.

The posterior pituitary (neurohypophysis) is composed of neuronal processes and glia and has three components: the neural lobe (pars nervosa, infundibular process) lying behind the anterior pituitary in the sella turcica; the pituitary stalk (infundibular stem) in which axons run from the brain above; and the median eminence (infundibulum), a funnel-shaped extension of the hypothalamus.

Embryologically, the anterior pituitary is thought to be derived from an outgrowth of the foregut endoderm called Rathke's pouch. This connects with a downgrowth of the developing hypothalamus, which forms the posterior pituitary and comes to lie in the base of the skull.

The vascular supply of the pituitary integrates the functions of the endocrine and nervous systems.

A special network of blood vessels (pituitary portal system, see Fig 14.3) carries hormones from the hypothalamus of the brain to stimulate or inhibit the hormone secretion of the anterior pituitary.

The major blood supply to the anterior pituitary is derived from vessels that run down the pituitary stalk. These are easily damaged in severe head injury, resulting in death of the anterior pituitary and consequent ablation of its endocrine function.

ANTERIOR PITUITARY

The anterior pituitary secretes several hormones into the bloodstream.

The anterior pituitary is served by a fine capillary network which, bringing blood from the hypothalamus, contains both stimulatory and inhibitory hormones (Fig. 14.4). These hormones control the neuroendocrine cells of the anterior pituitary. In turn their secretions diffuse back into the capillary network, which subsequently drains into the pituitary veins and thence into the carotid venous sinus and systemic circulation.

Fig. 14.3 Vascular supply of the pituitary.
The blood supply of the pituitary arises from three paired arteries originating from the internal carotid arteries. The superior hypophyseal arteries enter the median eminence and form the external plexus close to nerve endings from neuroendocrine cells in the hypothalamus. This gives way to a parallel capillary network which surrounds larger central muscular vessels and runs down the pituitary stalk to form the long portal vessels. Arising from the portal vessels, capillary vessels run forward into the anterior pituitary, providing a direct vascular link between the hypothalamus and the neuroendocrine cells of the anterior pituitary.
Additional blood supply to the posterior pituitary is derived from the small middle and inferior hypophyseal arteries. A minor blood supply to the periphery of the anterior pituitary is derived from small blood vessels in the capsule of the gland.

Fig. 14.4 Anterior pituitary cells and vessels.
Toluidine blue resin section showing pituitary endocrine cells (E) arranged in groups and surrounded by capillaries (C).

The anterior pituitary contains five distinct types of endocrine cell which vary in their distribution within the gland (Figs 14.5 and 14.6); each type has the same basic ultrastructure (Fig. 14.7). These cells are:

- somatotrophs (Fig. 14.8) which secrete growth hormone (GH);
- lactotrophs (Fig. 14.9), which secrete prolactin (PRL);
- corticotrophs (Fig. 14.10), which secrete adrenocorticotropic hormone (ACTH), β-lipotrophin (β-LPH), α-melanocyte stimulating hormone (α-MSH), and β-endorphin.
- thyrotrophs, which secrete thyroid stimulating hormone (TSH).
- gonadotrophs (Fig. 14.11), which secrete the gonadotropic hormones, follicle stimulating hormone (FSH) and luteinizing hormone (LH).

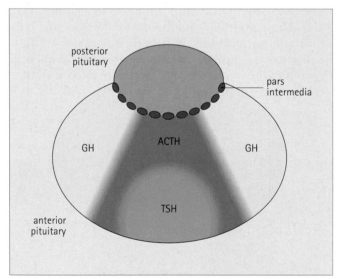

Fig. 14.5 Regional distribution of anterior pituitary cells.
Diagram of a horizontal cross-section of the distal lobe of the pituitary. The lateral wings contain mainly somatotrophs, which secrete GH, while corticotrophs, which secrete ACTH, β-lipotrophin, α-MSH and β-endorphin, are concentrated in the median portion of the gland just in front of the posterior pituitary. Thyrotrophs, which secrete TSH, are concentrated anteriorly. Lactotrophs secreting PRL and gonadotrophs secreting FSH and LH are uniformly scattered throughout the gland.

Fig. 14.6 Traditional methods for demonstrating cells of the anterior pituitary.
Traditionally cells of the anterior pituitary have been classified into three types: acidophils (cytoplasm staining with acidic dyes), basophils (cytoplasm staining with basic dyes and the periodic acid Schiff (PAS) method), and chromophobes (cells with no cytoplasmic staining). In the PAS orange-G hematoxylin stain shown here, acidophils (A) stain bright yellow, basophils (B) stain darkly, and chromophobes (C) do not stain. Nuclei are stained black by the hematoxylin.

It is now customary to classify cells according to their hormone content, which is demonstrable by immunohistochemical staining using antibodies to each hormone type. It is also possible to distinguish the cells of the anterior pituitary by electron microscopy.

These techniques have shown that acidophils are cells secreting GH or PRL (i.e. somatotrophs and lactotrophs), and that basophils are thyrotrophs, corticotrophs, and gonadotrophs. All of these cells contain abundant dense core granules. Basophils stain well with hematoxylin and PAS, which detect glycosyl groups, because TSH, LH and FSH are glycoproteins and the ACTH precursor protein is glycosylated. Chromophobes fail to stain because they contain very few granules, but may be lactotroph, somatotroph, thyrotroph, gonadotroph or corticotroph in nature. Some cells, which contain sparse dense-core granules with no recognizable immunostaining, have been termed null cells.

Fig. 14.7 Ultrastructure of anterior pituitary cells.
Electron micrograph of anterior pituitary cells showing their numerous hormone-containing dense-core granules (G).

Fig. 14.8 Somatotrophs.
Somatotrophs make up about 50% of the anterior pituitary and are generally large, ovoid or polygonal in shape, as shown in this section stained to show GH by an immunoperoxidase method.

Ultrastructurally, somatotrophs contain abundant randomly distributed electron-dense granules which measure from 300–600 nm in diameter, but the majority are between 350–450 nm. The rough endoplasmic reticulum is arranged in parallel stacks, many positioned parallel to the cell membranes. Tumors which are derived from somatotroph cells contain spherical bundles of intermediate filaments called fibrous bodies.

Fig. 14.9 Lactotrophs.
Lactotrophs make up about 25% of the anterior pituitary. While some are rounded and polygonal, most are compressed by adjacent cells into narrow angular profiles as shown in this section of gland stained by an immunoperoxidase method to show prolactin. They increase in size and number during pregnancy and lactation.

Ultrastructurally, lactotrophs have a prominent Golgi compared to all other anterior pituitary cells and their granules measure 200–350 nm in diameter. Interestingly, exocytosis may be seen at their lateral borders (misplaced exocytosis) as well as in the usual site adjacent to capillary basement membrane. This feature can be used in diagnostic assessment, as it is limited to lactotroph-derived tumors.

Fig. 14.10 Corticotrophs.
Accounting for 15–20% of the anterior pituitary, corticotrophs are large and polygonal in shape, as shown in this micrograph stained to show ACTH by an immunoperoxidase technique.

Many corticotrophs possess an unstained perinuclear vacuole called the enigmatic body, which is derived from secondary lysosomes. Granules in corticotrophs are large and typically measure 250–700 nm in diameter.

Large perinuclear bundles of intermediate cytokeratin filaments are prominent ultrastructurally and these become even more prominent in glucocorticoid excess, when they are visible under the light microscope as pink-staining inclusions (Crooke's hyaline).

Fig. 14.11 Gonadotrophs.
Constituting around 10% of anterior pituitary cells, gonadotrophs are scattered as single cells or small groups throughout the gland, as seen in this section which has been stained to show the β-subunit of FSH by an immunoperoxidase technique. Both FSH and LH may be evident within the same cell.

Ultrastructurally the granules are 150–400 nm in diameter. Following ablation of the ovaries or testes, gonadotrophs develop extensive cytoplasmic vacuolation. This is due to dilation of the endoplasmic reticulum by stored product and caused by the loss of feedback inhibition by gonadal steroids. Such cells, large, rounded, and vacuolated on light microscopy, are called castration cells.

The intermediate lobe of the anterior pituitary is relatively small in man.

The intermediate lobe of the anterior pituitary is located between the posterior pituitary and the distal lobe (see Fig. 14.2). It is poorly developed in humans compared to other mammals, consisting of a series of gland-like acini lined by a cuboidal epithelium. These cells are usually immunoreactive for corticotropic hormones and it has been suggested that they may be producing one of the minor subunits of the pre-pro-opiomelanocortic peptide such as β-LPH, α-MSH, or β-endorphin, rather than ACTH.

The tuberal lobe is an upward extension of the anterior pituitary around the pituitary stalk.

The tuberal lobe consists of a thin layer of cuboidal epithelial cells. Immunohistochemically most of the cells are gonadotrophs.

PITUITARY ADENOMA

Adenomas are benign tumors of pituitary neuroendocrine cells and are commonly functional, causing endocrine syndromes. They are usually treated by surgical removal.

Fig. 14.12 Pituitary adenoma.
Micrograph of pituitary showing proliferation of somatotrophs. The resulting excessive GH secretion caused acromegaly.

Occasionally nests of squamous cells can be seen, from which cysts and even tumors may develop. It has been assumed that these are embryological remnants of the endodermal Rathke's pouch.

POSTERIOR PITUITARY

The posterior pituitary is a continuation of the hypothalamic region of the brain.

The posterior pituitary extends down into the pituitary stalk and sella turcica (see Fig. 14.2) and secretes oxytocin and antidiuretic hormone (vasopressin).

It is composed of the axons of neuronal cells lying in the supraoptic and paraventricular nuclei of the hypothalamus, together with supporting glial cells termed pituicytes (Fig. 14.13). The axons terminate in the posterior pituitary adjacent to a rich network of capillary vessels.

Fig. 14.13 Posterior pituitary.
The posterior pituitary is composed of axons which originate from cells in the hypothalamus and possess numerous neurosecretory granules containing either oxytocin or vasopressin, together with a carrier protein termed neurophysin, and ATP. Where axons are adjacent to capillaries they form fusiform swellings filled with neurosecretory granules (Herring bodies). The posterior pituitary also contains specialized stellate-shaped glial cells called pituicytes.

In this micrograph the axons are seen as a pale fibrillary background in which the nuclei of pituicytes (P) and small capillary vessels are present.

HYPOTHALAMUS

__The actions of the endocrine and nervous systems are coordinated by the hypothalamus__.

The hypothalamus is a region of brain composed of several clusters of neurons that secrete hormones. These hormones act as either releasing or inhibiting factors for the hormones secreted by the anterior pituitary, and are transported to the pituitary gland by two routes as follows:

- a specialized system of blood vessels transports hypothalamic hormones to act locally on neuroendocrine cells in the anterior pituitary (Fig. 14.14);
- axons project down from the hypothalamus to form the pituitary stalk, which terminates as the posterior pituitary.

PITUITARY GLAND AND HYPOTHALAMUS

- anterior pituitary secretes prolactin, GH, ACTH, TSH, FSH, LH and others

- posterior pituitary stores and secretes oxytocin and ADH which are made in hypothalamic nuclei

- hypothalamus is in direct communication with posterior pituitary via pituitary stalk, and anterior pituitary via pituitary portal vessels

- hypothalamus produces hormones stimulating or inhibiting release of anterior pituitary hormones

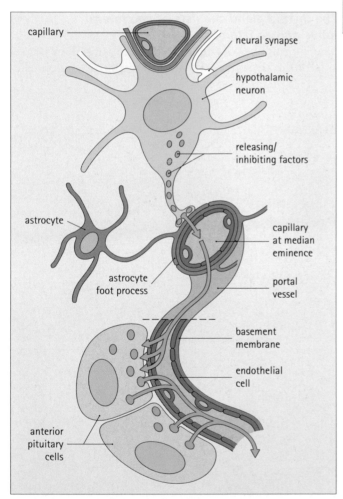

Fig. 14.14 Hypothalamic control of anterior pituitary hormone production.
Hypothalamic neurons secrete releasing/inhibiting factors in response to chemoreceptive and neural inputs. These hormones diffuse into capillaries at the median eminence and are carried to the anterior pituitary in the portal vessels. Astrocyte foot processes surrounding the capillary vessels form part of their diffusion barrier.

Hypothalamic hormones

At least eight hormones are known to be secreted by hypothalamic neurons. Two of these are the peptides **oxytocin** and **arginine vasopressin**, synthesized in the cell bodies of neurons in the supraoptic and paraventricular nuclei of the hypothalamus. They pass down axons into the posterior pituitary via the pituitary stalk and are released into the capillaries of the posterior pituitary.

The other hypothalamic hormones are inhibiting or releasing hormones controlling secretion of anterior pituitary hormones. They are transported via the pituitary portal vessels (see Fig. 14.14). These are:

- Thyrotropin releasing hormone (TRH) – mainly from dorsomedial nuclei

- Gonadotropin releasing hormone (GnRH) – mainly from arcuate nuclei and pre-optic area

- Growth hormone releasing hormone (GHRH) – mainly from arcuate nuclei

- Corticotropin releasing hormone (CRH) – from anterior part of paraventricular nuclei

- Growth hormone inhibiting hormone (GIH) – also known as **somatostatin** (SS) – from paraventricular nuclei

- Prolactin release inhibiting hormone (PIH) – also known as **dopamine** (DA)– from arcuate nuclei.

No single prolactin releasing hormone has been found, but other hormones have this action e.g. oxytocin, VIP and TRH.

PINEAL

The pineal gland secretes melatonin.

The pineal gland is located just below the posterior end of the corpus callosum of the brain. It is a flattened conical structure 6–10 mm long and 5–6 mm wide; it is covered by leptomeninges and composed of lobules of specialized cells which are separated by septa containing unmyelinated nerves and blood vessels (Fig. 14.15). The gland consists of two major cell types: pinealocytes and glial cells.

Pinealocytes are neuron-like cells that produce melatonin, which induces rhythmic changes in the secretions of the hypothalamus, pituitary and gonads, and is said to act as an endocrine transducer. They have pink-staining cytoplasm and dark-staining rounded nuclei, and are often arranged in rosettes, where several cells surround a central fibrillary area composed of cell processes directed towards a small capillary vessel.

Glial cells tend to be bipolar elongated cells that run between nests of pinealocytes. They are indistinct unless specially stained.

A common age-related change in the pineal is the accumulation of calcium particles, which are visible on a skull radiograph; thus the gland can be used as a radiologic midline landmark.

The pineal gland is innervated by sympathetic and parasympathetic nervous systems. In addition, signals from the retina arrive indirectly, as shown in Fig. 14.15a.

THYROID

INTRODUCTION

The thyroid gland secretes two hormones, thyroxine and calcitonin. Thyroxine has the major role in the regulation of the basal metabolic rate, while calcitonin is involved in calcium homeostasis.

The thyroid gland consists of two lateral lobes and an isthmus.

The lateral lobes of the thyroid are arranged on either side of the thyroid cartilage and upper trachea in the

Fig. 14.15 Pineal gland.
(a) Diagram to show the location of the pineal gland. Output of pineal melatonin is modulated by light through nervous pathways which input as sympathetic innervation to the gland.
(b) Low-power micrograph of a reticulin-stained section of pineal showing the septa (S) which divide it into discrete lobules (L) of pinealocytes.

(c) High-power micrograph of an H&E-stained section of pineal showing a single pineal lobule surrounded by septa composed of glial processes and small vessels. In the center of the lobule pinealocyte cell bodies are found in a background of pink-staining cell processes, some of which form a rosette structure.

anterior portion of the neck. These lobes are joined near their lower poles by the isthmus crossing in front of the lower larynx; occasionally a small triangular pyramidal lobe projects upwards from the midpoint of the isthmus.

Each lateral lobe is about 5 cm long, 3–4 cm wide and 2–3 cm deep. In the healthy adult, the thyroid weighs 15–20 g and is slightly heavier in males, though many factors influence its weight at any one time, for example pathological abnormalities.

The thyroid is enclosed by a thin collagenous capsule from which internal septa penetrate the parenchyma, dividing it into irregular lobules.

Embryologically the thyroid develops from a downgrowth of endoderm arising near the root of the tongue and called the thyroglossal duct, which atrophies and leaves a nodule of thyroid tissue at its correct anatomic site.

THYROGLOSSAL DUCT CYST

Occasionally the thyroglossal duct fails to atrophy completely, and thyroglossal duct tissue persists in the midline of the neck, usually as a cyst or a sinus track (thyroglossal duct cyst).

The thyroid gland contains colloid which is rich in thyroglobulin.

The glandular component of the thyroid is composed of epithelium arranged as tightly-packed spherical units called acini (Fig. 14.16).

Each acinus is lined by a single layer of specialized thyroid epithelium which rests on a basement membrane and encloses a lumen filled with thyroid colloid, a pink-staining (eosinophilic) homogenous proteinaceous material rich in thyroglobulin.

Thyroglobulin is the storage form of thyroxine and is an iodinated glycoprotein (Fig. 14.17). The size of an acinus depends on whether it is in a secretory or a storage phase.

During an active secretory phase the thyroid follicular cells show the following changes:
- the endoplasmic reticulum becomes more prominent;
- free ribosomes become more prominent;
- the Golgi enlarges;
- the surface microvilli increase in number and length;
- intracytoplasmic droplets appear (representing colloid in endocytotic vesicles generated by pseudopodial extensions of cytoplasm at the luminal surface).

The synthesis and breakdown of thyroglobulin is controlled by the hypothalamus and pituitary gland.

Low blood thyroxine levels stimulate the hypothalamus to produce thyrotropin releasing hormone (TRH), which then stimulates the anterior pituitary to produce thyroid stimulating hormone (TSH). In turn, TSH stimulates both thyroglobulin synthesis and breakdown, with a consequent increase in thyroxine release into the capillary circulation. When thyroxine levels rise, TRH and TSH production decreases.

Fig. 14.16 Thyroid.
Micrograph showing thyroid acinus composed of specialized thyroid epithelium (TE) resting on a basement membrane (BM). These epithelial cells enclose a lumen filled with thyroid colloid (TC), and are surrounded by a fine network of capillaries (C) associated with thin fibrous septa.

THYROID HORMONES

The two hormones are triiodothyronine (T3) and thyroxine, which is tetraiodothyronine (T4), both of which are iodinated derivatives of tyrosine. The thyroid follicular cells produce and secrete mainly T4 (only 5–10% of the thyroid's output in T3), but T3 is functionally much more potent than T4. Most of the active T3 is produced in other tissues by the removal of one iodine molecule from T4; kidney and liver are particularly important deiodinators of T4. In the plasma, both T3 and T4 are largely bound to a protein, thyroxine-binding globulin-TBG; probably only the free non-bound hormones are physiologically active.

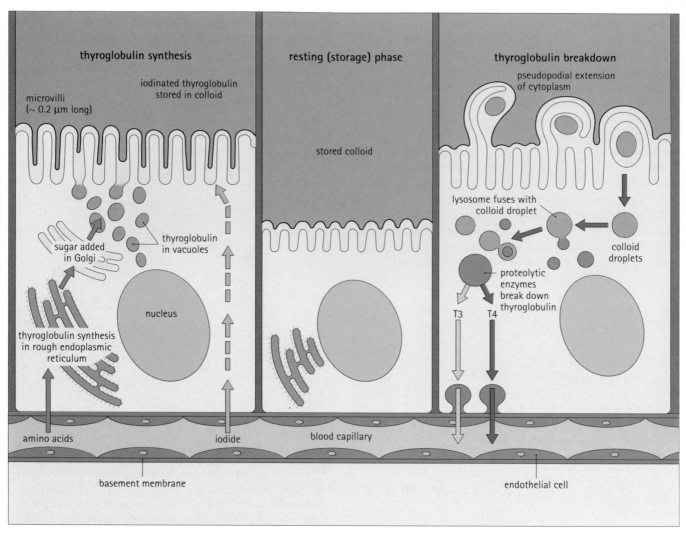

Fig. 14.17 Thyroid colloid.

(a) Thyroglobulin is produced by the thyroid epithelial cells, its protein component being synthesized in the rough endoplasmic reticulum and transported by the Golgi where most of its sugar component is added by glycolysation.

Thyroglobulin leaves the exit face of the Golgi in small vacuoles which are transported to the luminal surface. It is released into the lumen by exocytosis.

Shortly after this release iodine is added to its tyrosine component, the iodine having been formed in the epithelial cell cytoplasm by the oxidation of iodide. (The thyroid epithelial cell is not only able to transport iodide against a concentration gradient from the capillary blood into the lumen of the follicle, but is also able to convert iodide into iodine).

(b) Thyroglobulin acts as a reservoir from which thyroxine can be produced and secreted into the capillary circulation when required.

(c) To release thyroxine from the stored colloid, the thyroid epithelial cell extrudes pseudopodial extensions of cytoplasm from its luminal surface; these enclose small droplets of colloid which are then incorporated into its cytoplasm.

Lysosomes fuse with the small vacuoles and hydrolysis and proteolysis of the thyroglobulin occur, breaking it into smaller units, the most important of which is tetraiodothyronine (T4) or thyroxine. Another product is triiodothyronine (T3). Both are iodinated amino acids.

THYROTOXICOSIS

In thyrotoxicosis the thyroid epithelial cells increase in size and number and their work rate increases so that excessive thyroxine is produced (Fig. 14.18).

This is manifest clinically by weight loss and heat intolerance (due to an increased basal metabolic rate), tremor, rapid pulse, and bulging of the eyes (exophthalmos), due to an increase in the orbital support tissues.

Fig. 14.18 Thyrotoxic hyperplasia.
Micrograph showing the characteristic features of hyperplastic thyroid. An increased number of thyroid epithelial cells is shown by the development of papillary folds of acinar epithelium; in addition each epithelial cell is large and columnar and the edges of the colloid (C) are scalloped, indicating active removal of stored colloid for processing into thyroxine.

The thyroid also produces the hormone calcitonin.
Calcitonin inhibits calcium resorption from bones by osteoclasts, thus antagonizing the action of parathormone (see page 263), and lowering blood calcium levels. It may increase the rate of osteoid mineralization.

Calcitonin-producing cells (C cells) are scattered between the thyroid acinus (follicle) lining cells, but are occasionally seen in small clusters in the interstitial spaces between adjacent acini. The latter location, most common in animals such as the dog, explains the archaic name 'parafollicular cells'.

C cells are small pale-staining cells, which are difficult to see by routine light microscopy but can be identified either by electron microscopy, or by immunoperoxidase techniques (Fig. 14.19). Ultrastructurally they contain the dense-core neurosecretory granules that are characteristic of neuroendocrine cells.

Calcitonin secretion seems to be controlled directly by blood calcium levels.

Fig. 14.19 Thyroid C cells.
Micrograph showing the distribution of thyroid C cells (identified using an immunoperoxidase method for calcitonin) in the adult human thyroid; they are scattered between the thyroid acinus lining cells singly, in clumps, and as interstitial clusters. Cells in the acini tend to be sited on the basement membrane, apparently having no contact with the colloid–filled lumen.

THYROID

- thyroid acinar cells synthesize and release thyroxine

- thyroxine stored as thyroglobulin in colloid in thyroid acinar lumina

- thyroxine synthesis and release is controlled by hormones from anterior pituitary (TSH), in turn controlled by hypothalamic hormone, TRH

- C cells (mainly interstitial) secrete calcitonin in response to a high blood calcium level

PARATHYROID

The parathyroid glands secrete parathormone, which is involved in calcium homeostasis.

The parathyroid glands, of which there are at least four and in some people up to eight, are small, pale coffee-colored endocrine glands. They are usually ovoid in shape, but are occasionally flattened by moulding from adjacent organs or tissues.

Each gland is approximately 5 mm long, 3 mm wide and 1–2 mm thick, although size varies considerably with age and calcium metabolic status. In adults each gland weighs approximately 130 mg, those in women being slightly heavier than in men.

Parathyroid glands are sited in the neck in the region of the thyroid gland but their precise location is variable. They are derived from the third and fourth branchial pouches, the glands from the third pouch being located near the lower pole of the thyroid, while those from the fourth lie close to the upper pole, either behind it or at the cricothyroid junction; those behind the upper pole are often sited inside the thyroid capsule and are therefore apparently intrathyroidal.

The parathyroids at the lower pole have a much more variable location. Approximately half are sited on the anterior or posterior surface of the lower pole of the lateral lobes, the other half being located in the thymic tongue just beneath the lower pole. Occasionally parathyroid glands may be found in the mediastinum, within thymic remnants.

Three main histological cell types are seen in the parathyroid.

The normal adult human parathyroid is surrounded by a thin fibrous capsule and is composed of three cell types:
- adipocytes;
- chief cells, which produce parathormone;
- oxyphil cells.

Adipocytes appear in the parathyroid at puberty and gradually increase in number until about the age of 40, from then on remaining a fairly constant proportion of the entire gland, though their number may decrease in old age. They form a background stroma in which the chief and oxyphil cells are arranged in cords and nests close to a fine network of capillary vessels.

When there is a continuous increased requirement for parathyroid hormone, for example when the serum calcium level is persistently low in renal failure, the chief cells increase in number (hyperplasia) at the expense of the adipocytes.

Parathyroid chief cells are the active endocrine component of the gland.

Chief cells are about 8–10 μm in diameter and are roughly spherical in shape. Their nuclei are small, round, dark-staining and central, and their cytoplasm is usually pale pinkish-purple (Fig. 14.20), although at certain stages they become vacuolated with glycogen and lipid, when they are sometimes referred to as 'clear cells'.

Their ultrastructural appearance depends largely on whether they are in a resting, synthesizing or secreting stage of hormone response. They contain membrane-bound neuroendocrine granules of parathormone commonly arranged towards the periphery of the cell. In the synthesizing phase there are stacks of rough endoplasmic reticulum and an active Golgi. In the resting phase the neuroendocrine granules are still present but the Golgi is small and the rough endoplasmic reticulum less prominent; glycogen granules and small lipid droplets are also seen. This glycogen and lipid becomes less apparent during hormone synthesis but reappears when the cells are secreting the packaged hormone.

In the healthy adult with a normal calcium balance approximately 80% of the chief cells are in the resting phase. If hypercalcaemia develops, this proportion increases to 100% (and the cells contain numerous fine lipid droplets) but decreases with transient or permanent hypocalcaemia. At light microscopy, a synthesizing or secreting chief cell can be identified by its purplish cytoplasm and the absence of fine lipid droplets.

Parathyroid oxyphil cells are larger than chief cells and have abundant eosinophilic cytoplasm.

Parathyroid oxyphil cells are greater than 10μm in diameter) and the cytoplasm is markedly eosinophilic and granular due to the presence of many mitochondria. Their nuclei are small, spherical and dark-staining.

Ultrastructurally, oxyphil cell cytoplasm is packed with large active mitochondria, with intervening cytoplasm containing only scanty free ribosomes and glycogen granules; endoplasmic reticulum and neurosecretory vacuoles are uncommon, indicating that the cells are not endocrinologically active. Transitional cell forms with features of both oxyphil and active chief cells are occasionally seen.

Oxyphil cells are rare before puberty but appear in increasing numbers in early adult life, either singly or in clumps. In the elderly they are often numerous and sometimes form variably sized oval or rounded tumor-like nodules within a normal sized parathyroid.

Fig. 14.20 Parathyroid.

(a) Low-power micrograph of an H&E-stained section of parathyroid. Note the adipocytes (A), which are seen as non-staining areas.

(b) High-power micrograph of an H&E-stained section of parathyroid showing chief cells (C) and oxyphil cells (O).

(c) Electron micrograph of parathyroid showing the edge of an oxyphil cell and its nucleus (N). Note the scanty peripheral neurosecretory granules (G) and numerous mitochondria (M) in this resting phase cell.

DISORDERS OF PARATHORMONE SECRETION

Parathormone maintains the serum calcium level by mobilizing calcium from the pool located in mineralized bone. Thus excess parathormone has a destructive effect on bone. Such hyperparathyroidism may be primary or secondary.

Primary hyperparathyroidism results from a benign tumor (adenoma) of one of the parathyroid glands (Fig. 14.21) and produces hypercalcemia.

Secondary hyperparathyroidism is due to generalized hyperplasia of all of the parathyroid glands in response to a low serum calcium resulting from excessive loss of calcium in the urine. This is usually caused by a primary disease of the kidneys (renal hyperparathyroidism).

Persistent hypercalcaemia can produce severe systemic symptoms, including muscular weakness, dizziness, lethargy and extreme thirst. It predisposes to the deposition of calcium salts in the tissues (heterotopic calcification), particularly in blood vessel walls.

Hypocalcaemia is usually caused by surgical removal of most or all of the parathyroid glands, but can also result from excessive loss of calcium from the kidney or from inadequate dietary calcium absorption.

Fig. 14.21 Parathyroid adenoma.
Micrograph showing a benign tumor (adenoma) of the parathyroid gland. The tumor is composed of sheets of chief cells secreting parathormone.

Such tumors are treated by surgical removal.

ADRENALS

INTRODUCTION

The adrenal glands are located on the upper poles of the kidneys and combine two distinct endocrine systems within one organ. The adrenal cortex synthesizes and secretes steroid hormones produced from cholesterol. The adrenal medulla is a neuroendocrine component, synthesizing and secreting the vasoactive amines, epinephrine and norepinephrine

ADRENAL CORTEX

The adrenal cortex secretes steroid hormones.

The adrenal cortex, the outer layer of the adrenal gland in the adult, is composed of three distinct zones. These zones, the zona glomerulosa, zona fasciculata and zona reticularis, are bound externally by a thin fibrous capsule and internally by the adrenal medulla (Fig. 14.22).

The outer zona glomerulosa (Fig. 14.23) synthesizes and secretes mineralocorticoids, mainly aldosterone and deoxycorticosterone. The zona glomerulosa is the thin subcapsular zone of adrenal cortex that merges imperceptibly on its inner surface with the middle zona fasciculata. It is not always a complete layer and has a patchy distribution.

The middle zona fasciculata (Fig. 14.24) secretes glucocorticoids, mainly cortisol and corticosterone, and also small amounts of the androgenic steroid dehydroepiandrosterone (DHA). The zona fasciculata occupies most of the adrenal cortex and is composed of large rectangular cells with light-staining clear or finely vacuolated cytoplasm due to intracytoplasmic accumulation of

Fig. 14.22 Adrenal cortex (low power).
Micrograph showing the three distinct zones of the adrenal cortex, the zona glomerulosa (ZG), the zona fasciculata (ZF) and the zona reticularis (ZR), which are enclosed by a capsule (C).

Fig. 14.23 Zona glomerulosa.
The zona glomerulosa is composed of small compact cells (C) arranged in clumps and separated by stroma composed largely of thin-walled capillaries. The cells contain scanty lipid droplets associated with well developed smooth endoplasmic reticulum and comparatively little rough endoplasmic reticulum.

Fig. 14.24 Zona fasciculata.
ⓐ These cells are arranged in vertical columns, which are usually 2–3 cells wide, the columns being separated by capillaries (Cap).
ⓑ Ultrastructurally, the cells have prominent rough endoplasmic reticulum, characteristic small round or ovoid mitochondria with tubular cristae and extensive lipid vacuoles. The surfaces of cells adjacent to capillaries may show small microvilli extending to the capillary wall.

lipid droplets containing cholesterol and intermediate lipids, as well as formed glucocorticoids.

The inner zona reticularis (Fig. 14.25) produces androgenic steroids and some glucocorticoids, but normally only in small amounts. This inner zone of adrenal cortex is thinner than the zona fasciculata, but thicker than the zona glomerulosa. It is composed of cells with eosino-

Fig. 14.25 Zona reticularis.

philic cytoplasm arranged in an anastomosing network of clumps and columns with a capillary network closely apposed to the cell membranes. A characteristic feature of this layer when stained with H&E is the presence of brown pigment (lipofuscin). To the naked eye the layer appears pale brown, whereas the zona fasciculata is bright yellow.

Ultrastructurally, the cells possess prominent smooth endoplasmic reticulum and electron-dense irregular aggregations of lipofuscin, as well as lysosomes and oval or long mitochondria with tubular cristae similar to those seen in the cells of the zona fasciculata.

The adrenal in the fetus has an extra outer cell layer.

In the fetus and neonate, the adrenal cortex is proportionately much larger than in the adult and has an additional external cortical zone. This additional outer layer involutes after birth, the three layers of the adult cortex developing from the remaining cells. The cells that involute have the appearance of steroid-secreting cells, possessing a large Golgi and many lipid droplets; furthermore they have round mitochondria with tubular cristae very similar to those of the adult zona fasciculata.

Activity of the fetal adrenal cortex is partly controlled by the fetal pituitary through the feedback of cortisol on pituitary ACTH secretion, and partly controlled by the placenta.

DISORDERS OF THE ADRENAL CORTEX

The most common disorders of the adrenal cortex are hypoadrenalism and hyperadrenalism, resulting respectively from a deficiency or an excess of all of the adrenal cortical steroid hormones; their clinical manifestations are, however, largely due to the hormones produced by the zona fasciculata, the glucocorticoids.

The commonest cause of hypoadrenalism (Addison's syndrome) is destruction of both adrenals by disease, leaving insufficient adrenal cortex for hormone production. This usually results from autoimmune disease, but can also be due to tuberculosis.

In addition, hypoadrenalism can be induced by giving large doses of glucocorticoids therapeutically; this suppresses ACTH secretion by the pituitary so that the adrenal cortex produces no native steroid hormone. If the therapeutic steroid is suddenly discontinued, an acute hypoadrenal crisis may develop.

Hypoadrenalism is manifest clinically by hypotension, hyponatremia and brown skin pigmentation, and may present as a sudden collapse associated with severe shock.

Hyperadrenalism usually results from hyperplasia of the adrenal cortex or from a hormone-secreting tumor. If the tumor produces glucocorticoids, the patient develops Cushing's syndrome, whereas mineralocorticoid production results in Conn's syndrome.

CUSHING'S SYNDROME is manifest clinically by Cushingoid facies, hirsutism, acne, central obesity, striae, osteoporosis, diabetes mellitus, hypertension, hypokalemia, muscle weakness and mental disturbance.

CONN'S SYNDROME is associated with hypertension, hypokalemia causing polyuria and muscle weakness, and alkalosis.

ADRENAL MEDULLA

The adrenal medulla secretes catecholamines.

The adrenal medulla, the centre of the adrenal gland, is surrounded by adrenal cortex. The adrenal medulla is derived from the neural crest and is part of the neuroendocrine system, secreting epinephrine (adrenaline), norepinephrine (noradrenaline), and associated peptides, including enkephalins. Epinephrine and norepinephrine synthesis is controlled by sympathetic and parasympathetic nerve twigs present in the gland.

Adrenal medullary cells have large, commonly pale-staining nuclei and their cytoplasm is usually finely granular with a purplish staining reaction. They are usually polyhedral in shape, arranged in clumps, cords or columns, and surrounded by a rich network of capillaries (Fig. 14.26a).

Cells of the adrenal medulla contain neurosecretory granules.

Ultrastructurally, cells of the adrenal medulla contain neuroendocrine granules. These vary in size and appearance, ranging from 150–350 nm in diameter.

Cells secreting epinephrine have small spherical neuroendocrine granules, almost entirely occupied by electron-dense material with a narrow, clear halo between the central material and the thin surrounding membrane.

Cells secreting norepinephrine have larger neuroendocrine granules with a more obvious electron-lucent layer inside the membrane, the granules containing irregular and often angulated electron-dense material (Fig. 14.26b).

Adrenal medullary cells synthesize and store their respective peptide hormones, normally releasing only small amounts at a time, though during periods of acute stress or excitement larger quantities are secreted under the influence of the autonomic nervous system.

Because of their high catecholamine content, adrenal medullary cells develop an intense brown color when exposed to air or to a strong oxidizing agent, such as potassium dichromate, due to the formation of brown pigment when the amines are oxidized. This is the basis of their antiquated name 'chromaffin cells'.

There is a rich vascular supply to both cortex and medulla.

The adrenal glands receive a rich arterial supply which forms an arterial plexus of capsular arteries over their surface. Two types of vessel are derived from these arteries: cortical arterioles and medullary arterioles, supplying blood to the cortex and medulla respectively, although there is communication between the two systems at the interface between cortex and medulla. The vascular supply is shown in Fig. 14.27.

ADRENAL

- zona glomerulosa (narrow, subcapsular zone of cortex) secretes mineralocorticoids, mainly aldosterone

- zona fasciculata (broad, yellow mid-zone of cortex) secretes glucocorticoids, mainly cortisol and corticosterone

- zona reticularis (narrow inner zone of cortex) secretes mainly androgenic steroids

- adrenal medulla (central, enclosed by cortex, brown) is neuroendocrine and secretes epinephrine (adrenaline) and norepinephrine (noradrenaline)

Fig. 14.26 Adrenal medulla.
(a) Micrograph of adrenal medullary cells showing their large nuclei and finely granular cytoplasm.
(b) Electron micrograph showing large dense-core granules corresponding to norepinephrine (N) and epinephrine (A) granules.

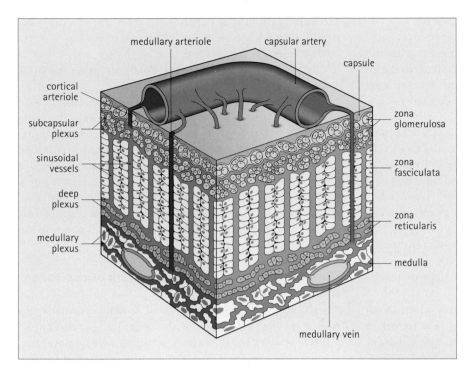

Fig. 14.27 Vascular anatomy of the adrenal gland.
Cortical arterioles form a subcapsular plexus. This gives rise to sinusoidal vessels running down between the columns of the zona fasciculata of the adrenal cortex before forming a further deep plexus in the zona reticularis. This deeper plexus communicates with the plexus of vessels supplying the medulla.

Medullary arterioles arise directly from the capsular arteries and run straight down through the cortex into the medulla where they form a medullary plexus. The deep medullary plexus drains by small venous vessels into the large medullary vein.

PANCREAS

INTRODUCTION

The neuroendocrine component of the human pancreas exists in three forms:

- islets of Langerhans are distinct structures accounting for most of the hormone-producing cells;
- isolated nests or clumps of neuroendocrine cells form a minority population of cells gathered into small groups, which are distinct from islets;
- single cells are scattered within the exocrine (see page 207) and ductular component of the pancreas and are demonstrable by immunocytochemical methods.

Pancreatic endocrine cells are grouped into clusters called islets of Langerhans.

Islets of Langerhans are discrete, rounded clusters of cells scattered throughout the pancreatic tissue. They are embedded in its exocrine component and are most numerous in the tail region. They vary considerably in size and in the number of cells they contain. Individual cells within the islets are smaller and paler than the exocrine cells and assume spherical or polygonal shapes from moulding by adjacent cells. Each islet has a capillary network which is in contact with each cell (Fig. 14.28).

Pancreatic islets develop as cellular buds from the same small ducts which ultimately supply the exocrine pancreatic components. Occasionally in man variably sized islets can be seen in association with a pancreatic duct in the supporting fibrous tissue.

Fig. 14.28 Islets of Langerhans.
(a) Medium-power photomicrograph of an islet of Langerhans (I) embedded in the exocrine component (E) of the pancreas. The islets, roughly spherical, are composed of much smaller cells than the exocrine pancreas, from which they are separated by a fine fibrocollagenous capsule (C).
(b) High-power micrograph showing islet cells. Note that each cell is in contact with the capillary network (C).

Each pancreatic islet contains a number of different neuroendocrine cells.

Each different cell type is mainly concerned with the secretion of a single hormone. The nomenclature of these individual cell types is confusing, and so here each cell type is identified by its main hormone, with other terms being given in brackets.

There are four main cell types and at least two minor ones. Of the total number of pancreatic endocrine cells, the proportions of the main cell types are as follows:

• approximately 70% are insulin and amylin-secreting cells (B or β cells) (Fig. 14.29);
• approximately 20% are glucagon-secreting cells (A or α cells) (Fig. 14.30);
• approximately 5–10% are somatostatin-secreting cells (D, δ or type III cells) (Fig. 14.31);
• approximately 1–2% are pancreatic polypeptide secreting cells (PP or F cells).

The PP cells, which are comparatively scanty when a random block of the pancreas is examined, are found in greater numbers in the posterior lobe of the pancreas, in the head and neck region. They are also found as scattered cells in duct walls. Their neurosecretory vacuoles are spherical with a central electron-dense core surrounded by a wide electron-lucent area.

The minor cell types are:
• vasoactive-intestinal peptide (VIP)-secreting cells (DI or type IV cells);
• mixed secretion cells (EC or enterochromaffin cells).

Minor cell types are present in small numbers in the islets and scattered in the exocrine and ductular components. The mixed secretion cells have been reported to produce a number of active peptides, including serotonin, motilin and substance P.

An apparent anomaly is that the gastric hormone, gastrin, is secreted in excess by some islet cell tumors, but has not been satisfactorily demonstrated in the normal pancreatic islet.

The islets contain a complex network of capillaries with fenestrated endothelium.

These capillaries arise from small arterioles outside the islet and, after penetrating the islet, merge with capillaries supplying the exocrine component of the pancreas. Fenestrated capillary endothelium is a common feature in endocrine tissue.

Fig. 14.29 Insulin–secreting cells.
(a) Immunocytochemical method for insulin.
(b) Immunocytochemical method for amylin (same islet).

Insulin/amylin-secreting cells occupy the central area of the pancreatic islets and are the most common cell type.

These cells have well-developed rough endoplasmic reticulum, a prominent Golgi, and numerous neurosecretory vesicles about 300 nm in diameter. The vesicles have a central electron-dense core in the form of a rhomboidal or polyhedral crystalline structure surrounded by an electron-lucent halo and bounded by a narrow membrane. In a few vesicles the core is missing, possibly due to the recent discharge of insulin (the central core is thought to be composed of insulin complexed with zinc). The peptide amylin is thought to modulate the action of insulin.

Pancreatic islets are innervated by the autonomic nervous system.

There are both sympathetic and parasympathetic twigs contacting the surfaces of about 10% of all the cells directly. There are well developed gap junctions between adjacent islet cells, which may provide the mechanism whereby the neural stimulus is passed to all cells. The autonomic nervous system also innervates the blood vessels and possibly affects perfusion.

Parasympathetic stimulation increases insulin and glucagon output, whereas sympathetic stimulation inhibits insulin release.

Fig. 14.30 Glucagon-secreting cells.
Glucagon-secreting cells are located mainly at the periphery of the pancreatic islets as shown in this micrograph of a section stained to show glucagon by an immunoperoxidase technique.

Glucagon-secreting cells possess similar ultrastructural features to those of insulin-secreting cells, except the secretory vesicles are smaller and have a more spherical electron-dense core which is usually eccentrically located.

Fig. 14.31 Somatostatin-secreting cells.
Somatostatin-secreting cells are a minority population and, in man, are scattered apparently randomly throughout the pancreatic islets, as shown in this micrograph stained to show somatostatin by an immunoperoxidase technique. Some islets contain substantial numbers of these cells while others contain none at all.

Somatostatin-secreting cells contain larger neurosecretory vesicles than insulin-secreting and glucagon-secreting cells, being up to 350 nm in diameter, and also their core is much less electron-dense.

OVARY AND TESTIS

Although their main function is to produce female and male gametes, the ovary and testis also act as endocrine organs (see Chapter 16, pages 309-319, and Chapter 17).

DIFFUSE NEUROENDOCRINE SYSTEM

INTRODUCTION

So far, only those neuroendocrine cells that are gathered together to form distinct endocrine glands have been discussed. There is, however, an extensive system of scattered neuroendocrine cells producing hormones and active peptides, many of which act on the local environment rather than having a distant systemic impact. Almost all of these cells belong to the so-called APUD or diffuse neuroendocrine system and have the following common characteristics:

- uptake and decarboxylation of amine precursor compounds, producing active amines, peptides and hormones (amine precursor uptake and decarboxylation, APUD cells)
- possession of characteristic cytoplasmic organelles, known as dense-core granules, neurosecretory vesicles, or rimmed vacuoles.

These have a common basic structure of a variably electron-dense core (usually spherical, but occasionally angulated), a clear electron-lucent halo around the dense core, a thin distinct membrane surrounding the halo, and, irrespective of the shape of the central dense core, the entire vesicle is usually spherical or oval. The vesicles vary in size (usually 100–600 nm in diameter), shape (spherical or oval), width of electron-lucent halo, and electron density of the central core, depending on the nature of the amine, peptide or hormone produced. In some cases their secretion is under neural control.

Examples of neuroendocrine cells have already been described in this chapter, for example, adrenal medullary cells (see page 266), calcitonin-secreting C cells (see page 261) and pancreatic islet cells (see page 268). Further examples occur in other chapters, for example renin-producing juxtaglomerular cells (see page 299).

The important cells of the diffuse neuroendocrine system are gut-associated endocrine cells and respiratory-associated endocrine cells.

Gut-associated endocrine cells are seen throughout the intestinal tract.

Throughout the alimentary tract the lining epithelium contains scattered endocrine cells termed gut-associated endocrine cells or enteroendocrine cells. Enteroendocrine cells are mainly concentrated in the stomach and small intestine (see Figs. 11.32 and 11.41). They are also present in the lower esophagus and large intestine, and in the ducts of organs draining into the gut (i.e. the bile and pancreatic ducts).

In general, enteroendocrine cells are small, with a spherical nucleus and pale-staining cytoplasm, and lie in contact with the basement membrane on which the mucosal epithelial cells sit (Fig. 14.32); many are not in contact with the lumen. Neurosecretory vesicles are concentrated mainly in the basal portion of these cells.

Enteroendocrine cells are difficult to identify by routine H&E staining, but can be highlighted by certain silver stains, which is why they were formerly termed argentaffin or argyrophil cells. Another old synonym, enterochromaffin cells, is based on their reaction with potassium dichromate to produce a brown pigment. Immunocytochemical methods have demonstrated many more enteroendocrine cells than are visible by silver methods; they also indicate the cells' main secretion. These methods, therefore, have effectively replaced silver methods for demonstrating such cells.

The ultrastructural features of enteroendocrine cells, particularly the size, shape and number of neurosecretory vesicles, vary according to the amine or peptide hormone produced, and more than 20 such products have been identified. Most of these hormones cannot be accurately matched with an ultrastructurally characteristic cell type, and it is likely that some or all of the cells can produce more than one active secretion.

Respiratory-associated endocrine cells are seen throughout the respiratory tract.

Pulmonary neuroendocrine cells in humans exist in two forms, scattered and aggregated.

Individual neuroendocrine cells are scattered throughout the trachea, intrapulmonary airways and occasionally in the alveolar wall. These cells are pale when stained by H&E and are difficult to distinguish without the aid of special methods such as immunocytochemical techniques. Most of the cell sits on the epithelial basement membrane in a manner similar to that of enteroendocrine cells (see Fig. 14.32a), but a cytoplasmic

Fig. 14.32 Enteroendocrine cell.

ⓐ Low-power electron micrograph showing enteroendocrine cells (E) in the base of a small bowel gland. This contrasts with a Paneth cell (P) (see Fig. 10.39).
ⓑ High-power electron micrograph showing neuroendocrine vesicles facing the basement membrane (BM) of the gland, and an adjacent capillary vessel (C).
ⓒ Micrograph showing enteroendocrine cells (E) demonstrated by an immunoperoxidase method to detect synaptophysin, a glycoprotein specific to the neuroendocrine vesicle membrane.

process extends towards the lumen between adjacent epithelial cells.

Small aggregates of neuroendocrine cells form small mounds protruding into the airway lumen or alveoli. These aggregates, which are particularly prominent where airways branch, receive unmyelinated axons from peribronchial and peribronchiolar nerves and have been called neuroepithelial bodies (see Fig. 10.11).

The cytoplasm of both individual and clumped pulmonary neuroendocrine cells contains numerous neurosecretory vesicles. Serotonin, bombesin, calcitonin and leu-enkephalin have all been demonstrated within these cells.

In humans, respiratory-associated neuroendocrine cells are most numerous and prominent at birth, decreasing rapidly thereafter, whereas in some other animals, particularly rodents, they remain in significant numbers throughout life.

PARAGANGLIA

The paraganglia are specialized neuroendocrine glands associated with the autonomic nervous system.

Paraganglia consist of prominent neuroendocrine cells containing neurosecretory vesicles. Those which have been adequately investigated have been shown to contain active amine or peptide hormones and are therefore regarded as part of the neuroendocrine system.

In many cases their precise function and the nature of their secretions is not clear, but it is known that some of the larger paraganglia in the thorax and neck (e.g. aortic body and carotid body) act as chemoreceptors.

Paraganglia vary in size from clumps of a few cells associated with nerves, visible only with microscopy, to structures up to 3 mm in diameter which are anatomically distinct. The largest paraganglia are the intercarotid paraganglia (carotid bodies) and the aortic sympathetic paraganglia (organ of Zuckerkandl).

Paraganglia are composed of chief cells, sustentacular cells and blood vessels.

Chief cells are neuroendocrine cells containing neurosecretory vesicles arranged into roughly round clumps or nests (zellerballen). Each clump is surrounded by an intimate network of capillaries with fenestrated endothelium and a basement membrane. The neuroendocrine cells are of two types.

Most are termed light cells and have pale vacuolated cytoplasm containing moderate numbers of spherical electron-dense neurosecretory vesicles about 100–150 nm in diameter.

A small proportion are termed dark cells and have darker staining cytoplasm containing large numbers of pleomorphic, often angulated, neurosecretory vesicles 50–250 nm in diameter.

Between the neuroendocrine cells and the capillaries are occasional flattened support cells, the sustentacular cells (Fig. 14.33).

Sustentacular cells, which account for 35–45% of paraganglion cells, have elongated spindle-shaped nuclei and pale-staining cytoplasm with ill-defined cell borders. Concentrated at the periphery of the clumps of neuroendocrine cells, they send cytoplasmic processes into the clumps and also around nerve axons, thus behaving in a similar manner to Schwann cells (see Chapter 6), which they closely resemble histologically and ultrastructurally.

Paraganglia are richly innervated by both the sympathetic and parasympathetic nervous systems.

The carotid and aortic bodies are important paraganglia.

A single oval carotid body lies in the fibrocollagenous support tissue between the bifurcation of each common carotid artery into internal and external branches. Each carotid body measures about $3 \times 2 \times 2$ mm and weighs 5–15 mg.

Carotid bodies are most prominent in children and teenagers, becoming progressively less obvious with increasing age, except in people with chronic hypoxia due to lung disease, or those living in low oxygen tension at high altitudes; in these people the carotid bodies increase in size as a result of hyperplasia (an increase in cell number) and may reach 40 mg in weight.

The carotid body has the general structure of all paraganglia (see Fig. 14.33) and in humans the main peptides identified in it are enkephalins. In other species, such as

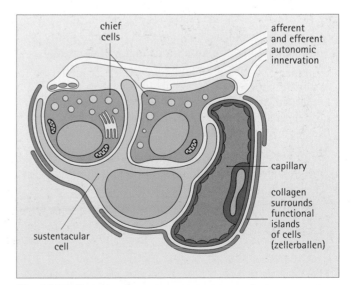

Fig. 14.33 Paraganglion.
Diagram to illustrate a paraganglion, showing that it is composed of chief cells arranged into clumps surrounded by sustentacular cells and capillaries.

the cat, other active peptides are also found, including VIP, substance P, and catecholamines.

Similar in structure to the carotid bodies, but smaller, are the aortic pulmonary paraganglia (aortic bodies), located on the concave surface of the arch of the aorta, close to where the right pulmonary artery passes beneath.

The carotid and aortic bodies act as chemoreceptors monitoring the arterial oxygen tension and pH of the blood, the precise mechanism of which is not known.

CAROTID BODY FUNCTION

The human carotid body contains a mixture of peptides, particularly methionine enkephalin and leucine enkephalin, with smaller amounts of neurotensin and bombesin. In addition, some of the neurosecretory vacuoles contain active amines, including epinephrine (adrenaline), norepinephrine (noradrenaline), serotonin and dopamine.

The carotid body acts as a peripheral chemoreceptor, responding to significant alterations in arterial blood gas tensions and in blood pH. Acute hypoxia is countered by an increase in the respiratory rate; this is thought to be mediated by the release of some of the above transmitters, which in turn stimulate afferent nerve terminals.

Chronic hypoxia (such as that seen physiologically in people living at high altitude and pathologically in patients with chronic lung disease or cyanotic congenital heart disease) leads to persistent enlargement of the carotid bodies, up to 2 or 3 times the normal size, due to hyperplasia of both sustentacular and chief cells.

With old age, the carotid bodies may show progressive lymphocytic infiltration and fibrosis.

Numerous aortic sympathetic paraganglia lie around the abdominal aorta.

Aortic sympathetic paragangila are mainly situated around the abdominal aorta from above the level of origin of the renal arteries to the iliac bifurcation and beyond. On the anterior surface of the aorta they are particularly numerous around the coeliac axis and around the origin of the inferior mesenteric artery. Although prominent in infants, they are much less obvious in adults and are rarely discernible with the naked eye. Collectively they are known as the organs of Zuckerkandl, particularly the cluster around the origin of the inferior mesenteric artery.

Histologically, aortic sympathetic paraganglia have the same general structure of paraganglia, but the neuroendocrine cells have larger neurosecretory granules than those in the carotid body and more closely resemble those of the adrenal medulla (Fig. 14.34).

Fig. 14.34 Aortic sympathetic paraganglion.
Low-power micrograph showing a small aortic sympathetic type paraganglion. Note the afferent nerve fibers (N) and the nests of neuroendocrine cells (NE).

Fig. 14.35 Thyroid.
Micrograph showing normal human thyroid composed of variable sized follicles (F) filled with pink-staining thyroid colloid. In this illustration, the thyroid follicles are in a storage phase, so the lining epithelium (E) is cuboidal or flat and the stored colloid fills the follicle. There is a complex intimate capillary network between adjacent follicles.

The details of the thyroid epithelial cell in an active phase are illustrated in Fig. 14.17, and the calcitonin-secreting component of the thyroid in Fig. 14.19.

Fig. 14.36 Parathyroid gland.
Micrograph showing a child's parathyroid gland (P) closely associated with lymphoid tissue (L). The gland is almost entirely composed of endocrine cells separated by fibrocollagenous septa (S) rich in blood vessels. With increasing age, progressively more adipose tissue develops in the parathyroid gland (see page 262). The details of the cell types present in the parathyroid are illustrated in Fig. 14.20.

Fig. 14.37 Pituitary gland.
Micrograph of human anterior pituitary (adenohypophysis) stained by the H&E method and showing clusters of endocrine cells with varying degrees of cytoplasmic staining by eosin. The cells with the strongest eosin staining (E) are responsible for the secretion of growth hormone; the identity of the other cell types can only be accurately established by immunocytochemical methods (see Figs. 14.8–14.11), although other special staining methods enable some to be classified further (see Fig. 14.6).

The spaces between clumps of pituitary endocrine cells are occupied by a complex capillary network (C).

Fig. 14.38 Adrenal gland.

(a) Low-power micrograph showing adrenal cortex (C) and medulla (M). Three distinct zones can be seen in the cortex, the zona glomerulosa, (ZG), zona fasciculata (ZF) and zona reticularis (ZR).

(b) Micrograph showing the adrenal cortex at higher magnification. Note the zona glomerulosa, (ZG), zona fasciculata (ZF) and zona reticularis (ZR). The zona fasciculata is the middle zone, and is composed of pale-staining cells rich in lipid droplets. The histological details of the cells in these zones are shown in greater detail in Figs. 14.23–14.25.

(c) Medium- power micrograph of adrenal medulla, which is composed of irregularly shaped cells with granular cytoplasm. These cells contain abundant neuroendocrine vesicles and secrete epinephrine and norepinephrine (see Fig. 14.26). There is an intimate capillary supply.

1. THE EPITHELIAL CELLS OF THE THYROID ACINUS

(a) synthesize and secrete calcitonin
(b) can convert iodide into iodine
(c) can break down thyroglobulin with the release of active thyroid hormones
(d) are controlled by TSH from the hypothalamus
(e) may proliferate and produce a hyperthyroid state

2. THE PARATHYROID GLANDS

(a) are always four in number
(b) secrete parathormone in response to a high serum calcium
(c) contain chief cells which are the main hormone secretors
(d) contain a variable amount of adipose tissue
(e) may develop benign tumors which lead to bone destruction

3. MATCH THE COMPONENTS OF THE ADRENAL WITH THE RELEVANT MAJOR SECRETION

(a) zona reticularis
(b) medulla
(c) zona fasciculata
(d) zona glomerulosa

    i. cortisone   iii. androgens
    ii. aldosterone   iv. (nor)epinephrine

4. THE PITUITARY GLAND

(a) is divided into two parts, the anterior (neurohypophysis) and posterior (adenohypophysis)
(b) is supplied by blood vessels which run from the hypothalamus
(c) secretes ADH from the adenohypophysis
(d) has most of the GH-secreting cells in the lateral wings of the adenohypophysis
(e) is sited in the sella turcica

15. Urinary System

INTRODUCTION

The main function of the urinary system is the production, storage and voiding of urine.

Urine is an aqueous solution of excess anions and cations and many of the breakdown products of the body's metabolic processes, particularly those which would be toxic if allowed to accumulate.

The most important toxic metabolites are the nitrogen containing products of protein breakdown, such as urea and creatinine. The composition and concentration of urine can be varied to maintain internal homeostasis.

Urine production and the control of its composition, is the responsibility of the kidneys, while storage and voiding is performed by the bladder.

The pelvicalyceal systems and ureters transfer urine from the kidneys to the bladder and the urethra is the channel through which stored urine is voided from the bladder.

The pelvicalyceal systems, ureters, bladder and urethra have a relatively uncomplicated structure (see page 305). The kidney, however, performs a wide range of biochemical and physiologic tasks during the production of urine and its structure is accordingly complex.

OUTLINE OF THE URINARY SYSTEM

The general arrangement of the of the urinary system is illustrated in Figure 15.1.

The kidneys are solid, bean-shaped organs located high on the posterior abdominal wall beneath the peritoneum.

The concave aspect of each bean faces toward the midline, where the major channel of arterial supply (the aorta) and venous drainage (the inferior vena cava) run. This concave area is called the hilum. It is the site of entry of the renal arterial supply, and of the emergence of the renal venous drainage and urine transport system.

The pelvicalyceal system and ureters are hollow muscular tubes lined by a specialized epithelium.

The epithelium is resistant to damage by the variable osmolarity of urine and by the concentration of toxic solutes within it. The walls of the tubes are composed of smooth muscle capable of pushing the fluid towards the bladder by alternate coordinated contraction and relaxation; this process is called peristalsis.

The bladder acts as both a reservoir and a pump.

The bladder has basically the same structure as the pelvicalyceal system and ureters but its arrangement of muscle fibers is more sophisticated to allow it to act as both a capacious reservoir for urine and as a pump to force out the urine through the urethra under voluntary control.

Fig. 15.1 Urinary system.
Photograph of dissected urinary system from a term male stillbirth demonstrating the interrelationship between the aorta (A), inferior vena cava (IVC), kidneys (K), ureters (UR), bladder (B), and urethra (U). In the adult the bladder is more spherical.

KIDNEY STRUCTURE

The kidney is divided into cortex and medulla.

Each kidney has two distinct zones, an outer cortex and an inner medulla (Fig. 15.2).

The cortex forms an outer shell and also forms columns (the so-called columns of Bertin) which lie between the individual units of the medulla.

The medulla is composed of a series of conical structures (medullary pyramids), the base of each cone being continuous with the inner limit of the cortex and the pointed peak of the pyramid protruding into part of the urine collecting system (the calyceal system) towards the hilum of the kidney. This pointed tip of the medullary pyramid is known as the papilla.

Each human kidney bears 10–18 medullary pyramids, thus 10–18 papillae protrude into the collecting calyces.

Each medullary pyramid, with its associated shell of cortex, comprises a functional and structural lobe of the kidney. This lobar architecture is clearly visible in the fetal kidney (see Fig. 15.1) but becomes less obvious as the kidney increases in size with increasing age.

KIDNEY FUNCTION

The kidney is essential for fluid, electrolyte and acid–base balance and also has an endocrine function.

Urine is produced in the kidney by the selective removal of substances from the blood plasma. Subsequent controlled reabsorption of water, ions, salts, sugars and other carbohydrates, and small molecular weight proteins allows the kidney to produce urine, the composition of which is appropriate to the body's internal environment and requirements at the time.

For example, if the plasma volume is expanded and diluted by a substantial ingestion of water, the kidney will then excrete the excess water by producing large quantities of a dilute urine. Conversely, if fluid ingestion is restricted, the kidney will produce a small amount of highly concentrated urine.

Whatever the quantity and concentration of the urine, it will contain the required amount of waste products and ions to maintain internal biochemical homeostasis.

An inability to produce concentrated or dilute urine is an important feature of kidney failure, as is evidence of inadequate excretion of nitrogenous waste products and other substances, for example potassium ions (see page 300).

It is important to realize that the kidneys (and lungs) differ from most other organs in one important respect. In most organs, the vascular supply is the servant of the parenchymal tissues, providing them with oxygen and other raw materials required for the tissue's metabolic processes, and carrying synthesized cell products and waste materials away from the organ. In the kidney, however, the parenchymatous components of the organ are the servants of the blood supply, since the function of the kidney, in broad terms, is the filtration and cleansing of the blood.

Thus, the parenchymal unit of the kidney, the nephron, which is composed of the glomerulus and cortical and medullary tubular systems, can be regarded as an appendage of the renal blood vascular system, attached to it for servicing purposes. It is not surprising, therefore, that the blood vascular system of the kidney is both substantial and structurally unusual, reflecting its central role. The two kidneys receive 25% of the total cardiac output. Consequently, most of the important and common diseases of the kidney result from abnormality in the blood vascular component (see page 300).

The kidney also produces the hormones erythropoietin and renin.

Fig. 15.2 Adult human kidney.
Photograph of adult human kidney cut longitudinally to show the arrangement of the cortex (C), medulla (M), and papillae (P).

KIDNEY VASCULATURE

Arteries supplying the kidney branch within the renal substance to supply distinct regions.

In most cases, the arterial supply to each kidney comes from a single renal artery, which is a substantial, direct lateral branch of the abdominal aorta. A common variant is the presence of a separate artery arising directly from the aorta and supplying one or other pole.

The renal artery runs towards the concave hilum of the kidney and divides into two main branches, one anterior, one posterior (Fig. 15.3), each of which divides into a number of interlobar arteries that run between the medullary pyramids, one branch to each developmental lobe.

At about the midpoint of the thickness of the kidney parenchyma, where the cortex abuts on the broad base of the medullary pyramid (the corticomedullary junction), the interlobar artery divides into several lateral arcuate arteries, which run laterally.

The arcuate arteries then give rise to a series of side branches (interlobular arteries), which run vertically upwards into the cortex.

Interlobular arteries give rise laterally to a series of arterioles, called afferent arterioles, usually directly, but sometimes via a short intralobular artery. These arteries terminate at the periphery of the kidney, just beneath the capsule, supplying a stellate subcapsular arteriolar and capillary plexus.

Thus far, the arterial supply has been anatomically unremarkable. From the afferent arterioles onward, however, the renal vascular system becomes unique.

Fig. 15.3 Arterial system of the kidney.

ⓐ Arteriogram of a whole postmortem human kidney showing the division of the main renal artery (MRA) into two branches, a comparatively minor posterior branch (PRA), and a more substantial anterior branch (ARA).

The posterior branch supplies the lower pole, while the larger anterior branch divides, in this case, into four segmental arteries, which together supply the mid-zone and upper pole of the kidney.

ⓑ In this section the posterior (PRA) and anterior (ARA) branches of the renal artery can be seen, although some segments are missing due to the tortuosity of the arteries at the hilum.

Note the interlobar arteries (IL), the arcuate arteries (ArcA), and the fine network of interlobular arteries (ILA).

The faint haziness (AA) in some areas of the cortex indicates filling of the afferent arterioles.

RENAL MICROCIRCULATION
The renal microcirculation contains two capillary systems.

In almost every other organ, the capillary network lies between the terminal part of the arterial/arteriolar system and the proximal part of the venular/venous system, and is the major site of oxygen/carbon dioxide exchange. In contrast, the renal vascular system has a highly specialized preliminary capillary network, the glomerular tuft, which receives blood from an afferent arteriole, and which is the site of filtration of waste products from plasma, together with a second capillary system arising from the efferent arteriole, which varies in structure and function according to its location within the kidney (Fig. 15.4).

In most cases, after leaving the glomerulus, the efferent arteriole divides into a complex capillary system which runs in the interstitial spaces between the components of the system of cortical tubules. Each capillary is in intimate contact with these tubules, and is thus ideally placed to take up any substances reabsorbed from the glomerular filtrate by tubular epithelial cells (see page 289).

However, the capillary system originating from efferent arterioles leaving glomeruli situated deep in the cortex, close to the corticomedullary junction (juxtamedullary glomeruli), is different (see Fig. 15.4). These efferent arterioles divide into a series of long, thin-walled vessels, the vasa recta, which run straight down into the medulla alongside the medullary components of the tubular systems. These vessels play an important role in the ionic and fluid exchanges occurring in the medulla (see page 295). Some vasa recta arise as direct, vertically running side branches of the arcuate artery.

The first capillary system, the glomerular tuft, does not transfer its contained oxygen to the tissues, nor does it take up a significant amount of carbon dioxide. The major exchange of dissolved gases takes place in the second capillary system. Oxygen is supplied to the cortical and medullary parts of the renal parenchyma which have the highest demand because of their high metabolic activity.

The venous drainage of the kidney mirrors the arterial supply.

In general, the renal venous drainage mirrors the arterial supply, except that there is no venous equivalent of the glomerular capillary tuft. The subcapsular arteriolar and capillary plexus drain into a subcapsular venular and venous plexus of stellate veins which form the origin of the interlobular veins. As they proceed towards the corticomedullary junction the interlobular veins receive venous tributaries from the peritubular capillary network, and, as the juxtamedullary zone is approached, from some of the venous tributaries from the medulla, which are the venous equivalent of the arterial vasa recta.

Many of the medullary venous vessels drain directly into the arcuate veins, which run laterally with the equivalent artery at the corticomedullary junction. These in turn drain into large interlobular veins lying between adjacent medullary pyramids and then into the major vein tributaries at the renal hilum. The major renal vein opens end-to-side into the inferior vena cava.

NEPHRON

The functional unit of the kidney parenchyma which serves the blood supply is called the nephron.

The nephron has two main components:
- the glomerulus, which is associated with the first capillary system;
- the cortical and medullary tubular systems, which are associated with the second capillary system.

The glomerulus is the site of initial blood filtration and the tubular systems are the site where the concentration and chemical content of blood returned to the general systemic circulation, and hence the concentration and content of the urine to be voided from the body, is controlled.

Within the renal cortex, the nephrons are organized in a distinct repeated lobular pattern. The glomeruli, and proximal and distal tubules, are aligned mainly on either side of the interlobular arteries which supply them with blood (see Fig. 15.4).

At the midpoint between adjacent interlobular arteries is a vertically running arrangement of tubules and ducts known as the medullary ray (see Fig. 15.31c), at the centre of which is a main collecting duct which collects all of the largely unconcentrated urine from the nephrons on either side. The other tubular components of the medullary ray are the straight collecting tubules carrying urine from the end of the distal tubule to the main cortical collecting duct. The duct systems of the medullary ray run vertically downward into the medulla.

The subunit of cortex, comprising a centrally placed medullary ray and the nephrons on either side of it, is called the renal lobule and each interlobular artery runs upward in the cortex between adjacent lobules. This lobular arrangement and the medullary ray system can be seen in Figure 15.31.

Fig. 15.4 Renal microcirculation.

(a) Diagram illustrating the principles of the renal microcirculation. The afferent arteriole, which is a branch of the interlobular artery, enters the glomerular capillary tuft at the vascular hilum. The emerging vessel, the efferent arteriole, normally divides into a complex system of capillaries, the peritubular capillary network, which surrounds the cortical tubules.

The venous tributaries arising from the peritubular capillary network drain into small veins opening into the interlobular vein, which runs vertically alongside the interlobular artery and drains into the arcuate vein running alongside the arcuate artery at the corticomedullary junction.

Close to the corticomedullary junction some of the efferent arterioles give rise to vertically running vessels, the vasa recta, which pass down into the medulla alongside the medullary duct and tubular systems. Some vasa recta arise as direct branches of the arcuate artery and drain directly into the arcuate vein.

(b) A carmine-gelatin injection specimen showing a vertically running interlobular artery (ILA) in the renal cortex, with glomerular capillary tufts (G) arising from lateral branches of the artery, and the afferent arterioles (AA). Some peritubular capillary networks (PCN) can also be seen.

(c) A carmine-gelatin injection specimen showing the interlobular artery (ILA), the afferent (AA) and efferent arterioles (EA), the glomerular tuft (G), and the peritubular capillary network (PCN).

(d) A carmine-gelatin injection specimen of the corticomedullary junction. Note the arcuate artery (ArcA), an interlobular artery (ILA), glomeruli (G), and a number of peritubular capillary networks (PCN) in the cortex. The medulla contains parallel bundles of straight blood vessels, the vasa recta (VR), some of which arise as direct vertical branches of the arcuate artery and others from the efferent arterioles of some glomeruli close to the corticomedullary junction.

GLOMERULUS

The first functional component of the nephron encountered by the microcirculation is the **glomerulus**, which is the site of initial filtration of the blood arriving by the afferent arterioles.

The afferent arteriole enters the glomerulus at the vascular pole.

The afferent arteriole, which enters the glomerulus immediately, splits up into about five main branches. Each branch then subdivides into its own capillary network (see Fig. 15.4), the short main branch and its capillaries being supported by its own strip or stalk of mesangium (see page 281).

The division of the glomerular capillary network into about five independent segments gives the glomerular tuft an implicit lobulation which is rarely apparent by routine light microscopy in health but becomes evident in some forms of primary glomerular disease, particularly when the mesangial component of each segment is enlarged (see Fig. 15.14). The independence of each glomerular segment is also demonstrated by disease affecting only one segment (e.g. segmental glomerulonephritis).

The glomerular capillaries converge to form a single efferent arteriole which leaves the glomerulus at the same vascular pole as the afferent arteriole enters.

The glomerulus is a complex structure in which capillaries are in intimate contact with a specialized epithelium.

In simple terms, the structure of the glomerulus is best conceived as a globular capillary network intruding into a hollow sphere of epithelial cells called Bowman's capsule, which represents the bulbous, distended, closed end of a long hollow tubular system (Fig. 15.5). This means that the glomerular capillary system, which is lined internally by endothelial cells, acquires an outer layer of epithelial cells that is continuous at the vascular pole with the cells lining Bowman's capsule.

The epithelial cells of Bowman's capsule are flat and simple, except near the opening of the tubular system, where they become more cuboidal and acquire some of the cytoplasmic organelles of the proximal convoluted tubule epithelial cells (see page 289).

In contrast, the epithelial cells coating the glomerular capillary tuft are larger and have a highly specialized and unusual structure which has led to their being named podocytes (see page 284).

The epithelial-lined space between the coated glomerular capillary network and the parietal shell of Bowman's capsule is called the urinary space, and is continuous with the lumen of the long tubular system of the nephron.

As well as the outer epithelial (podocyte) coating, the glomerular capillary network has other unusual features, including the possession of an unusually thick basement membrane (the glomerular basement membrane) and the presence of a supporting strip or stalk, analogous to the mesentery of the small bowel, called the mesangium (Fig. 15.6 and see page 286).

Blood enters the glomerular capillary network from the afferent arteriole. Ultrafiltration of the blood then occurs in the glomerular capillary network and the filtrate passes into the urinary space before passing down the tubular system. The partly filtered blood leaves the glomerulus via the efferent arteriole and flows onward to provide an oxygenated blood supply to the tubular systems.

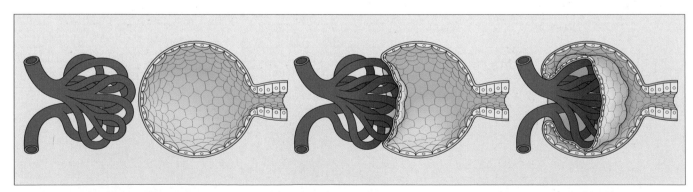

Fig. 15.5 Relationship between the glomerular capillary tuft and Bowman's capsule.
Although the glomerulus and Bowman's capsule do not in fact develop in this way, the relationships between the two are best conceived by imagining the intrusion of the glomerular tuft into the spherical, distended and closed end of the tubular system.

This is particularly helpful in conceptualizing the glomerular tuft with its outer coating of epithelial cells which is continuous with the cells lining Bowman's capsule.

Fig. 15.6 Normal human glomerulus.

(a) An H&E paraffin section of normal human kidney which has been inflation fixed to distend the blood vessels. Note the afferent arteriole (AA) and efferent arteriole (EA) at the vascular pole.

Opposite the vascular pole is the tubular pole (TP) where the urinary space (US) empties into the first part of the tubular system.

Although fine details of the glomerular structure are not apparent in this micrograph, the suggestion of glomerular lobulation is evident. The flattened epithelial lining of Bowman's capsule (BC) is easily seen.

(b) A thin epoxy resin section of a normal human glomerulus stained with toluidine blue. This technique permits much greater resolution of the structure of the glomerulus. The dilated capillary loops contain red blood cells (RBC) and are supported by the darkly stained mesangium (M).

(c) High-power micrograph of a thin epoxy resin section of a segment of the glomerular tuft stained with toluidine blue. At this magnification, details of the glomerular capillary wall, endothelial and epithelial cells, and mesangium become apparent.

The capillary loops are supported by darkly stained mesangial stalks comprising acellular matrix (Mx) and nucleated mesangial cells (Mc). The capillary basement membrane is lined internally by endothelial cytoplasm and endothelial cell nuclei (E) are apparent.

External to the glomerular basement membrane are the epithelial podocytes (P).

GLOMERULAR FILTRATION BARRIER

The barrier between circulating blood and the urinary space is the glomerular filtration barrier (Fig. 15.7).

It is composed of:

- the capillary endothelial inner layer;
- the unusually thick glomerular capillary basement membrane;
- the podocyte (the outer epithelial) layer.

An additional component of the functional barrier is a high polyanionic charge on some of the above structural components.

Glomerular capillary endothelial cells are attenuated and fenestrated.

The endothelial cells in the renal glomeruli are adapted for their specialized filtration role. The cytoplasm forms a thin sheet broken by numerous small circular pores or fenestrations, each about 70 nm in diameter. Their nuclei are usually located near the mesangium. Normal glomerular capillary endothelium is shown ultrastructurally in Figure 15.7. A diagrammatic representation, illustrating the structure of the endothelium and its relationships with other glomerular components, is shown in Figure 15.13b.

Fig. 15.7 Glomerular capillary wall.

(a) Electron micrograph showing the relationship between the glomerular basement membrane (GBM), capillary lumen (L), endothelial cytoplasm (EnC) and the epithelial podocyte (EP) with its primary (P1) and secondary (P2) foot process system.

(b) High-power electron micrograph of the glomerular filtration barrier, comprising fenestrated endothelial cytoplasm (EnC), glomerular basement membrane and podocyte foot processes. Note the filtration slit membrane (FSM, see page 284).

GLOMERULAR ENDOTHELIAL ABNORMALITIES

In some primary glomerular diseases there is a great increase in the size and number of the endothelial cells, and the glomerular capillary lumina become blocked (Fig. 15.8). This produces the acute nephritic syndrome, which is characterized by:

- an increase in blood pressure due to the increased peripheral resistance following blockage of the vast glomerular capillary network;
- a rise in the blood levels of nitrogenous waste products due to the failure of filtration by the abnormal glomeruli;
- hematuria (loss of red blood cells in the urine), the mechanism of which is not known.
- edema (fluid accumulation in support tissues).

Primary structural abnormalities of the glomerulus, such as that illustrated here, are known by the name glomerulonephritis. The micrograph shows an example of acute endocapillary glomerulonephritis.

Fig. 15.8 Acute nephritic syndrome.
This paraffin section of kidney from a child with acute nephritic syndrome has been stained by the Jones methenamine silver technique to highlight the basement membranes and mesangium of the glomerular capillary loops (brown-black). The capillary lumina are obliterated by proliferation of cells within the basement membrane, which are therefore largely endothelial cells. If this occurs in all of the glomeruli, as is usually the case, blood flow through the glomerular capillary network is reduced.

The glomerular basement membrane is divided into three distinct zones.

Glomerular basement membrane is much thicker than normal capillary basement membranes elsewhere. It measures approximately 310–350 nm in healthy young adults, being slightly thicker in males. Both the inner endothelial and outer epithelial cell populations contribute to its production. It has three layers:

- a central electron-dense lamina densa;
- electron-lucent lamina rara interna on the endothelial or capillary lumen side;
- electron-lucent lamina rara externa on the epithelial podocyte, or urinary space side.

This layered structure is clearly seen in rodents and children but becomes less apparent in most adults.

The lamina densa is partly composed of type IV collagen (see page 55), and the fibril network acts as a physical barrier to the passage of large molecules from the blood into the urinary space.

The lamina rara layers, and the surfaces of some podocyte secondary foot processes, contain fixed negatively charged (polyanionic) sites, composed of glycosaminoglycan (see page 56). In the basement membrane this is heparan sulfate, and on the foot process surfaces it is a sialic acid-rich substance named podocalyxin. When demonstrated ultrastructurally using a cationic substance such as ruthenium red or polyethylenimine (Fig. 15.9), such sites appear to be organized to form fairly regular lattice with a spacing of approximately 60 nm.

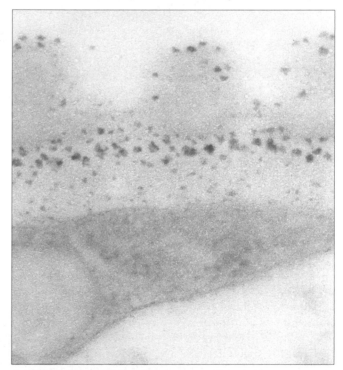

Fig. 15.9 Glomerular basement membrane–polyanionic sites (polyethylenimine method).
Electron micrograph of the glomerular filtration barrier identifying the sites of high polyanionic charge in both the basement membrane and on the surfaces of the podocyte foot processes. Loss of this surface anionic charge leads to leakage of excess protein.

It is thought that the polyanionic sites act as a charge barrier, preventing the passage of cationic molecules.

The combination of layers in the glomerular basement membrane produces both a physical and electrical barrier to the passage of large molecules (i.e. over 70 kD) and highly cationic molecules of many sizes. Nevertheless, certain large molecules, including some proteins, may pass through into the urinary space and require reabsorption in the tubular system.

The full thickness of the glomerular basement membrane does not completely surround the circumference of the capillary wall, but instead occupies about three-quarters of it, being partly deficient at the site of the attachment of the capillary to the mesangium. The lamina rara interna continues as an ill-defined layer between the endothelial cytoplasm and the cytoplasmic and matrix components of the mesangium (see Fig.15.13b).

BASEMENT MEMBRANE ABNORMALITIES IN GLOMERULAR DISEASE

Abnormalities in the structure of the glomerular basement membrane are responsible for some important kidney diseases which are characterized by an excessive loss of protein in urine (proteinuria). Sometimes so much is lost in the urine that the capacity of the liver to synthesize fresh protein (particularly albumin) is outstripped. The patient then develops a low blood albumin (hypoalbuminemia), and edema due the low oncotic pressure of the blood.

The combination of proteinuria, hypoalbuminemia and edema is called the **nephrotic syndrome**.

There are many causes of the nephrotic syndrome, but all appear to be related to a structural or functional abnormality of the glomerular basement membrane.

Diseases in which the abnormality is structural include diabetes mellitus and membranous nephropathy.

In nephrotic syndrome associated with diabetes mellitus the glomerular basement is thickened 3–5 fold and the demarcation into three laminae is lost (Fig. 15.10a). In membranous nephropathy, the basement membrane is damaged by the deposition of antigen-antibody complexes (Fig. 15.10b).

Although in these examples the basement membrane is physically thickened, it is functionally leaky and many large molecules pass into the urinary space, including large molecular weight proteins.

Fig. 15.10 Patterns of basement membrane thickening in disease.
ⓐ Electron micrograph of a uniformly thickened basement membrane from a patient with diabetes mellitus who presented with the nephrotic syndrome. Photographed at same magnification as Fig. 15.7a.
ⓑ Electron micrograph of a basement membrane thickened by deposition of antigen-antibody complexes on the epithelial side. It is taken from a patient with membranous nephropathy who presented with the nephrotic syndrome. Photographed at same magnification as Fig. 15.7a.

The podocyte layer lies on the outer surface of the glomerular capillaries.

The podocyte layer is composed of specialized epithelium which is continuous at the vascular hilum with the flat, relatively inert epithelium lining Bowman's capsule. It is highly specialized in structure, and presumably in function as well, though much of its functional detail is not known.

The podocyte is so named because the main body of the cell hovers above the external surface of the glomerular capillary and sends down cytoplasmic extensions (foot processes) which make contact with the basement membrane (see Figs 15.7 and 15.11).

Between adjacent foot processes on the glomerular basement membrane is a fairly consistent gap of 30–60 mm, the filtration slit. A thin membrane, the filtration slit membrane, bridges the gap between adjacent foot processes.

The functional aspects of this complex cytoplasmic arrangement are not understood, but it obviously plays an important role in preventing certain molecules from passing into the urinary space. Loss of the podocyte foot process pattern in some renal diseases is associated with such excessive protein loss (mainly albumin) that the patient develops the nephrotic syndrome (see above).

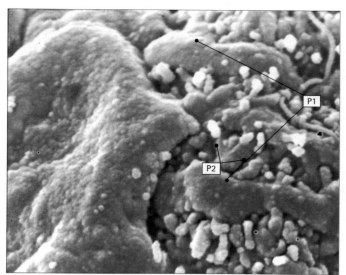

Fig. 15.11 Epithelial podocyte.
Scanning electron micrograph of the epithelial podocyte and its foot processes in a healthy human adult.

Arising from the main cell body of each epithelial cell are a number of broad cytoplasmic processes, the primary processes (P1), which extend along and wrap around the capillary, giving rise at regular intervals to a series of smaller processes, the secondary processes (P2), which rest on the glomerular basement membrane. There is interdigitation of secondary processes so that adjacent foot processes may be derived from different podocytes. The foot process pattern in the adult human is not so neatly arranged as it is in the neonate or the rodent.

PODOCYTE ABNORMALITIES IN GLOMERULAR DISEASE

In children, the most common cause of the nephrotic syndrome is the so-called minimal change nephropathy. By light microscopy the glomerulus appears normal but electron microscopy reveals loss of the foot process pattern, with the outer surface of the glomerular capillaries being covered by an almost continuous sheet of podocyte cytoplasm, probably representing primary process remnants (Fig. 15.12). The abnormality is usually only temporary; structure and function return to normal in time. The podocyte abnormalities are associated with loss of the polyanionic charge (see page 284), which possibly explains the protein leak.

Fig. 15.12 Foot process fusion.
Compare the foot process arrangement in this electron micrograph with that seen normally (Fig. 15.7). In this kidney from a child with the nephrotic syndrome due to minimal change nephropathy, the complex secondary foot process arrangement is lost and the primary foot processes (P1) lie directly on the basement membrane (BM). Minimal change nephropathy is the commonest cause of the nephrotic syndrome in childhood and spontaneously resolves with no long term renal impairment.

MESANGIUM

The mesangial support to the glomerular capillary network has two components, mesangial cells and extracellular mesangial matrix. The role of the mesangium as a support for the glomerular capillary system can be seen in Figure 15.6, while Figure 15.13 illustrates the details of the structure of the mesangium, and its relationship to the glomerular capillary and the glomerular basement membrane.

Mesangial cells are irregular in shape and have a number of cytoplasmic processes.

The mesangial cell processes run in an apparently haphazard fashion through the extracellular mesangial matrix. The mesangial cell nucleus is round or oval and is larger than the endothelial cell nucleus (see Fig. 15.6). There is a dense rim of nuclear chromatin inside the nuclear membrane and numerous small chromatin clumps are scattered throughout the nucleoplasm.

The mesangial cell cytoplasm contains myosin-like filaments and bears angiotensin II receptors. In the

Fig. 15.13 Mesangium.

(a) Electron micrograph of mesangium (M) and its relationship with the glomerular capillary (GC).

The capillary wall is deficient in basement membrane (BM) at the site of attachment to the mesangium, the wall being composed of endothelial cell cytoplasm (EnC) lying directly on mesangial matrix (MM).

The basement membrane continues over the surface of the mesangium to the next capillary loop.

(b) The podocytes with their foot processes (green) are separated from the fenestrated endothelium (red) by the glomerular basement membrane. Note the supporting role of the mesangium (matrix-beige, cytoplasm-brown).

The lamina densa (purple) and lamina rara externa (blue) of the basement membrane (see Fig. 4.11) are not continuous around the capillary, but are reflected over the mesangial surface to the next capillary.

The lamina rara interna (beige) appears to blend with the mesangial matrix where the capillary is attached to the mesangium.

experimental animal, contraction of mesangial cell filaments has been shown to be stimulated by angiotensin II.

Mesangial matrix is an acellular material produced by the mesangial cell.

The mesangial matrix largely encloses the mesangial cells but is permeated by mesangial cell cytoplasmic processes. Ultrastructurally it is of variable electron density, the more electron-lucent parts closely resembling the lamina rara interna of the glomerular basement membrane with which it is in continuity where the glomerular capillary and mesangium meet.

The mesangium may have roles in phagocytosis, maintaining basement membrane and glomerular blood flow.

The precise mechanisms of action of the mesangium in humans are not known. It has four postulated functions:

- support of the glomerular capillary loop system;
- possible control of blood flow through the glomerular loop by the myosin-angiotensin mechanism described above;
- possible phagocytic function;
- possible maintenance of the glomerular basement membrane.

Intravenously injected particulate matter (e.g. colloidal carbon, ferritin etc.) in the experimental animal, and circulating immune complexes in man, appear in the mesangium in some disease states. The incompleteness of the basement membrane over the area of attachment to the mesangium would facilitate phagocytic function.

Note the close resemblance and continuity of mesangial matrix and lamina rara interna. The importance of the mesangium in human glomerular disease suggests that it is a vital functional component of the glomerulus and that its significance has been overlooked.

MESANGIAL ABNORMALITIES

Abnormalities of the mesangium are an important component of many glomerular diseases.

In some forms of immunological damage to the glomerulus there is a proliferation of mesangial cells which leads to compression of the glomerular capillaries (mesangial glomerulonephritis); this is often associated with the deposition of immune complexes within the mesangium (Fig. 15.14).

In diabetes mellitus, the mesangial cells of one or more of the glomerular segments produce excessive amounts of acellular matrix to form spherical nodules known as Kimmelstiel-Wilson nodules (Fig. 15.15).

In permanently damaged glomeruli, whatever the cause, excessive formation of mesangial matrix in all segments eventually converts the glomerular tuft into an acellular spherical mass (hyalinization, see end-stage kidney, Fig.15.30).

Fig. 15.14 Mesangial glomerulonephritis.
A paraffin section of kidney showing proliferation of the mesangial cells (M) and excessive production of mesangial matrix (Mx) expanding the lobules of the glomerular tuft and beginning to compress the glomerular capillary lumina. This pattern of disease is called mesangial glomerulonephritis.

Fig. 15.15 Kimmelstiel–Wilson nodule.
An H&E-stained paraffin section of kidney from a patient with diabetes mellitus showing a localized nodule of mesangial matrix (Kimmelstiel-Wilson nodule, K) in two of the glomerular lobules.

THE GLOMERULUS

- the glomerulus is the site of ultrafiltration of blood

- filtration occurs across the highly specialized glomerular capillary wall, with filtrate entering the urinary space enclosed by Bowman's capsule

- the filtration barrier comprises glomerular capillary endothelium, glomerular basement membrane (GBM) and epithelial podocyte attached to outer surface of GBM

- further physicochemical barrier is the high polyanionic charge on the outer surface of GBM and podocyte surface, preventing passage of cationic molecules

- initial glomerular filtrate passes down tubular and collecting duct systems, where controlled reabsorption and further excretion of small molecules (including water) occurs

- filtered blood leaving glomerulus via efferent arteriole enters a second capillary system around the tubules

TUBULAR AND COLLECTING SYSTEM

INTRODUCTION

The glomerular filtrate leaves the urinary space at the tubular pole of the glomerulus and enters a tubule which modifies its composition. The names of the different parts of this tubule and the course of the glomerular filtrate after leaving the glomerulus on its way to being excreted is illustrated in Fig. 15.16.

The convoluted parts of both proximal and distal tubules are found close to the glomeruli, which are usually clustered around the ascending interlobular arteries from which their afferent arterioles are derived.

In contrast, the straight parts of the tubular system and the cortical parts of the collecting duct system are concentrated together in the segments of cortex virtually devoid of glomeruli; these segments are inaccurately called medullary rays.

Such zoning divides the cortex into lobules. Each lobule is the segment of cortex between adjacent interlobular arteries and has a medullary ray at its centre.

Fig. 15.16 Tubular and collecting system of the nephron.
The first part of the tubular system is the proximal tubule, which is a continuation of Bowman's capsule and initially pursues a convoluted course (the proximal convoluted tubule), remaining close to the glomerulus from which it arises.

The proximal tubule then straightens and descends toward the medulla (proximal straight tubule, or the thick descending limb of the loop of Henle), merging with a thin-walled part of the tubular system (thin limb of the loop of Henle). This runs down in the cortex, and then in the medulla, toward the papillary tip (descending thin limb). It then loops back on itself (ascending thin limb) and re-enters the cortex. The wall then becomes thicker, forming the straight segment of the distal tubule (the thick ascending limb of the loop of Henle or the distal straight tubule).

In the cortex, close to the glomeruli, the distal tubule becomes convoluted (distal convoluted tubule), and empties into a collecting tubule, which in turn empties into a collecting duct lying within the medullary ray.

The collecting ducts descend into the medulla where a number converge to produce large-diameter ducts in the papillae (papillary ducts or ducts of Bellini). These ducts open into the calyces at the tips of the papillae, the concentration of the openings producing a sieve-like surface appearance to the papillary tip (the area cribrosa).

The lengths of the various components of the tubular system vary, mainly according to the location of the glomerulus from which each is derived. The main variation in length occurs in the thin ascending and descending limbs of the loop of Henle. The proximal convoluted tubule is longer than the distal convoluted tubule.

The proximal tubule is vital for reabsorption of glomerular filtrate.

In the proximal tubule there is extensive reabsorption of various components of the glomerular filtrate (Fig. 15.17).

The cells that line the proximal tubule are continuous with the cells lining Bowman's capsule and there is an abrupt transition of cell form at the tubular pole of the glomerulus.

The proximal tubule lining cells are adapted for fluid and ion exchange.

Proximal tubule cells are cuboidal or columnar and have a centrally placed nucleus and a well-developed luminal brush border. The brush border is composed of numerous closely packed microvilli about 1 mm in length. At the base of the microvillous brush border are pinocytotic vesicles which lie close to lysosomes. Each cell rests on a basement membrane which is continuous with the basement membrane of Bowman's capsule.

The basal membrane of each tubule cell shows extensive basal interdigitation and some lateral interdigitation which

Fig. 15.17 Functional aspects of proximal convoluted tubule cells.

In the proximal tubule there is extensive reabsorption of components of the glomerular filtrate. The apical microvilli of the proximal tubule cells provide an immense surface area for absorption and the mitochondria, which are particularly numerous and prominent in the convoluted portion, provide the energy for the active transport of various components against gradients.

The reabsorption of water is largely a secondary osmotic consequence of the active transport of Na^+ ions into the lateral spaces between adjacent tubule cells, which is followed by passive diffusion of Cl^- ions. This increases the hydrostatic pressure in the lateral intercellular space and watery fluid is forced through the tubule basement membrane into the interstitial tissue and thence into the peritubular capillary network. The active transport of Na^+ ions into the intercellular space is mediated by the Na^+/K^+ ATPase pump, which is active in the region of lateral cell membranes.

Proteins, polypeptides and amino acids are also reabsorbed from the glomerular filtrate in the proximal tubule region. Soluble amino acids probably pass through with the water under the influence of the Na^+ ion pump.

In contrast, large molecular weight proteins and polypeptides are reabsorbed by endocytosis (see Fig. 2.4).

It is presumed that proteins and polypeptides are broken down by lysosomal enzymes (see page 21) into amino acids which then enter the circulation via the intercellular space, interstitial support tissue and capillaries under the influence of the Na^+ pump.

Glucose is reabsorbed by the Na^+ pump mechanism, whereas larger carbohydrate molecules may follow the same route as the larger protein molecules.

Enzymes capable of breaking down proteins and the larger molecular weight sugars can be demonstrated at the microvillous surface.

makes the lateral borders irregular and difficult to define except apically, where the intercellular space is sealed off from the tubule lumen by a tight junction (Fig. 15.18).

Although the lateral intercellular space of proximal tubule cells is narrow and difficult to define throughout its length from apex to base, it is often easy to see places where the space is distended into roughly spherical saccules.

In the lower half of each proximal tubule cell, numerous elongated mitochondria are closely associated with the basal interdigitations from adjacent cells and are arranged in parallel with the interdigitating basal cytoplasmic membranes.

The membrane and cytoplasmic specializations are most developed in the convoluted part of the proximal tubule. In the straight descending portion, as the thin loop of Henle is approached, the microvilli become smaller and less numerous, the degree of basal and lateral interdigitation less marked, and mitochondria and lysosomes fewer. The cells also become more cuboidal.

Fig. 15.18 Proximal convoluted tubule.
(a) Diagram showing the microvillous surface, the complex basal interdigitations, and the lateral interdigitations of proximal convoluted tubule cells.
(b) High-power micrograph showing the microvillous brush border (MV) lining the lumen of the azan-stained proximal tubule.
(c) High-power electron micrograph of the microvillous brush border (MV) and the system of pinocytotic vesicles (PV).
    Note the tight junction (TJ) joining adjacent cells near the base of the brush border.
(d) Electron micrograph showing the system of basal interdigitations (BI) at the site of attachment of the proximal convoluted tubule cell to its basement membrane (BM). Note the abundant large mitochondria (M) and the proximity of an interstitial capillary (C).
(e) Scanning electron micrograph of the lumen of a proximal convoluted tubule showing the complex system of microvilli.

The Loop of Henle is divided into thick and thin parts.

Traditionally, the loop of Henle is regarded as having thick descending and ascending components, and a thin-walled section in between. It is better, however, to regard the thin-walled part as a distinct functional and structural entity for the following two reasons.

Firstly, the thick descending and ascending components are ultrastructurally closely identifiable with the proximal and distal convoluted tubules.

Secondly, the transitions between thick and thin tubules are abrupt, whereas the thick ascending and descending parts merge gradually with the proximal and distal convoluted tubules.

The thin limbs of the loop of Henle are lined by a flat epithelium and vary in length.

The thin limbs of the loop of Henle vary in length. Those associated with juxtamedullary glomeruli are long and extend deep into the medulla towards the papillary tip, whereas those associated with mid-cortical or subcapsular glomeruli extend only partway into the medulla. Thus thin Henle loops may be found in the cortex and medulla, and in the human kidney a few loops of Henle are located entirely within the cortex.

The thin limbs, both ascending and descending, have flat lining epithelium showing very little cytoplasmic specialization (Fig. 15.19). At its simplest, the thin loop resembles a dilated capillary by light microscopy and can be difficult to distinguish in routine paraffin sections.

In other areas, however, the epithelium, though flat, is rather more prominent, and ultrastructurally has short microvilli and some of the basal and lateral interdigitations seen to a greater degree in proximal tubules. In some rodents this taller, more specialized epithelial pattern is consistently found in the descending thin limb of short-looped nephrons from more superficial glomeruli, but such consistent placement is not apparent in man.

The thin limb of the loop of Henle maintains an osmotic gradient in the renal parenchyma.

The thin limb of loop of Henle creates a gradient of hypertonicity. The gradient is from the corticomedullary junction to the tip of the renal papilla, and is effected by the variable passage of sodium and chloride ions between the lumen of the Henle loop and the interstitium. This gradient allows concentration of the urine in the collecting duct system as it passes through the medulla. The widely accepted explanation of this mechanism is called the countercurrent multiplier hypothesis (Fig. 15.20).

Fig. 15.19 Loop of Henle.
This electron micrograph shows the structural simplicity of the thin loops of Henle (H) in the medulla.

Fig. 15.20 Countercurrent multiplier hypothesis.
The descending thin limb of the loop of Henle is freely permeable to water, Na⁺ and Cl⁻ ions, whereas the ascending thin limb, which is impermeable to water, actively pumps Cl⁻ ions out of the lumen into the interstitium, whereupon Na⁺ ions follow to maintain ionic neutrality.

Thus the ascending limb discharges Na⁺ and Cl⁻ ions into the interstitium but retains water within its lumen. Some of the Na⁺ and Cl⁻ ions diffuse back into the tubular lumen at the descending thin limb but are pushed out again when they reach the ascending limb.

This produces the multiplier effect and leads to hypertonicity of the interstitial tissue in relation to the fluid in the tubular lumen, particularly near the papillary tip. The fluid emerging from the end of the ascending limb of the loop of Henle into the distal tubule system is hypotonic.

The distal tubule starts after the loop of Henle.

The ascending thin limb of the loop of Henle opens into the short straight part of the distal tubule, which passes into the cortex running in a medullary ray and then becomes convoluted before opening into the collecting tubule. At about the junction between the straight and convoluted parts, the distal tubule runs close to the glomerular hilum to form a specialized segment called the macula densa (see page 299).

The cells lining the distal tubule are adapted for fluid and ion exchange.

The distal tubule is lined by cuboidal epithelial cells with extensive basal and lateral interdigitations. These are similar to those seen in the proximal tubule but the microvilli on the luminal surface are less well formed and comparatively scanty (Fig. 15.21). Mitochondria are numerous and mainly situated close to the lateral and basal interdigitations. There are none of the luminal invaginations and vesicles seen close to the microvillous border in the proximal convoluted tubule.

The structure of the distal tubule is virtually identical in the convoluted and straight segments (ascending thick limb of loop of Henle), but the macula densa shows a local variation in structure.

Fig. 15.21 Distal tubule.
Electron micrograph showing the features of a distal convoluted tubule cell. Note that it exhibits similar basal interdigitations (BI) to those of the proximal convoluted tubule cell, but that the luminal microvilli (MV) are scanty and poorly formed. Compare with Fig. 15.7.

The distal tubule is crucial to the control of acid–base balance, and is also important in urine concentration.

As can be deduced from its rich mitochondrial content, the distal tubule cell has the ability to pump ions against concentration gradients.

In the distal tubule:

- sodium ions are reabsorbed from the dilute urine in the lumen and potassium ions are excreted;
- bicarbonate ions are reabsorbed and hydrogen ions are excreted, thus rendering the urine acidic.

These functions are dependent on the presence of the hormone aldosterone, a mineralocorticoid secreted by the adrenal cortex (see page 264).

Antidiuretic hormone controls the permeability of the distal tubular epithelium to water.

Antidiuretic hormone (ADH) secreted by the posterior pituitary acts on the last part of the distal convoluted tubule. Its effect is to increase the permeability of the tubule, thus permitting the absorption of water to produce a more concentrated urine.

ADH also acts on the collecting ducts in a similar manner, permitting the absorption of water from the duct lumen into the hypertonic interstitium, and thence into the blood system (vasa recta). This movement of water is dependent on the countercurrent exchanger system (see Fig. 15.25).

Abnormalities of tubular function

The renal tubular and duct system is almost entirely dependent for its oxygen supply on the integrity of the glomerular capillary network and the arterial vessels supplying the glomeruli, since they receive oxygen from the peritubular capillary networks which are branches of the efferent arterioles leaving the glomeruli (see Fig. 15.4).

Thus the tubular epithelial cells can become significantly hypoxic if there is arterial or glomerular disease that

DIABETES INSIPIDUS

In the permanent absence of ADH, as occurs in the disease diabetes insipidus, vast quantities of dilute urine are formed because of the failure of water reabsorption at the distal convoluted tubule and collecting ducts

Fatal body water depletion is only prevented by drinking large quantities of water, which is stimulated by a constant feeling of thirst.

reduces the blood flow into the efferent arterioles. For example, obliteration of the glomerular capillary lumina by proliferation of the lining endothelial cells (see Fig. 15.8) leads to impaired oxygenation of the tubular epithelial cells. The clinical and biochemical picture is however usually dominated by features resulting from retention of nitrogenous waste products and the increase in peripheral vascular resistance (acute nephritic syndrome, see page 283).

If such damage to the glomeruli persists, then the tubular epithelial cells become so starved of oxygen that their enzyme systems and various pumping mechanisms are unable to function, and biochemical abnormalities develop as a result of the loss of the sensitive homeostatic mechanisms.

The most important biochemical abnormalities resulting from impaired tubular function are due to failure of excretion of H^+ and K^+ ions. The blood therefore contains a high concentration of H^+ ions (acidosis) and K^+ ions (hyperkalemia). These, along with the retention of nitrogenous waste material due to failure of glomerular function, are features of renal failure (see page 300).

METABOLIC DISORDERS OF TUBULES

Several functional disorders of renal tubular transport are described, which lead to metabolic disturbances. Some of these are acquired secondary to tubular damage, whereas others are inherited metabolic diseases.

Failure to resorb water is seen in chronic renal failure, nephrocalcinosis, and hypokalemia. It is also seen in nephrogenic diabetes insipidus (a rare disease).

Fanconi's syndrome is a generalized disorder of renal tubular transport, in which there is glycosuria, aminoaciduria and renal tubular acidosis. Although it may be primary, it is more often seen secondary to tubulointerstitial diseases such as toxic tubular damage.

Aminoaciduria syndromes result in excretion of abnormal amounts of amino acids in the urine. This may be due to elevated blood levels, but may be caused by primary defects in tubular transport as, for example, in cystinuria.

Renal tubular acidosis Type I results in defective function of distal tubules and failure to acidify urine. This may be acquired, being seen in tubulointerstitial diseases, or (rarely) may be inherited as a disorder of metabolism.

Renal tubular acidosis Type II results in defective function of the proximal tubule due to defective bicarbonate resorption. It is usually seen as part of Fanconi's syndrome.

ACUTE TUBULAR NECROSIS

Failure of tubular function due to poor oxygenation can also occur in the absence of any significant disease of arteries or glomeruli. The most common cause is a central failure of blood circulation due to poor cardiac output, which in turn is usually due either to low blood volume (hypovolemia), for example, following massive blood loss through hemorrhage, or to low blood pressure (hypotension), for example, following a myocardial infarction.

Poor perfusion through the peritubular capillary network leads to inadequate oxygen supplies for the tubular epithelial cells, and this leads to failure of enzyme systems and pump mechanisms, with consequent biochemical abnormalities, particularly acidosis and hyperkalemia. Because the glomeruli are not being perfused with arterial blood at an adequate pressure, little filtration takes place, so the production of urine falls or may even cease. The syndrome of acute renal failure comprises:

- oliguria or anuria (partial or total cessation of urine production);
- hyperkalemia (raised K^+ level in the blood);
- acidosis (raised H^+ level in the blood).

When the tubular failure is due to a central cause such as hypovolemia or hypotension, the tubular epithelial cells degenerate (Fig. 15.22). Their histologic appearance is due to accumulation of water within the cytosol.

If hypovolemia or hypotension are treated promptly, tubular epithelial cells can recover normal structure and function, otherwise, the tubular epithelial cells die (acute tubular necrosis). If adequate oxygenation is reestablished, the tubules become repopulated with epithelial cells. In renal grafting, the tubular epithelial cells of the donor kidney die almost immediately after the kidney is removed. When the kidney is transplanted (usually many hours after its removal) and its arterial supply is reestablished, the tubules are eventually repopulated with functioning epithelial cells, and normal homeostatic control is established.

Fig. 15.22 Acute tubular damage.
Micrograph of and H&E-stained paraffin section from a patient with early acute renal failure.

The proximal convoluted tubule epithelium shows early degenerative changes resulting from inadequate oxygenation following a prolonged fall in blood pressure. The individual cells are swollen with water as a result of failure of the Na^+/K^+ ATPase pump at the lateral walls of the cells, leading to inadequate excretion of water into the interstitium. Note that the microvilli are largely lost. Compare with Fig. 15.18.

The collecting tubules and ducts start after the distal tubule.

The convoluted segment of the distal tubule opens into the collecting system of tubules and ducts. This transition is not abrupt as there is a variable segment (sometimes called the connecting segment) where the epithelial lining contains both distal tubule and collecting tubule cell types in an apparently random fashion.

The collecting tubules are lined by two cell types.

The collecting tubule (Fig. 15.23) is lined by two types of cell: clear cells (the majority) and intercalated dark cells.

The clear cells are cuboidal or rather flat in the proximal part of the collecting system; they have light, poorly staining cytoplasm, which contains few cytoplasmic organelles (mainly randomly arranged small round mitochondria). Basal membrane infoldings are present in the proximal part of the collecting system but become less apparent further along, while microvilli are short and sparse.

Fig. 15.23 Collecting tubule.
Electron micrograph of collecting tubule which connects the end of the distal convoluted tubule and the collecting duct in the medullary ray of the cortex. Note the intercalated dark cell (DC), which is rich in mitochondria, and the sparse, short microvilli (MV) of the clear cells (CC).

The intercalated or dark cells are richer in cytoplasmic organelles, possessing numerous mitochondria. Their luminal surface has a well-developed microvillous system, with vesicles in the cytoplasm at the base of the microvilli. Normally there are no basal infoldings.

The collecting tubules in the cortex pass towards the medullary rays and open into collecting ducts.

The collecting ducts run vertically within the rays into the medulla. All of the medullary collecting ducts merge near the papilla to form large straight papillary ducts which run to the tip of papilla where they open out into the pelvicalyceal system.

The collecting ducts are lined initially by epithelium that is identical in type to that of the collecting tubules. As they pass down the medullary rays and into the medulla, however, the number of intercalated dark cells decreases and the clear cells become progressively taller and more prominent, so that, as the papilla is approached, the ducts are lined by regular straight-sided columnar clear cells (Fig. 15.24).

In humans, the basement membrane of the collecting duct system becomes progressively thicker as it nears the papillary tip. This feature becomes exaggerated with age.

The collecting tubules and ducts play an important role in the final concentration of urine.

The collecting tubules and ducts are not solely conduits for the transfer of urine into the pelvicalyceal system but are instrumental in concentrating urine to a degree appropriate to the level of blood hydration. This is achieved by interplay between the collecting tubules and ducts, the interstitium and the vasa recta, to produce a countercurrent exchanger system (Figs 15.25 and 15.26). Controlled water

transport is made possible by the variable permeability of the collecting duct under the influence of ADH (see page 293). The amount of ADH released depends on the body's requirement for water excretion or retention.

In the presence of high levels of ADH, water is lost from the collecting duct lumen into the interstitium, from where it passes into the blood circulation via the ascending vasa recta. This results in the production of a small amount of highly concentrated urine. When low levels of ADH are present, water remains within the collecting duct lumen and is lost in the form of copious dilute urine.

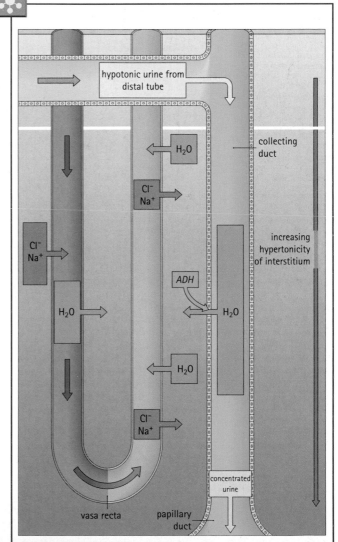

Fig. 15.25 Countercurrent exchanger system.
Dilute urine in the collecting tubule and duct system is progressively concentrated by the osmotic transfer of water from the lumen into the hypertonic medullary interstitial tissue, whence it is reabsorbed into the vasa recta. The hypertonicity is due to the high concentration of Na^+ and Cl^- ions in the medulla, resulting from the countercurrent multiplier activity of the loops of Henle. Thus, an increasingly concentrated urine is produced.

Fig. 15.24 Collecting duct.
Electron micrograph of a large collecting duct in the medulla. Note the lining of regular cuboidal or columnar clear cells and the sparsity of organelles.

The vascular networks of the vasa recta also play a role in the concentration of urine in the medulla.

On the descending (arterial) side of the looped vessels, the walls are permeable to water and salts; water passes out into the interstitium and sodium and chloride ions pass in. Thus, blood in the vasa recta is more or less in equilibrium with the hypertonic medullary interstitium.

On the ascending (venous) side of the vascular loop, sodium and chloride ions pass from the vessel lumen to the interstitium and water is reabsorbed into the venous blood from the interstitium.

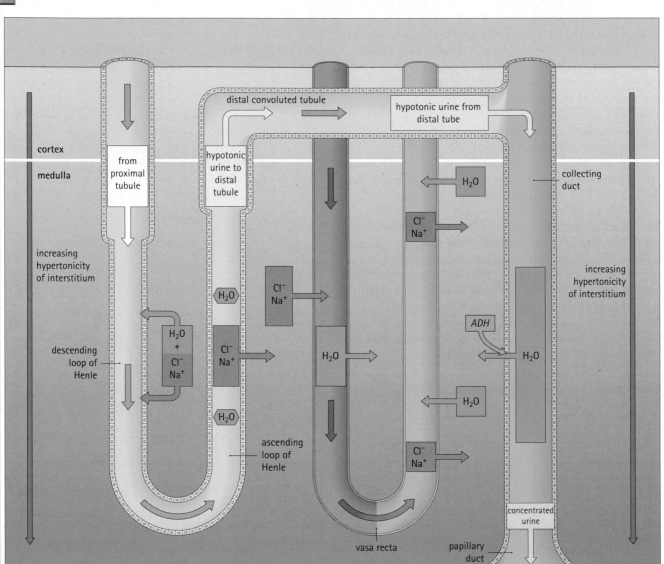

Fig. 15.26 Interrelationships between countercurrent multiplier and exchanger systems.

Movement of water ions across the walls of the thin loops of Henle (countercurrent multiplier, see Fig. 15.20) creates a hypertonic milieu in the interstitium, the tonicity increasing progressively as the tip of the papilla is approached.

The resulting hypertonicity of the interstitium encourages the absorption of water from the dilute urine passing down the collecting duct (countercurrent exchanger, see Fig. 15.25). The amount of water absorbed, and hence the final concentration of the urine excreted, is controlled by the level of circulating antidiuretic hormone (ADH), which regulates the collecting ducts permeability to water.

TUBULAR AND COLLECTING DUCT SYSTEM FUNCTIONS

- proximal convoluted tubule – reabsorption of water, glucose and amino acid by Na+/K+/ATPase pump, while larger molecules reabsorbed by endoyctosis

- thin loop of Henle – creates gradient of hypertonicity to allow concentration of urine in collecting duct system

- distal tubule – Na+ and HCO_3^- ions reabsorbed from urine in exchange for K+ and H+ which are excreted, dependent on aldosterone

- collecting tubules and ducts – control final concentration of urine by regulated reabsorption of water from urine under influence of hypertonicity gradient and antidiuretic hormone

DISORDERS OF COLLECTING DUCTS

The most important disorders of the collecting ducts are:
- infection, which usually results from the ascent of bacteria into the kidney from an infection in the bladder;
- papillary necrosis, in which the tips of the papillae undergo necrosis and drop off;
- deposition of insoluble crystals, which may occur in gout (urate crystals) or in hypercalcemia (calcium crystals).

RENAL INTERSTITIUM

The renal interstitium contains vessels and specialized interstitial cells.

In the cortex of the human kidney the interstitial space is small and largely occupied by small blood vessels and lymphatics. In the medulla, the interstitium becomes a significant component, both in bulk and in function. The interstitium increases in both size and importance as the tip of the papilla is neared (see Figs 15.35 and 15.36).

Ultrastructurally, the medullary interstitium is largely composed of loose electron-lucent acellular material, partly protein and partly glycosaminoglycans, in which collagen fibers, lipid droplets and basal lamina-like material are scattered. Variable numbers of interstitial cells are also present (Fig. 15.27).

In humans, the most frequently seen interstitial cell is irregular in outline with narrow, stellate cytoplasmic processes extending in all directions into the interstitial matrix. In rodents, these cell processes can often be seen to contact thin loops of Henle and adjacent medullary capillaries, sometimes seeming to act as a bridge between the two, but this is rarely apparent in man.

The cytoplasm of interstitial cells in man contains mitochondria, lysosomes, lipid droplets and small runs of rough endoplasmic reticulum.

Another type of interstitial cell, which is often spindle-shaped and contains abundant rough endoplasmic reticulum, resembles a fibroblast.

The importance of the medullary interstitium in salt and water homeostasis has already been described in relation to the functions of the loops of Henle, vasa recta and collecting ducts. The function of the interstitial cells is, however, not known. Although the renal medulla is known to be an important site of prostaglandin synthesis, it is currently believed that the epithelial cells of the collecting ducts, and not the interstitial cells, are responsible.

Fig. 15.27 Medullary interstitial cell and matrix.
Electron micrograph showing a typical human medullary interstitial cell (IC) located in the loose matrix near to the loop of Henle (H). The characteristic cytoplasmic feature is the presence of electron-dense spherical lipid droplets (LD); there is abundant rough endoplasmic reticulum and a few mitochondria.

JUXTAGLOMERULAR APPARATUS

The juxtaglomerular apparatus is involved in maintaining blood pressure and volume by the production of the hormone renin. It is a specialized adaptation of vascular and tubular tissues which allows blood flow to affect renin output. The juxtaglomerular apparatus comprises:

- renin-producing cells located in the walls of the afferent and efferent arterioles at the vascular hilum of the glomerulus;
- lacis cells;
- the macula densa area of distal tubule (Fig. 15.28).

Renin-secreting cells contain neuroendocrine granules.

In man, renin-producing cells are concentrated mainly in the walls of the afferent arteriole, although small numbers are present in the efferent arteriole.

Renin-producing cells have the ultrastructural features of highly specialized myoepithelial cells, with some

Fig. 15.28 Juxtaglomerular apparatus.
(a) Diagram of the juxtaglomerular apparatus, which consists of the macula densa, lacis cells, and the afferent and efferent arterioles. Within the walls of the arterioles are granular renin-secreting cells.
(b) Masson trichome stain showing the macula densa (MD) and afferent arteriole (AA) with prominent muscle cells (M) containing renin granules.

The efferent vessel and lacis cells are not visible in this section.
(c) Electron micrograph of human juxtaglomerular apparatus. Note the macula densa (MD), renin-producing cells (R), lacis cells (L), glomerular mesangial cells (G), and urinary space (US).
(d) High-power electron micrograph of the renin-secreting granular cells in the afferent arteriole wall. Note the protogranules (PG) (Type I) and mature granules (MG) (Type II).

contractile filaments. They also contain neuroendocrine granules of many shapes and sizes, although two distinct types can be recognized.

Type I granules are irregular in shape and contain rhomboidal crystalline bodies (protogranules) which are believed to be the precursors of the other types of granules.

Type II granules are larger, spherical, uniformly electron-dense and have an ill-defined membrane; they are thought to represent the mature renin-secreting granules.

The lacis cells resemble mesangial cells.

Lacis cells have a network (lacis) of thin interwoven processes which are separated by an acellular matrix of basement membrane-like material. Lacis cells occupy the triangular region bordered by the macula densa at the base and the afferent and efferent arterioles at the sides; the apex is formed by the base of the glomerular mesangium.

Because of their apparent continuity with the glomerular mesangium at the vascular pole of the glomerulus, these cells have also been called extraglomerular mesangial cells. Their function is not known.

The macula densa is a specialized adaptation of distal tubular epithelium.

The macula densa is a specialized zone of the distal tubule where it is in close contact with the vascular hilum of the glomerulus.

In this region the epithelial cells of the distal tubule are taller and more tightly packed than elsewhere in the tubule and the nuclei lie closer to the luminal surface; the Golgi is located between the nucleus and the basement membrane.

The precise function of this specialized zone of distal tubule is not known but it may act as a sensor, regulating juxtaglomerular function by monitoring sodium and chloride levels in the distal tubule lumen.

Renin converts angiotensinogen to active angiotensin, which then causes the adrenals to secrete aldosterone.

Renin produced in the juxtaglomerular apparatus catalyzes the conversion of inactive angiotensinogen. Angiotensinogen is an α_2-globulin produced in the liver, converted by renin to the decapeptide angiotensin I. Angiotensin I is then converted to angiotensin II, which stimulates the secretion of aldosterone by the zona glomerulosa of the adrenal cortex (see page 264).

Aldosterone is a mineralocorticoid hormone which regulates body sodium and potassium ion levels through its effect on the sodium pump mechanism at cell membranes.

In the distal tubule of the kidney, aldosterone promotes the reabsorption of sodium ions and water from the glomerular filtrate (Fig. 15.29), and thereby contributes to the maintenance of plasma volume and blood pressure.

Fig. 15.29 Renin–angiotensin–aldosterone system.
(a) Renin secreted by the juxtaglomerular apparatus (JGA) catalyzes the production of angiotensin I from its inactive precursor, angiotensinogen. Angiotensin I is then converted in the lung into the active octapeptide, angiotensin II, which stimulates the release of aldosterone from the adrenal cortex. Aldosterone mediates the absorption of sodium and water from the glomerular filtrate at the distal tubule.

The feedback control of renin secretion is not known.
(b) Immunocytochemical method for renin (brown) showing its location at the vascular hilum in relation to the afferent (AA) and efferent (EA) arterioles. Note the macula densa (MD).

Renin synthesis may be modulated by sodium concentration or blood pressure.

Two possible mechanisms have been proposed for the feedback control of renin synthesis and release, and it is probable that both may operate.

One is that the macula densa cells monitor the sodium concentration (or some other parameter) in the distal tubule lumen contents and effect some form of control over renin release by the granulated juxtaglomerular cells in the arteriole walls. The other postulated mechanism is that the juxtaglomerular cells act as sensory receptors by monitoring arteriolar stretching caused by an increase in blood volume.

ERYTHROPOIETIN SYNTHESIS

The kidney secretes erythropoietin but the site and mechanism are unknown.

Another function which has been ascribed to the juxtaglomerular apparatus is the synthesis of the erythrocyte-stimulating hormone, erythropoietin. There is no substantial evidence for this, other than the proven neuroendocrine function of the apparatus.

Despite the application of modern techniques, the precise site of erythropoietin formation within the kidney remains unknown. Based on tissue culture studies, claims have been made for its synthesis by mesangial cells, but gene probe analysis seems to indicate that erythropoietin messenger RNA is confined to the cortical tubules and interstitium.

KIDNEY FAILURE

Since the blood circulatory system in the kidney is its most important component, it is not surprising that many renal diseases are the result of abnormalities in this system. Common vascular diseases, such as systemic hypertension, diabetes mellitus and atherosclerosis, frequently damage the kidney, leading to impaired excretory and homeostatic functions.

Chronic renal failure

Decreased blood flow through the glomerular capillary system because of thickening of the arterial and arteriolar walls, and the consequent reduction in the lumina of these vessels, produces chronic ischemia of the tubular system and reduces glomerular filtration. If prolonged, this leads to disuse shrinkage of the components of the glomerulus (glomerular hyalinization) and atrophy of the tubules (Fig. 15.30). When these changes affect most of the glomeruli and their associated tubular systems, all of the functions of the kidney are impaired, and the patient develops symptoms of chronic renal failure.

Failure of the kidney's excretory function leads to retention in the blood of toxic metabolic waste materials, particularly urea and creatinine, from the endogenous breakdown of body protein. This is called **uremia**; the accumulation of urea and creatinine can be measured chemically. Eventually, without treatment, this intoxication leads to coma, fitting, and death. Failure of homeostatic functions carried out by the renal tubules leads to a loss of control of the body's water and electrolyte concentration; hydrogen and potassium ions accumulate in the blood, producing acidosis and hyperkalemia.

The kidneys are unable to produce a urine with a concentration or dilution commensurate with the body's needs. Instead a urine of constant specific gravity is produced, irrespective of the degree of hemoconcentration or hemodilution.

These biochemical disorders are the result of inexorable destruction of all of the activities of all nephrons. Chronic renal failure is irreversible.

Acute renal failure

In acute renal failure there is a sudden transient cessation of all nephron activity, which is usually due to damage to all tubules, or all glomeruli, or both. Depending on the cause, some recovery is usually possible if the patient can be sustained through the period of intense metabolic upset while the nephrons are inactive.

Fig. 15.30 End-stage kidney failure.
This H&E section shows the kidney from a patient with long-standing chronic renal failure due to progressive disease of the renal arterial supply. Little remains of the normal structure of the nephron. The glomeruli have been converted into acellular spheres containing no capillary network and the tubules have atrophied, the epithelial cells being flattened or cuboidal.

Fig. 15.31 Anatomy of adult kidney.

ⓐ Photograph of sectioned adult kidney, which has been fixed in formalin and the near natural color restored in alcohol. Note the cortex (C), the medullary pyramid (M) culminating in the papillary tip (P), which protrudes into the lumen of a calyx (Ca). Interlobar arteries (IA) and arcuate arteries (ArcA) can also be seen. Little detail of cortical structure is visible with the naked eye but the vertical linearity of the components of the medulla is highlighted by clusters of prominent blood vessels (vasa recta).

ⓑ In this H&E- stained paraffin section the distinction between cortex (C) and medulla (M) is easily seen. This section also shows the vertical linearity of the components

of the medulla, both tubules and vessels.

At this low magnification, glomeruli can be seen as small dots in the cortex. Note that some areas of the cortex are free of glomeruli, but contain vertically running duct systems; these areas are known as medullary rays and represent the sites where cortical tubules drain into the collecting ducts.

ⓒ In this micrograph of cortex at a higher magnification than in b it can be seen that the medullary ray (MR) area is devoid of glomeruli and that the interlobular arteries (ILA) run in the glomeruli-rich area.

ⓓ Renal cortex – glomerulus (G) and cortical tubules (T).

Fig. 15.32 Glomerulus.

ⓐ The details of the structure of the glomerular tuft are not easily seen in routine paraffin sections without the assistance of special stains to delineate capillary basement membranes. In this high- power micrograph occasional capillary lumina (CL) can be seen, but it is difficult to distinguish clearly between endothelial, mesangial and epithelial podocyte cells.

ⓑ A glomerulus stained by the Jones methenamine silver method to show the mesangium and capillary basement membranes. Clear delineation of the capillary basement membrane permits the recognition of endothelial cells (inside the membrane) and epithelial podocytes (outside the membrane). Note that this fortuitous section shows both the vascular (VP) and tubular (TP) poles.

Fig. 15.33 Cortical tubules.

In this high-power micrograph of cortical tubules, the proximal tubules (PT) are most numerous and prominent, having tall epithelium and small lumina. Distal tubules (DT) are smaller, have a cuboidal epithelium and proportionately larger lumina. Note the intimate capillary network (CN). Collecting ducts on their way to the medullary ray and thick and thin loops of Henle are also visible.

Fig. 15.34 Juxtaglomerular apparatus.

Any glomerulus sectioned through the vascular hilum may show part of the juxtaglomerular apparatus (JGA), though the detailed structure is rarely apparent. The most easily seen component in a paraffin section is the macula densa (MD), and the afferent and efferent arterioles are sometimes visible. Without the assistance of special stains, the juxtaglomerular and lacis cells cannot be specifically identified.

Fig. 15.35 Medulla.

In the medulla, all the various tubules, ducts and vessels run in the same direction, toward the papillary tip. The appearance on histologic examination depends on whether the section has been cut longitudinally to the axis of the tubules (in which case the tubules and ducts are cut in longitudinal section) or transversely. In most randomly selected tissue blocks, the section is usually oblique to the longitudinal plane of the medulla to a greater or lesser extent.

ⓐ In this micrograph of outer medulla, just below the corticomedullary junction, the tubules and ducts are seen in transverse section. The outer medulla contains a mixture of thick descending and ascending portions of Henle loops (HT), which are histologically very similar to proximal and distal convoluted tubule, thin loops of Henle (HL), small collecting ducts (CD) and vasa recta (VR). In this region there is a small amount of interstitium in which a few interstitial cells (IC) can be seen.

ⓑ Micrograph of the same area of outer medulla shown in a sectioned almost longitudinally.

Fig. 15.35ⓒ In this micrograph of lower medulla note the difference in the content of tubules and ducts to that of outer medulla shown inⓐandⓑ. There are now no thick portions of Henle loops but thin Henle loops (HL) are numerous as are thin-walled capillaries (C).

The collecting ducts (CD) are larger and lined by distinct, clear-celled cuboidal epithelium. The pale-staining interstitium now forms a substantial part of the tissue, and scattered small stellate and spindle-shaped interstitial cells (IC) are numerous. In this micrograph the Henle loops, vessels and collecting ducts are in transverse section.

ⓓ Micrograph of same area of lower medulla shown inⓒ sectioned longitudinally. Note the prominent straight collecting ducts running down towards the papilla; the nearer the tip of the papilla, the larger the ducts become.

Fig. 15.36 Papilla.
The large collecting ducts (CD) are few in number as a result of fusion; they open into the calyx (C) at the papillary tip. At the papilla, the distal medulla consists almost entirely of large collecting ducts embedded in bulky interstitium (I), with very few thin Henle loops and a number of vasa recta vessels. Interstitial cells are numerous.

LYMPHATIC DRAINAGE AND NERVE SUPPLY OF THE KIDNEY

The importance of the lymphatic drainage and nerve supply of the kidney in normal function is probably minimal, since both are destroyed during renal transplantation with no obvious serious side-effects.

Lymphatics in the kidney run with blood vessels.

The lymphatic drainage of the cortex of the kidney is mainly by a series of lymphatics which run in parallel with the cortical blood vessels. The main channels follow the interlobular, arcuate and interlobar blood vessels and emerge at the kidney hilum. A minor lymphatic system runs in the renal capsule and receives small tributaries from the outer cortex. There is some communication between these two systems within the cortex.

The kidney is supplied by autonomic innervation.

The nerve supply to the kidney arises mainly from the coeliac plexus. Both adrenergic and cholinergic fibers have been demonstrated. In general, these nerves have been seen to follow the course of blood vessels throughout the cortex and the outer medulla.

LOWER URINARY TRACT

The lower urinary tract is a series of conduits and reservoirs for urine.

The lower urinary tract is a functional rather than a geographical entity, since it extends from an intrarenal component high in the loins to the tip of the urethra. It comprises:

- the calyceal collecting system into which the large collecting ducts of Bellini in the medullary papillae discharge the urine;
- the renal pelvis, which is the reservoir at the hilum of the kidney into which the various calyces pass the urine;
- the ureter, which is a long muscular tube that conducts urine down to the bladder;
- the bladder, which acts as a major reservoir, holding the urine until it can be voided;
- the urethra, through which the urine stored in the bladder is voided to the exterior.

At various points there are sphincters capable of closing off parts of the lower urinary tract so that it can act as a reservoir. The most important of these muscular sphincters are located at the junction between the bladder and urethra and are under voluntary control.

These excretory passages have essentially the same basic structure, being hollow tubes with muscular walls.

With the exception of part of the urethra, they are lined by a specialized epithelium that is capable of withstanding contact with a fluid of variable concentration containing a number of toxic substances. This specialized lining is a form of stratified epithelium known as transitional epithelium or, in this site, the urothelium (Fig. 15.37).

The lower urinary tract is lined by specialized transitional epithelium termed urothelium.

The urothelium is a multilayered epithelium which varies in thickness at various sites in the lower urinary tract. In the small calyces it is only 2–3 cell layers thick, but in the empty bladder it can usually be seen to contain up to 5 or 6 layers; presumably this reflects the different degrees of distension to which the two components are usually subjected. As these epithelial cells have the ability to stretch, shift on each other, and flatten, a distended bladder may appear to be lined by only a 2–3 cell layer of stretched, flat cells.

In the non-distended state, urothelium has a rather compact, cuboidal basal layer, polygonal-celled middle layers, and a surface layer composed of tall, rather columnar cells, which are often binucleate, with a convex luminal surface bulging into the lumen.

Fig. 15.37 Basic structure of lower urinary tract.
Low-power micrograph of a transverse section of human ureter showing the basic structure of the lower urinary tract. The walls are muscular and there is an internal lining of specialized urothelium.

By light microscopy the luminal surface of urothelium often appears fuzzy in the undistended bladder due to the relaxation of the complex and convoluted cell surface membrane (Fig. 15.38).

Urothelial cells have specialized plaques in the apical cell membrane.

Ultrastructurally, the surface layer of urothelium is highly specialized. The luminal aspect of each cell is convoluted, with deep clefts running down into the cytoplasm, which also contains fusiform vesicles lined by cell membrane identical to that seen on the luminal surface (Fig. 15.39).

It is not yet clear whether all these vesicles communicate with the lumen (i.e. represent clefts which have been sectioned obliquely) or whether they represent reserve segments of surface membrane which can be incorporated into the surface layer when the lumen is distended with urine and a greater surface area is required.

In conditions of distension, the tall cells of the surface layer become flattened and lose their convex apical bulge, while ultrastructurally the deep clefts and multilaminate vesicles largely disappear. Throughout most of the lower urinary tract the urothelium stands on a thin, indistinct basement membrane supported by a variable layer of dense subepithelial support tissue which is mainly collagen (the lamina propria).

The lamina propria and muscle layers are external to the urothelium.

The urothelium is supported by a vascular lamina propria. Beneath the lamina propria are the layers of smooth

Fig. 15.38 Urothelium.
(a) High-power micrograph showing the characteristic appearance of the H&E-stained urothelium in the undistended state. When the lumen is distended with urine the cells flatten and form a thinner layer. Note the 5-6 layers, the occasional binucleate surface cell, and the indistinct luminal surface (LS).
(b) Masson trichrome stain showing the lateral cell borders of urothelium and its stratified nature. Note the indistinct luminal membrane (LS).

Fig. 15.39 Urothelial cell surface.
Electron micrograph of a non-distended human bladder post mortem, showing something of the unique structure of the surface of the urothelial cell. The luminal surface shows areas of a three-layered cell membrane (asymmetric membrane), most clearly seen in the invagination forming membrane plaques.

The membrane has a central lucent lamina between a thick electron-dense outer lamina and a thinner dense inner lamina. Immediately beneath the surface, the cytoplasm contains numerous round or oval vesicles (multilaminate vesicles) lined by identical trilaminar membrane. These vesicles become incorporated into the luminal surface by fusing with the frequent invaginations as the bladder fills and the surface urothelium stretches.

muscle which, in the pelvicalyceal system and ureters, are responsible for the peristaltic contractions forcing urine down into the bladder in one direction only.

The ureter has a spiral arrangement of smooth muscle in its wall.

In the simple tubular ureter there appear to be two distinct layers of muscle: an inner longitudinal layer and an outer circular layer (see Fig. 15.37). However, three-dimensional studies suggest that both muscle layers are in fact helical arrangements, with a loosely spiraled internal helix and a more tightly spiraled outer helix (Fig. 15.40), which appear to be longitudinal and circular, respectively, when the ureter is sectioned transversely.

In the architecturally more complex pelvicalyceal system, and in the virtually spherical bladder, arrangement of the muscle layers is less clearly defined.

The urinary bladder has three layers of smooth muscle.

The bladder is considered to have three muscle layers:

- an inner layer continuous with the inner longitudinal layer of the ureter;
- a middle layer continuous with the outer circular layer of the ureter;
- an additional outer layer in which the fibers run in approximately the same direction as the innermost layer (i.e. approximately longitudinal).

Since the bladder is roughly spherical instead of cylindrical, and the bladder musculature is, in any case, a distorted continuation of the helical arrangement seen in the ureter, the terms longitudinal and circular have little meaning.

The arrangement of muscle often appears rather haphazard in histologic sections, except at the narrow bladder neck where the layers again become more distinct (Fig. 15.41).

A functional 'valve' prevents urine reflux during micturition.

In the normal ureter, which is a narrow-bore tube, urine is forced downward by peristalsis to prevent reflux back toward the kidney. In the larger spherical bladder, however, this cannot be achieved, since the lumen of the fully distended reservoir is too large for a segment of it to be closed off by muscle contraction; thus, when the bladder musculature contracts during micturition, urine could reflux back up the open ureters and damage the kidney.

Although there are no anatomic valves at the junction of the ureters and bladder, potentially damaging reflux is prevented by a physiologic valve, which results from the oblique path by which the ureters enter the postero-lateral bladder wall musculature.

As the bladder distends and enlarges, the ureteric openings close, partly due to compression of the ureter lumen by extrinsic pressure from the musculature of the bladder wall and partly by acute angulation at the site of opening produced by bladder distension.

At the junction between the bladder and the urethra is a muscular sphincter, the internal sphincter, which when closed permits the bladder to act as a reservoir of urine. When this sphincter relaxes micturition occurs.

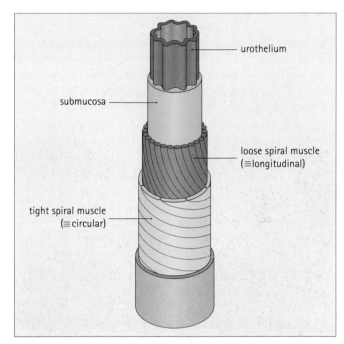

Fig. 15.40 Musculature of the lower urinary tract.
The arrangement of the muscle layers in the ureter is shown, emphasizing that the muscles are not truly circular and longitudinal, but are tight spirals and loose spirals.

Fig. 15.41 Bladder wall.
Beneath the urothelium is a fibrocollagenous submucosal region. The bulk of the wall is composed of smooth muscle which is loosely organized into three layers. This arrangement is most clearly seen at the bladder neck, as in this micrograph.

The bladder is supplied by autonomic innervation.

The bladder nerve supply is from the autonomic nervous system, and both sympathetic and parasympathetic nerves are found.

Sensory fibers from the bladder transmit signals as to the degree of bladder distension to the sacral spinal cord.

Parasympathetic fibers ending in the muscles and adventitia of the bladder act as the effector nerves for micturition.

Sympathetic nerves innervate the blood vessels to the bladder.

The urethra conducts urine from the bladder to be voided.

The urethra is the final conduit through which urine passes to the exterior. The anatomy of the urethra differs in the male and female.

The human female urethra is short, being approximately 5 cm long. It runs from the bladder and opens to the exterior in the midline of the genital vestibule just between the clitoris and superior border of the vaginal introitus.

The urethra is lined mainly by stratified squamous epithelium and its lamina propria contains many vascular channels as well as a few small mucus-secreting glands.

Although the urethral muscular wall is a continuation of the involuntary smooth muscle of the bladder, there is a sphincter, the external sphincter. This is composed of striated muscle and is under voluntary control; it is found around the mid-portion of the urethra where it passes through the striated muscles of the pelvic floor.

The male urethra is 20–25 cm long and is more complex than the female urethra since it serves two purposes. Not only is it the final conduit of the urinary system, but it is also the terminal conduit of the male reproductive system (see Fig. 16.1). It can be divided into three segments: the prostatic urethra, the membranous urethra, and the penile urethra.

The prostatic urethra begins at the bladder neck and runs through the prostate gland, from which many periurethral glands open into it through short ducts. It also receives the openings of the ejaculatory ducts.

The membranous urethra is the short segment (i.e. approximately 1 cm long), which runs through the pelvic floor muscles. This is the site of voluntary control of micturition since it is here that the external sphincter, of striated muscle, surrounds the urethra.

The penile urethra is the distal part of the urethra, and runs through the corpus spongiosum of the penis, opening to the exterior at the external meatus of the glans penis; small mucous glands, analogous to those in the female, open into the penile urethra.

The male urethra is lined proximally by transitional epithelium similar to that in the remainder of the lower urinary tract, but this becomes progressively less urothelial in character in the membranous and penile segments, where it changes to a rather non-specialized, pseudostratified, columnar epithelium. This finally changes to a stratified squamous epithelium at the distal penile urethra close to the external urinary meatus, where the epithelium merges with the stratified squamous epithelium of the glans penis.

1. THE GLOMERULAR FILTRATION BARRIER COMPRISES

(a) endothelial cells
(b) podocyte cytoplasm
(c) attenuated Bowman's capsule epithelium
(d) capillary basement membrane
(e) polyanionic charge barrier

2. PROXIMAL CONVOLUTED TUBULE EPITHELIUM

(a) shows extensive microvilli on luminal surface
(b) shows extensive basal interdigitation
(c) reabsorbs water from glomerular filtrate
(d) excretes glucose into the glomerular filtrate
(e) is partly controlled by the level of antidiuretic hormone (ADH) secreted by the posterior pituitary

3. THE JUXTAGLOMERULAR APPARATUS

(a) is located in the glomerular mesangium
(b) contains highly specialized myoepithelial cells which also contain neuroendocrine granules
(c) secretes angiotensin
(d) secretes renin
(e) is important in maintaining plasma volume and blood pressure

4. IN THE LOWER URINARY TRACT

(a) the renal pelvis, ureter and bladder are lined by transitional epithelium
(b) the ureter has two muscle layers
(c) the bladder has two muscle layers
(d) the male urethra is lined by a pseudostratified columnar epithelium throughout its length
(e) the female urethra is lined mainly by a stratified squamous epithelium

16. Male Reproductive System

INTRODUCTION

The male reproductive system is responsible for:
* production, nourishment and temporary storage of the haploid male gametes (spermatozoa);
* intromission of a suspension of spermatozoa (semen) into the female genital system;
* production of male sex hormones (androgens).

Whereas the first two functions are important only during the years of sexual maturity, hormone production is required throughout life, even in utero.

The male genital system (Fig. 16.1) comprises:
* testes, which produce spermatozoa, and synthesize and secrete androgens;
* epididymis, vas deferens, ejaculatory duct and part of the male urethra, which form the ductal system responsible for the carriage of spermatozoa to the exterior;
* seminal vesicles, the prostate gland and the bulbo-urethral glands (of Cowper), which are secretory glands providing fluid and nutrients to support and nourish the spermatozoa, and forming the bulk of the semen;
* penis, which is an organ capable of becoming erect for insertion into the female vagina during sexual intercourse.

The testes, epididymis, and vas deferens are located in the scrotal sac, which is a skin-covered pouch enclosing a mesothelium lined cavity continuous with the peritoneal cavity at the inguinal canal.

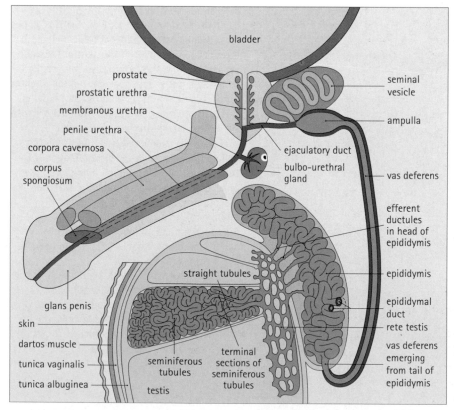

Fig. 16.1 Diagram of the male genital system.

Spermatogenesis occurs in the seminiferous tubules; the resulting spermatozoa pass into the rete testis at the hilum (mediastinum) of the testis.

From the rete testis, spermatozoa are transported by about a dozen efferent ductules into the head of the epididymis, where the ductules fuse to form the single, highly coiled epididymal duct. Within this duct they acquire their motility.

The spermatozoa then pass into a long straight tube, the vas deferens, which transports them from the scrotal sac into the short ejaculatory duct, receiving abundant secretions from the seminal vesicles.

The ejaculatory ducts from the right and left side run through the tissue of the prostate gland and open into the prostatic urethra.

Prostatic secretions and the secretions of the bulbourethral glands accompany or precede the semen along the penile urethra.

TESTES

ANATOMY AND DEVELOPMENT

The testes are paired organs located outside the body cavity in the scrotum.

The location of the testes in the scrotum (Fig. 16.2) means that they are maintained at a temperature approximately 2–3°C below body temperature; this lower temperature is essential for normal spermatogenesis.

Embryologically, the testes develop high on the posterior abdominal wall and migrate to the scrotum, usually arriving there in the seventh month of intrauterine life. When the testes fail to migrate into the scrotum (cryptorchidism) they fail to produce spermatozoa.

Each mature adult testis is a solid ovoid organ, approximately 4–5 cm long, 3 cm deep and 2.5 cm wide, and usually weighs 11–17 g. The right testis is commonly slightly larger and heavier than the left.

Each testis has an epididymis (see page 318) attached to its posterior surface and is suspended in the scrotal sac by the spermatic cord containing the vas deferens (see page 319), the arterial supply, and the venous and lymphatic drainage.

Fig. 16.2 Scrotum and tunica vaginalis.
ⓐ The scrotum is covered externally by skin with oblique hair follicles (producing curly hair) and numerous eccrine sweat glands.

In the deeper layers of the skin, smooth muscle fibers arranged in a rather haphazard manner form the poorly defined dartos muscle, contraction of which produces wrinkling of the scrotal skin.

Beneath the dartos muscle lies fibrocollagenous fascia (Colles' fascia), the deepest layer being compacted to form the dense parietal layer of tunica vaginalis, which is lined internally by flattened mesothelial cells similar to those lining the peritoneal cavity with which it is continuous. This smooth mesothelial-coated parietal tunica vaginalis forms the inner layer of the scrotal sac and is separated from the external surface of the testis by a potential space containing a watery fluid. This fluid acts as a lubricant, allowing the testis to move smoothly within the scrotal sac without friction.

The testis is covered externally by a thick collagenous capsule, the visceral layer of the tunica vaginalis (the tunica albuginea), the outer surface being coated with flattened mesothelial cells. Beneath the tunica albuginea lies a narrow variable layer of loosely arranged collagen containing superficial blood vessels; internal to this are the seminiferous tubules.
ⓑ Micrograph of the tunica albuginea of the testis. Note the scrotal cavity (C), the collagenous tunica albuginea (T) covered externally by small mesothelial cells, the narrow vascular layer (V), which is sometimes called the tunica vasculosa, and the seminiferous tubules (S).

Common causes of scrotal swelling are hydrocele, hematocele and inguinal hernia.

A hydrocele results when excessive fluid forms or accumulates within the scrotal cavity.

After trauma, bleeding into the scrotal cavity may produce a hematocele.

An inguinal hernia occurs when loops of intestine pass into the sac through the inguinal canal.

Judicious manipulation of the swelling usually allows the loops of intestine to be returned to the peritoneal cavity (i.e. reducible inguinal hernia).

Occasionally an inguinal hernia cannot be returned to the peritoneal cavity. In this situation (irreducible inguinal hernia), the venous drainage of the small intestinal loop may be compromised, leading to ischemic damage to the trapped loop of bowel (strangulated inguinal hernia).

Fig. 16.3 Testis.
Low-power micrograph of a sagittal section through testis stained by the van Gieson method, which colors collagen red. Note the tunica albuginea (T), which is thickened posteriorly to form the mediastinum testis (M). From the mediastinum, fibrous septa (S) enter the testis, separating it into lobules.

The testis is completely enclosed by the tunica albuginea, which is thickened posteriorly to form the mediastinum of the testis, projecting some way into the body of the testis (see Fig. 16.3). Blood and lymphatic vessels, and the channels carrying spermatozoa pass through this area (rete testis, see page 317). Fibrous septa from the mediastinum divide the body of the testis into 250–350 lobules, each lobule containing 1–4 seminiferous tubules.

SEMINIFEROUS TUBULES

A seminiferous tubule is a coiled, non-branching closed loop, both ends of which open into the rete testis.

The rete testis is a system of channels located at the posterior hilum of the testis, close to the mediastinum.

Each seminiferous tubule is approximately 150 μm in diameter, and 80 cm long. It has been calculated that the combined total length of all the seminiferous tubules in each testis is 300–900 m.

In a sexually mature adult, each seminiferous tubule has a central lumen lined by an actively replicating epithelium, the seminiferous or germinal epithelium, mixed with a population of supporting (sustentacular) cells, the Sertoli cells.

The lining cells sit on a well-defined basement membrane lying inside a collagenous layer containing fibroblasts and other spindle-shaped cells. These are contractile myoid cells containing intermediate filaments and desmin, like smooth muscle cells. In some animals these myoid cells form a continuous peritubular layer and contract rhythmically, possibly propelling the non-motile spermatozoa towards the rete testis (spermatozoa only acquire their motility after they have passed through the epididymis). In human testis, the myoid cells form a less distinct layer and are not usually circumferential.

The outer wall of the tubule, comprising basal lamina, collagen layer and myoid cell layer, is sometimes called the tunica propria.

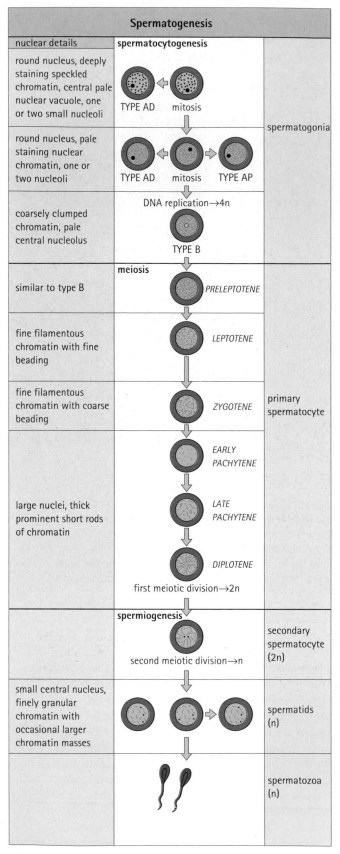

Spermatogenesis

nuclear details	spermatocytogenesis	
round nucleus, deeply staining speckled chromatin, central pale nuclear vacuole, one or two small nucleoli	TYPE AD ← mitosis	spermatogonia
round nucleus, pale staining nuclear chromatin, one or two nucleoli	TYPE AD ← mitosis → TYPE AP	
coarsely clumped chromatin, pale central nucleolus	DNA replication→4n TYPE B	
	meiosis	
similar to type B	*PRELEPTOTENE*	
fine filamentous chromatin with fine beading	*LEPTOTENE*	
fine filamentous chromatin with coarse beading	*ZYGOTENE*	primary spermatocyte
	EARLY PACHYTENE	
large nuclei, thick prominent short rods of chromatin	*LATE PACHYTENE*	
	DIPLOTENE first meiotic division→2n	
	spermiogenesis second meiotic division→n	secondary spermatocyte (2n)
small central nucleus, finely granular chromatin with occasional larger chromatin masses		spermatids (n)
		spermatozoa (n)

Blood vessels and clusters of hormone-producing interstitial (Leydig) cells are found between adjacent seminiferous tubules (Fig. 16.4).

GERMINAL EPITHELIUM AND SPERMATOGENESIS The germinal epithelium lining the seminiferous tubules produces the haploid male gametes (spermatozoa) by a series of steps called, in sequence, spermatocytogenesis, meiosis and spermiogenesis (Fig. 16.5).

Fig. 16.4 Seminiferous tubules and interstitium.
Micrograph showing seminiferous tubules (T) cut in transverse, longitudinal and oblique section, lined by germinal epithelium and enclosed by tunica propria. In the interstices are blood vessels and clumps of Leydig (interstitial) cells (L).

Fig. 16.5 Spermatocytogenesis and meiosis.
Spermatocytogenesis begins with the development of spermatogonia, of which three types are recognized: the type A dark (Ad) cell, the type A pale (Ap) cell, and the type B cell.

It is thought that the Ad cells are the precursor cells, which divide to produce new Ad cells and some Ap cells, the latter giving rise to type B cells, which subsequently pass through a meiotic phase to produce spermatocytes.

The B cells pass through several stages of maturation before the first meiotic division, and in these early stages are known as primary spermatocytes. The preleptotene cell is similar to the type B cell, but is not in contact with the basement membrane of the seminiferous tubule. The cell then undergoes its first meiotic division to produce a secondary spermatocyte which is smaller than its parent primary spermatocyte and has fine granular chromatin. This immediately undergoes a second meiotic division to produce the haploid spermatids from which the spermatozoa will develop.

The spermatids are located toward the lumen of the seminiferous tubule and have spherical central nuclei with finely granular chromatin and occasional larger chromatin masses. Their nuclear diameter is about half that of the primary spermatocytes from which they are derived.

In spermatocytogenesis, the stem cells (spermatogonia) undergo mitosis.

This mitotic division (see Fig. 2.26) produces not only more spermatogonia but also cells that differentiate into primary spermatocytes (Fig. 16.6).

In man, spermatogonia can be divided into three groups according to their nuclear appearances: type A dark (Ad) cells, type A pale (Ap) cells, and type B cells. It is thought that type Ad spermatogonia are the stem cells of the system, their mitotic division producing more type Ad cells and some type Ap cells, which further replicate by mitosis to form clusters of daughter cells linked to each other by cytoplasmic bridges. These type Ap spermatogonia mature into type B cells, which divide mitotically to produce further type B cells; these cells then mature in a cluster to produce primary spermatocytes.

Primary spermatocytes replicate their DNA shortly after their formation (i.e. they are 4n). Primary spermatocyte formation marks the end of spermatocytogenesis.

Meiotic division occurs at the spermatocyte stages.

Meiosis is described on page 29. Primary spermatocytes pass through a long prophase lasting about 22 days, during which changing patterns of nuclear chromatin enable preleptotene, leptotene, zygotene, pachytene and diplotene stages to be identified (see Fig. 16.5).

The first meiotic division occurs after the late pachytene/diplotene stages, with the formation of diploid secondary spermatocytes which rapidly (i.e. within a few hours) undergo the second meiotic division to produce haploid spermatids.

Spermiogenesis is the process by which haploid spermatids are transformed into spermatozoa.

Spermiogenesis can be divided into four phases, all of which occur while the spermatids are embedded in small hollows in the free luminal surface of the Sertoli cells (see page 316). These four phases (Fig. 16.7) are:

- the Golgi phase;
- the cap phase;
- the acrosome phase;
- the maturation phase.

The details of these phases are shown diagramatically in Fig. 16.7 on page 314.

Fig. 16.6 Spermatocytogenesis and spermiogenesis in seminiferous tubules.

Spermatogenesis occurs in waves along the length of the seminiferous tubules, and thus adjacent areas of the same tubule show spermatocytogenesis and spermiogenesis at various stages.

(a) Micrograph showing spermatogonia of various types including Ad and B types and preleptotene (PreL), zygotene/pachytene (Z/P) stages of primary spermatocytes. Some spermatids (St) are also present.

(b) Micrograph showing a later stage in which there is spermiogenesis as well as spermatocytogenesis. Ad spermatogonia, preleptotene (PreL) and zygotene/pachytene (Z/P) stages of primary spermatocytes, and spermatids (St) are shown, as well as developing spermatozoa (Sz) embedded in Sertoli cell cytoplasm. Sertoli cells are poorly defined in light microscopic sections of human testis.

MATURE SPERMATOZOON The mature spermatozoon comprises a head and a tail region, the latter being composed of a neck, a middle piece, a principal piece and an end piece (Fig. 16.8).

The head of a mature spermatozoon is composed of the nucleus covered by the acrosomal cap.

The spermatozoon head is flattened and pointed, and the chromatin of the nucleus is condensed and broken only by occasional clear nuclear vacuoles.

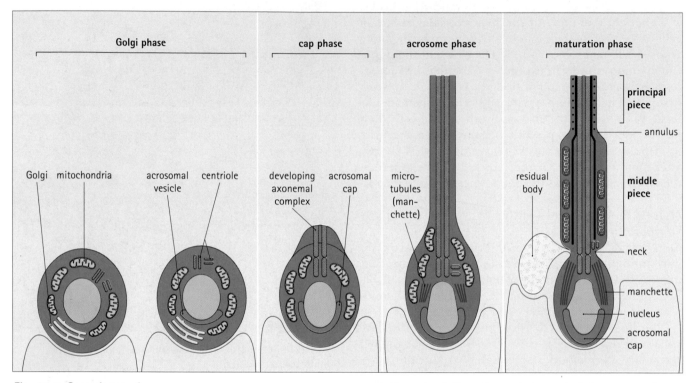

Fig. 16.7 Spermiogenesis.

In the Golgi phase, PAS-positive granules (pre-acrosomal granules) appear in the Golgi apparatus and fuse to form a membrane-bound acrosomal vesicle close to the nuclear membrane. This vesicle enlarges and its location marks what will be the anterior pole of the spermatozoon.

The two centrioles migrate to the opposite (posterior) pole of the spermatid, the distal centriole becoming aligned at right angles to the cell membrane. It then begins the formation of the axoneme complex of the sperm tail.

In the cap phase, the acrosomal vesicle changes shape to enclose the anterior half of the nucleus and become the acrosomal cap. The nuclear membrane beneath the acrosomal cap thickens and loses its pores and the nuclear chromatin becomes more condensed.

In the acrosome phase, the increasingly dense nucleus flattens and elongates; an anterior pole, capped by the acrosomal cap, and a posterior pole closely related to the developing axonemal complex can be identified. With the changed shape of the nucleus, the cytoplasm between the acrosomal cap and the anterior cell membrane migrates to the posterior part of the cell.

The entire cell orients itself so that the anterior pole is embedded in the luminal surface of the Sertoli cell, pointing down toward the base of the seminiferous tubule; the cytoplasm-rich posterior pole of the spermatid protrudes into the tubule lumen. At the same time, a sheath of microtubules, called the manchette, extends from the posterior part of the acrosomal cap toward the developing tail.

The centrioles (see Fig. 2.22), which have migrated posteriorly, from the neck of the developing spermatozoon, which is the connecting piece between the head (containing the nucleus and acrosomal cap) and the developing tail.

One centriole continues to synthesize the axonemal complex of the sperm tail, producing a regular tubular complex comprising two central microtubules surrounded by a ring of nine peripheral doublets. In the neck region, nine coarse fibers are produced which extend down into the tail around the microtubules of the axonemal complex.

Prominent mitochondria aggregate in and below the neck to surround the nine coarse fibers; this forms the segment known as the middle piece. The mitochondria finish abruptly at a ring (annulus) demarcating the middle piece from the main parts of the tail (the principal piece and end piece).

The maturation phase is characterized by the pinching off of surplus cytoplasm, particularly from the neck and middle piece regions, and its phagocytosis by Sertoli cells. The immature spermatozoa then become disconnected from the Sertoli cell surface and lie free in the seminiferous tubule lumen, marking the end of spermiogenesis. The immature male gametes are later modified in the ductular systems leading to the penis.

The duration of spermatocytogenesis from spermatogonium type Ad to released immature spermatozoon is about 70 days.

The acrosomal cap covers the anterior two-thirds to three-quarters of the nucleus; it is a glycoprotein containing numerous enzymes, including a protease, acid phosphatase, neuraminidase and hyaluronidase, and can be regarded as a specialized giant lysosome.

The acrosomal enzymes are released when the spermatozoon contacts the ovum; they facilitate penetration of the corona radiata and zona pellucida of the ovum (see Chapter 17) by the spermatozoal nuclear head.

The tail region of a mature spermatozoon is composed of the neck region, and middle, principal and end pieces.

Running throughout the tail is the axoneme which is responsible for spermatozoon motility; it is essentially a long, specialized cilium, with nine outer doublet tubules around a central tubule pair (see Fig 3.17)

The proximal part of the tail is the neck. This is a short narrow segment containing the pair of centrioles and connecting piece which form the nine fibrous rings surrounding the axoneme.

The axoneme runs through the centre of the middle piece and is surrounded by the nine coarse longitudinal fibers from the connecting piece in the neck and an outer zone of tightly packed, elongated mitochondria. The lower limit of the middle piece is marked by a sudden narrowing sometimes associated with an annular thickening of the cell membrane, the annulus.

The principal piece is the longest part of the tail and comprises the axoneme surrounded by the nine coarse longitudinal fibers which are in turn enclosed by numerous external sheath fibers orientated circumferentially. As one of the anterior and one of the posterior longitudinal fibers are fused with the circumferential fibers, the

Fig. 16.8 Mature human spermatozoon.
Diagram of a mature spermatozoon accompanied by electron micrographs confirming its structure.

remaining seven fibers are distributed asymmetrically, four in one lateral compartment and three in the other.

At the junction between the principal piece and the short end piece, the longitudinal and circumferential fibers cease. Thus the end piece is composed of axoneme only.

SERTOLI CELLS

The Sertoli cell sits on a basement membrane with its irregular apex extending into the lumen of the seminiferous tubule.

Sertoli cells are tall, columnar cells (Fig. 16.9) and are the main cell type until puberty, after which they comprise only about 10% of the cells lining the seminiferous tubules. In elderly men, however, a decrease in the number of germinal epithelial cells is common, so Sertoli cells again become a significant component of the tubule cell population.

Sertoli cells are not affected by any of the factors that injure the sensitive germinal epithelium. For example, they do not degenerate when exposed to normal body temperature and can therefore survive in the undescended testis.

The cell nucleus is irregular with deep folds, but tends towards an oval shape, with the long axis at right angles to the basement membrane. The nucleus has a vesicular chromatin pattern and a prominent nucleolus.

The Sertoli cell outline is irregular, with many ramifying cytoplasmic extensions which make contact with those from neighboring Sertoli cells to form a meshwork of cytoplasm. This encloses the developing cells of the germinal epithelium and forms tight junctions (see Fig. 3.6) which roughly divide the seminiferous tubule lining into basal and adluminal compartments.

Other forms of intercellular junctions (see Chapter 3) between Sertoli cells, including gap junctions and (occasionally) desmosomes, have been described, and intercellular junction-like structures have been seen between Sertoli cells and developing germinal epithelial cells.

Sertoli cell cytoplasm is eosinophilic and finely granular; it may contain lipid vacuoles. Ultrastructurally, it has abundant endoplasmic reticulum, often arranged as flat-stacked cisternae (annulate lamellae) with associated ribosomes. The lipid vacuoles are usually found close to the larger cisternae.

Endoplasmic reticulum is also prominent in the cytoplasmic processes interdigitating between the developing germ cells, while clusters of free ribosomes are numerous at the base of the cell. Microfibrils and microtubules are common in areas of cytoplasm close to the developing spermatids.

Spermatogonia and preleptotene spermatocytes occupy the basal compartment, while remaining primary spermatocytes, secondary spermatocytes and spermatids are located in the adluminal compartment.

Fig. 16.9 Sertoli cells.
Sertoli cells (SC) are rarely clearly identifiable in the lining of seminiferous tubules (S) in which active spermatogenesis is occurring, but form the entire lining of the tubule for a short distance at its distal end shortly before it drains into the rete testis system (R) at the mediastinum testis. This micrograph is taken from such an area.

These compartments are clearly distinguishable in some animal species, including primates, but not in man.

Sertoli cells have supportive, phagocytic and secretory functions.

Sertoli cells were originally thought to be supporting or sustentacular cells, but are now known to be polyfunctional.

Supportive functions probably include the provision of nutrients to developing germinal cells via their intimate cytoplasmic processes and the transport of waste materials from spermiogenesis to the blood and lymph vascular systems surrounding the seminiferous tubules.

It has long been assumed that Sertoli cells phagocytose any residual cytoplasm (residual bodies) shed by maturing spermatids during spermiogenesis. They may also phagocytose any effete cellular material derived from degenerate germinal cells that fail to complete spermatogenesis.

Secretory functions vary with sexual maturity. In the male embryo at about the 8th or 9th week of fetal development, Sertoli cells secrete Müllerian inhibitory substance (MIS), which is thought to suppress further development of the Müllerian duct system. In the prepubertal testis they may secrete a substance preventing meiotic division of the germinal epithelial cells.

In the mature testis, Sertoli cells secrete androgen binding protein (ABP), which binds testosterone and hydroxytestosterone produced outside the seminiferous tubule; high concentrations of these hormones are required within the germinal epithelium and tubule lumen for normal germ cell maturation.

ABP secretion is dependent on follicle stimulating hormone (FSH) secretion by the pituitary and FSH receptors are present on Sertoli cells. FSH promotes spermatogenesis, probably by inducing Sertoli cells to produce varying amounts of ABP.

Sertoli cells also secrete the hormone inhibin, which inhibits the secretion of FSH by the pituitary gland and therefore plays an important feedback role in controlling the rate of spermatogenesis.

Fig. 16.10 Leydig (interstitial) cells.
Micrograph showing a cluster of Leydig cells (L) situated in the interstitium between seminiferous tubules (ST). They have abundant eosinophilic cytoplasm, and some of the cells contain Reinke's crystalloids (RC).

The testicular interstitium contains hormone-secreting Leydig (interstitial) cells.

The interstitial tissue lying between the seminiferous tubules is a loose network of fibrocollagenous tissue composed of:

- fibroblasts;
- collagen, in which occasional macrophages and mast cells are present;
- blood and lymphatic vessels;
- clumps of interstitial or Leydig cells.

Leydig cells synthesize testosterone and, although they are most common in the tubular interstitium, they can occasionally be found in the mediastinum of the testis, the epididymis, or even in the spermatic cord. They are often closely related to nerves, like their female equivalent, the hilus cells of the ovary (see Chapter 17).

Leydig cells have round vesicular nuclei with prominent nuclear membranes and one or two nucleoli. Some of the cells are small and spindle shaped, and are thought to be immature forms, but most are round or polygonal.

Leydig cells have granular eosinophilic cytoplasm containing lipases, oxidative enzymes, esterases and a number of steroid dehydrogenases.

A characteristic feature of Leydig cells is Reinke's crystalloid, which is an intracytoplasmic, eosinophilic, elongated, rectangular or rhomboid mass, approximately 3 μm thick and up to 20 μm long (Fig. 16.10).

Reinke's crystalloids are not seen before puberty. They increase in number during the years of sexual maturity, becoming most common in old age.

Yellow-brown lipofuscin pigment is present in most Leydig cells.

The rete testis is a complex arrangement of interconnecting channels located at the mediastinum of the testis.

Spermatozoa formed in the seminiferous tubule loops pass to the terminal portions, which are lined entirely by Sertoli cells (see Fig. 16.9), and thence via the short straight tubules into the rete testis (Fig. 16.11) embedded in a fibrous stroma continuous with the tunica albuginea.

Fig. 16.11 Rete testis.
The rete testis is a network of interconnecting channels (C) into which the seminiferous tubules (T) empty. Spermatozoa are transferred from the rete testis to the epididymis via the efferent ductules.

Both straight tubules and rete testis are lined by a simple epithelium of cuboidal or low columnar cells bearing microvilli on their luminal surface. Most of the rete testis epithelial cells bear a single long central flagellum.

Channels of the rete testis fuse to form about a dozen efferent ductules.

These emerge from the upper end of the mediastinum of the testis, penetrating the tunica albuginea (see Fig. 16.1) and entering the head of the epididymis. Here they gradually merge to become a single tube, the epididymal duct.

The efferent ductules are lined by a mixed epithelium of tall ciliated columnar cells and non-ciliated cuboidal or low columnar cells with microvilli on their luminal surface (Fig. 16.12). The cilia beat toward the epididymis and propel the spermatozoa onward while the non-ciliated cells absorb some of the testicular fluid which is the transport medium for the immature and still immotile spermatozoa.

The efferent ductules are highly convoluted and have a narrow sheath of circumferential smooth muscle cells interspersed with elastic fibers; peristaltic contractions of this muscle enhance the progression of the spermatozoa.

Fig. 16.12 Efferent ductules.
Note the mixed columnar and cuboidal epithelium (E), the typical fringed internal lumen, and the circumferential ring of smooth muscle (SM) fibers.

EPIDIDYMIS

The epididymal duct (ductus epididymis) is formed by the fusion of the efferent ductules.

The epididymal duct is a single highly convoluted tube about 5 m long. It is embedded in a loose vascular supporting stroma of fibroblasts, collagen and glycosaminoglycan matrix, and is surrounded by a dense fibrocollagenous capsule, to form the comma-shaped body called the epididymis.

The epididymis can be divided into head, body and tail regions, with the efferent ductules entering the head and the distal end of the epididymal duct emerging at the tail to become the vas deferens.

The human epididymis is usually 5 cm long and 1 cm wide, and, as the entire 5 m of epididymal duct is contained within it, it is clear that the duct is enormously convoluted.

The epididymal duct is lined by a tall columnar epithelium bearing numerous very long, atypical microvilli.

These giant microvilli (Fig. 16.13) are largely immotile and are inaccurately named stereocilia; they neither contain the internal microtubular structures of cilia (see Fig. 3.17) nor function like cilia. They are about 80 μm long in the epididymal head and 40 μm long in the tail. The cells also possess coated vesicles and lysosomes, rough

Fig. 16.13 Epididymal duct.
ⓐ Micrograph of epididymal duct lined by tall columnar epithelium with basal nuclei; the lumina contain clumps of spermatozoa (S).
ⓑ High-power micrograph showing a single duct. Note the unusually tall microvilli (MV), the scattered small round cells at the base of the columnar epithelium (RC) and the narrow band of circular muscle fibers (M).

endoplasmic reticulum and a prominent Golgi. They have the following absorptive/phagocytic and secretory functions:

- absorption of testicular fluid commenced by the efferent ductules;
- phagocytosis and digestion of degenerate spermatozoa and residual bodies;
- secretion of glycoproteins, sialic acid and a substance called glycerylphosphorylcholine, which is believed to play a role in the maturation of the spermatozoa, though the precise mechanism is unknown. The glycoproteins bind to the surface membranes of the spermatozoa, but their function is also unknown.

In addition to the tall columnar cells, there is a population of small round cells with a high nucleus/cytoplasm ratio which lie on the epithelial basement membrane and are thought to be the precursors of the tall cells.

The entire epididymal duct is surrounded by a narrow sheath of circular muscle similar to that in the efferent ductules, but in the tail there is also a longitudinal layer internal to the circular layer, and an outer longitudinal layer.

All of the muscle layers thicken within the epididymal tail, becoming significant layers where the duct emerges to become the vas deferens.

VAS DEFERENS

The ductus (vas) deferens is a straight tube running vertically upward behind the epididymis within the spermatic cord.

The spermatic cord also contains arteries, veins, lymphatics and nerves. The veins form a complex anastomotic plexus called the pampiniform plexus. Externally the spermatic cord contains longitudinal fibers of voluntary striated muscle, the cremaster muscle.

The vas deferens has a thick, muscular wall composed of a middle circular, and outer and inner longitudinal layers. Internal to the inner layer is a fibroelastic lamina propria covered with a tall columnar epithelium almost identical to that of the epididymis but thrown up into longitudinal folds by the lamina propria; this produces a small stellate lumen (Fig. 16.14). Peristalsis of the thick muscular wall propels spermatozoa forward during emission.

Each vas deferens enters the pelvic cavity via the inguinal canal and then passes downward and medially to the base of the bladder. Near its distal end, close to the base of the bladder, each vas deferens has a dilatation (the ampulla) where the muscle layer becomes thinner; the mucosal layer in the ampulla appears thicker because the folds, some of which are branched, are taller.

At the distal end of the ampulla the vas deferens is joined by a short duct from the seminal vesicles.

Fig. 16.14 Vas deferens.
(a) Low-power micrograph showing the three muscle layers (a central circular (C) layer between outer (OL) and inner longitudinal (IL) layers) and the stellate lumen (SL).
(b) High-power micrograph showing the tall ciliated columnar epithelium (E), the basal layer of small regular round cells (RC), and the pattern of folds.

SEMINAL VESICLES

Each seminal vesicle is a highly convoluted, unbranched tubular diverticulum of the vas deferens.

The seminal vesicle is 15 cm long but is coiled on itself to form a body about 5–6 cm long. This tube is surrounded by an inner circular and an outer longitudinal smooth muscle layer, with an external layer of fibro-collagenous tissue containing many elastic fibers.

Seminal vesicle mucosa is composed of a fibroelastic lamina propria thrown up into tall, narrow complicated folds (Fig. 16.15), covered by non-ciliated, tall columnar epithelial cells and a population of non-specialized basal round cells similar to those seen in the proximal ducts and ductules. The tall cells have the characteristics of secretory cells, with large secretory vacuoles near their luminal surface and abundant rough endoplasmic reticulum; they may also contain small, yellow-brown lipofuscin granules.

The complexity of the mucosal folding produces a vast surface area for secretion and 70–80% of the human ejaculate is a thick, creamy-yellow secretion of the seminal vesicles. This secretion contains abundant fructose and other sugars, prostaglandins, proteins, amino acids, citric acid and ascorbic acid. Fructose is the major nutrient of spermatozoa.

Contraction of the seminal vesicle smooth muscle propels accumulated secretion into the ejaculatory duct.

The ejaculatory duct is formed by the merging of the short duct from the seminal vesicle with the vas deferens distal to the ampulla.

Each ejaculatory duct is only 1 cm long and is lined by an epithelium of tall columnar and small round cells identical to that of the ampulla; there is no smooth muscle in its wall. The right and left ejaculatory ducts run through the prostate gland and open into the prostatic urethra at the prostatic utricle.

PROSTATE
INTRODUCTION
The prostate is composed of secreting glands that open into the urethra, which runs through its body. These prostatic glands and ducts are embedded in a supporting stroma of fibroblasts, collagen and smooth muscle.

The entire prostate gland is surrounded by a fibro-collagenous capsule from which septa extend part way into its body, dividing it into ill-defined lobes.

The prostate gland progressively enlarges from about 45 years of age and may become very large in elderly men.

The prostatic glands are arranged in three concentric groups.

A small group of mucosal glands open directly into the urethra; a larger group of submucosal glands open into the urethra via short ducts; a substantial outer group of so-called main prostatic glands open into the urethra via long ducts (Fig. 16.16).

The ducts of the submucosal and main prostatic glands open posteriorly into the urethral sinuses on either side of a longitudinal ridge called the urethral crest.

The epithelium lining the prostate glands is thrown up into complex folds accompanied by a narrow supporting lamina propria. There are two types of epithelial cell:

- tall columnar or cuboidal cells with pale foamy cytoplasm and basal pale-staining nuclei;
- scanty flat basal cells with small dark-staining nuclei in contact with the basement membrane (Fig. 16.17).

Fig. 16.15 Seminal vesicle.
ⓐ Micrograph of seminal vesicle showing part of the muscular surround (M) and the pattern of tall mucosal folds. The lumen contains blobs of eosinophilic secretion (ES).
ⓑ Micrograph showing the tall columnar secretory epithelium at high magnification.

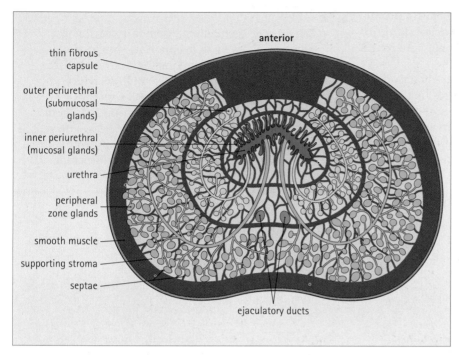

Fig. 16.16 Prostate.
The prostate is surrounded by a thin fibrous capsule internal to which is a substantial layer of smooth muscle giving rise to septa (mainly muscular but with a fine fibrocollagenous component) which penetrate the organ to provide an intimate stroma supporting and demarcating the glandular elements. Division into central and peripheral zones is indistinct.

The inner periurethral (mucosal) glands are small and open directly into the urethra around its entire surface; the outer periurethral glands are more numerous and open into the urethra through short ducts that enter the posterolateral urethral sinuses on their posterior surface on either side of the central ridge, the urethral crest. These two groups of glands comprise the central zone.

The glands of the peripheral zone empty their secretions into the urethra by way of long ducts opening alongside the urethral crest.

Fig. 16.17 Prostatic glands.
(a) Micrograph of prostatic mucosal glands (M) opening directly into the urethra (U).
(b) Micrograph showing the general architecture of a typical prostatic gland with its papillary pattern of ingrowths. Note the smooth muscular and fibrocollagenous stroma (S).
(c) Micrograph showing the cytologic detail of prostatic gland lining epithelium. It is composed of tall, pale-staining columnar cells (C) and occasional small basal cells (B) with darker staining nuclei.

Note the delicate supporting stroma of the papillary ingrowth (P) and the narrow periglandular layer of smooth muscle fibers (SM).

The lumen contains an uncalcified, concentrically laminated corpus amylacea (CA).

Ultrastructurally, the tall columnar cells have a prominent Golgi located between the basal nucleus and the luminal surface, lysosomes, secretory granules and rough endoplasmic reticulum are numerous.

The secretory products of these cells include acid phosphatase (produced in large quantities by the lysosomes), citric acid, fibrinolysin, amylase and other proteins. The gland lumina usually contain some stored secretions; in older men small spherical corpora amylacea, which are mainly condensed glycoprotein and often calcified, are found.

The ducts of the prostate gland may also be lined by tall columnar epithelium, but as they near the urethra this becomes progressively more cuboidal, and even transitional, like that of the urethra itself.

The prostatic epithelium depends on adequate testosterone levels to maintain its structural and functional integrity; any inadequacy is manifest by a change of epithelium from tall secretory to cuboidal, with loss of, or reduced, secretory activity. This change is seen increasingly from the middle years onward, and in extreme cases the epithelium may be converted to a stratified squamous pattern, often with keratin formation.

BENIGN PROSTATIC HYPERPLASIA

The commonest disorder of the prostate is benign prostatic hyperplasia, and occurs in eldery men. This is characterized by considerable enlargement of the prostatic glands in the mucous and submucosal gland groups due to an increase in the number and size of the glands and ducts, and an increase in the bulk of the supporting fibromuscular stroma. Many glands are over-distended with secretion (Fig. 16.18).

The increase in bulk of the prostatic tissue leads to compression of the urethra and micturition difficulties, including retention of urine.

Fig. 16.18 Benign prostatic hyperplasia.
Micrograph showing the low-power view of typical benign prostatic hyperplasia. There is nodular overgrowth of the periurethral glands (PUG), which is causing compression and distortion of the urethra (U). Note that the peripheral zone glands (PZG) are not involved.

CARCINOMA OF PROSTATE

Cancer in the prostate gland almost always originates in the main glands arranged around the periphery and is often advanced before symptoms arise due to blockage of the urethra (Fig. 16.19).

Fig. 16.19 Adenocarcinoma of the prostate.
Micrograph showing cancerous transformation of the prostatic glands. Those on the left have a normal arrangement with regular tall columnar epithelium. The cancerous prostatic glands on the right have lost their tall columnar pattern as well as their regular architecture.

BULBOURETHRAL GLANDS

Seminal fluid enters the prostatic urethra from right and left ejaculatory ducts, passing through the short membranous urethra and the penile urethra before entering the vagina during sexual intercourse. Opening into the membranous urethra are the long narrow ducts from the paired small bulbourethral glands.

The bulbourethral glands are lined by tall mucus secreting epithelium.

The bulbourethral glands are about 5 mm in diameter and the epithelium produces a watery, slightly mucoid fluid containing abundant sugars (mainly galactose) and some sialic acid. This fluid precedes the thicker semen along the penile urethra during emission and may have a lubricating function.

PENIS

The penis is composed of erectile tissue and contains part of the male urethra.

The erectile tissue is arranged into two dorsal cylinders (corpora cavernosa) and a smaller central ventral cylinder (corpus spongiosum) through which the penile urethra runs. The cylinders are each surrounded by a dense fibrocollagenous sheath, the tunica albuginea, which also holds them together (Fig. 16.20).

The erectile tissues are essentially interconnecting vascular spaces which are empty when the penis is flaccid (Figs. 16.21 and 16.22) but fill with blood during erection to form an enlarged, rigid organ.

The blood supply to the penis is provided by the dorsal and the deep arteries. From the deep arteries arise arteries supplying the tunica albuginea, and the helicine

Fig. 16.20 Penis.
Transverse section of penis showing the arrangement of the vascular erectile tissue into two dorsal corpora cavernosa (CC) and a single ventral corpus spongiosum (CS) through which the penile urethra (U) runs.

Small mucus glands in the corpus spongiosum are particularly concentrated around the penile urethra into which they open.

The corpora are enclosed within, and divided by, a broad fibrocollagenous capsule (C). The erectile core is surrounded by a sheath of skin to which it is connected by a very loose subcutis containing a number of blood vessels, including the small paired dorsal arteries and the midline superficial and deep dorsal veins.

Fig. 16.21 Corpus spongiosum.
Micrograph of corpus spongiosum showing large, irregular interconnecting vascular channels (C) lined by flat endothelium and separated by a fibrocollagenous stroma (S) containing some smooth muscle bundles.

Fig. 16.22 Corpora cavernosa.
(a) Micrograph of part of the corpora cavernosa (CC) with the central deep artery (A).

(b) Micrograph showing the system of interconnecting vascular channels (V) of the corpora cavernosa in the non-erectile state.

arteries, which supply the erectile tissue.

The helicine arteries are so named because they are spiral in the flaccid penis but during erection they straighten and dilate, filling the corpora with blood.

This filling effect is partly due to closure of the arteriovenous shunts existing between the helicine arteries and deep veins, which constitute the normal route of helicine artery blood flow in the flaccid state.

Parasympathetic nerve discharges cause the closure, leading to diversion of the helicine artery blood into the cavernous spaces, while increased pressure in the corpora compresses the thin-walled veins, preventing emptying.

After ejaculation the parasympathetic stimulation ceases, the arteriovenous shunts open and blood passes from the corpora into the veins.

During erection the two corpora cavernosa become more turgid than the corpus spongiosum. The pressure exerted by the corpus spongiosum on the urethra running through it is not sufficient to prevent passage of the semen, which is forcibly ejected by contraction of the smooth muscle, but is usually sufficient to prevent successful, pain-free micturition.

The erectile component of the penis is surrounded by skin, which has a very loose subcutis, permitting it to move considerably during intercourse.

At the distal end of the penis the corpus spongiosum terminates on the glans penis, which is covered with non-keratinizing squamous epithelium containing sebaceous glands.

The penile urethra opens to the exterior at the meatus at the centre of the glans penis.

For most of its length the penile urethra is lined by non-secreting columnar epithelium into which small mucus glands embedded in the corpus spongiosum drain. Within the glans penis, however, the urethra dilates (navicular fossa) and becomes lined by non-keratinizing stratified squamous epithelium identical to that covering the glans.

The end of the penis is normally covered by an overlap of penile skin (the prepuce), which is rich in elastic fibers permitting it to retract over the glans penis during intercourse.

ENDOCRINE CONTROL

The male sex hormone testosterone is essential for the male reproductive system to function successfully.

In the embryo, testosterone and other androgens produced by the immature testes are responsible for development of the penis and accessory sex glands, such as the prostate and epididymis.

With the onset of puberty, male secondary sexual characteristics develop under the influence of testosterone. This hormone also induces maturation and division of spermatogonia in the seminiferous tubules, leading eventually to full spermatogenesis with the production of mature spermatozoa.

In addition, testosterone is responsible for the maturation of the characteristic epithelia of the male genital ducts and the accessory glands which discharge secretions into them.

In the adult male, continued production of spermatozoa, and maintenance of the normal structure and function of the ducts and accessory glands, is dependent on continued testosterone production.

Failing testosterone production in old age leads to partial or complete cessation of spermatogenesis and alteration of the specialized secretory, absorptive and microvillose epithelium of the ducts and accessory glands to a more simplified cuboidal or squamous epithelium, which is unable to perform its previous functions.

Thus testosterone is the hub of the structure and function of the male genital system. It is produced by Leydig (interstitial) cells from cholesterol under the influence of luteinizing hormone secreted by the gonadotroph cells of the pituitary (see page 255).

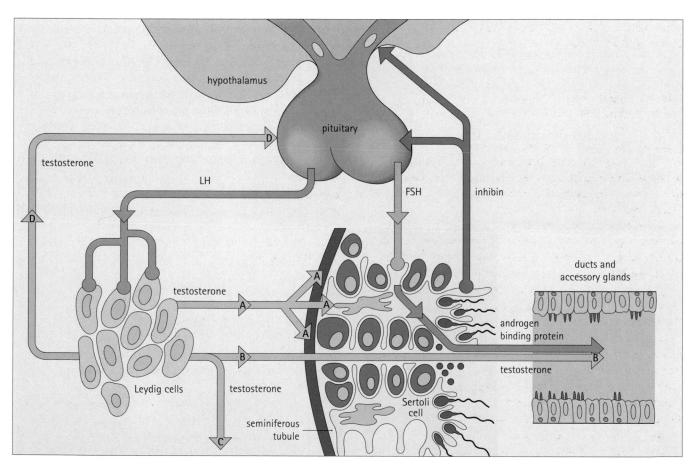

Fig. 16.23 Hormonal control of the male reproductive system. Testosterone stimulates spermatogenesis in seminiferous tubules (A), maintains structure and function of the ducts and accessory glands (B), stimulates and maintains secondary sexual characteristics (C), and provides a feedback mechanism (D) controlling pituitary output of luteinizing hormone (LH). Secretion of testosterone by Leydig cells is stimulated by LH. Sertoli cells secrete androgen-binding protein (ABP) under the influence of follicle stimulating hormone (FSH) from the pituitary, and also produce inhibin, which is responsible for feedback control.

1. IN THE TESTES, THE GERMINAL EPITHELIUM

(a) lines the seminiferous tubules and rete testes
(b) produces haploid male gametes
(c) is dependent on testosterone for its functional integrity
(d) is supported by Sertoli cells
(e) is an example of a renewing stem cell population

2. THE SPERMATOZOON

(a) contains the haploid nucleus in the head region
(b) has an acrosomal cap which contains several enzymes believed to help with penetration of the ovum
(c) contains an axoneme which is based on actin filaments
(d) is rich in mitochondria in the middle piece
(e) is formed by maturation of spermatids and takes place adjacent to the luminal surface of Leydig cells

3. THE PROSTATE GLAND

(a) discharges its secreted products into the seminal vesicles
(b) has three zones of glands termed mucosal, submucosal and main prostatic glands
(c) has both glandular and fibromuscular components
(d) has glandular elements lined by transitional epithelium
(e) is sensitive to endocrine stimulation, especially from testosterone

4. IN THE PENIS

(a) there are two dorsal corpora spongiosa and one ventral corpus cavernosum
(b) blood is supplied to the erectile tissue by the helicine arteries
(c) the urethra runs through the corpus spongiosum
(d) the urethra is lined by squamous epithelium in its distal portion in the glans penis
(e) there are small mucous glands which secrete into the urethra

17. Female Reproductive System

INTRODUCTION

The female reproductive system:
- produces haploid female gametes (ova);
- receives haploid male gametes (spermatozoa) prior to fertilization;
- provides a suitable environment for fertilization of ova by spermatozoa;
- provides a suitable physical and hormonal environment for implantation of the embryo;
- accommodates and nourishes the embryo and fetus during pregnancy;
- expels the mature fetus at the end of pregnancy.

The structure of the human female reproductive system changes considerably from childhood into reproductive maturity, and later the menopause, under the control of tropic hormones.

Furthermore, the various components undergo structural and functional modification at different stages in the monthly cycle.

The system (Figs. 17.1 and 17.2) comprises the ovaries, uterine tubes, uterus and vagina (collectively referred to as the **internal genitalia**), together with the mons pubis, vulva (labia majora and labia minora) and clitoris (referred to as the **external genitalia**).

Unlike many other mammals, the human female ovulates at regular intervals (approximately every 28 days) throughout the year.

As tissues from other animals do not accurately reflect the changes seen in the human, only human tissues are described and shown in this chapter.

MONS PUBIS, LABIA MAJORA AND LABIA MINORA

The mons pubis, labia majora and labia minora all consist of modified skin (see Chapter 18) as follows.

The mons pubis (mons veneris) is skin superimposed on a substantial pad of subcutaneous fat.

The mons pubis is the area overlying the symphysis pubis. It is characterized by the presence of unusually oblique hair follicles which produce the coarse, curly pubic hair common to most races. Underneath the skin is a pad of fat.

The labia majora are posterolateral extensions of the mons pubis on either side of the vaginal introitus.

The labia majora are similarly richly endowed with subcutaneous fat and oblique hair follicles (Fig. 17.1c). There are smooth muscle fibers in the subcutaneous fat.

The accumulation of subcutaneous fat and the development of the oblique hair follicles and pubic hair is hormone-dependent and begins with the onset of sexual maturity, usually between the ages of 10–13 years.

This area is also rich in apocrine glands and prominent sebaceous glands, both of which mature and become active at the onset of sexual maturity, while eccrine sweat glands, which are present from birth, show no change.

The labia minora are thin flaps of skin devoid of adipose tissue but with abundant blood vessels and elastic fibers.

Although hair follicles are absent, there are many sebaceous glands which open directly onto the epidermal surface (Fig. 17.1d).

The epidermis of both the labia majora and minora becomes pigmented by melanin with the onset of puberty. The outer, lateral aspect of the labia minora is usually more pigmented than the inner medial aspect and the epidermis has a well developed rete ridge system.

On the inner aspect, the melanin pigmentation becomes progressively reduced as the vaginal introitus is approached and the keratinized, stratified, squamous epithelium becomes thinner, with flattening of the rete ridges and thinning of the keratin layer.

This keratinized epithelium extends into the vaginal vestibule as far as the hymen, which is a thin fibrous membrane that is rarely completely intact and usually appears as an irregular 'frill' in the lining of the lower vagina, the hymeneal tegmentum. On its exterior (vulval) surface, the hymen is covered with the keratinized stratified squamous epithelium, whereas the inner (vaginal) surface is covered with non-keratinized, stratified, squamous epithelium, rich in glycogen, which is similar to that lining the vagina (see Fig. 17.3).

The hymen can be regarded as the junction between the internal and external genitalia.

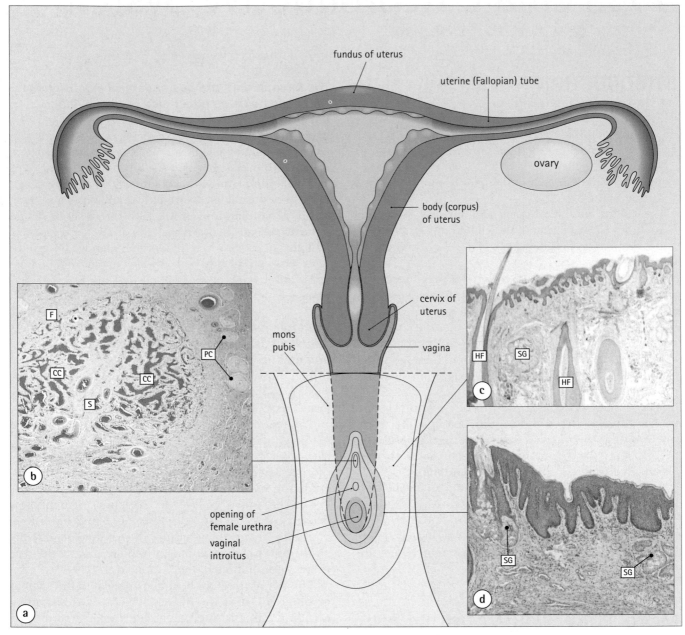

Fig. 17.1 Internal and external genitalia

(a) Diagram showing the relationship between the external and internal genitalia.

(b) Micrograph of clitoris; note the two corpora cavernosa (CC), arranged side by side and engorged with blood, the incomplete central septum (S), and the fibrocollagenous sheath (F), outside which are prominent nerve endings (mainly Pacinian touch corpuscles (PC), see Chapter 18).

(c) Micrograph of labia majora. The skin contains many hair follicles (HF), sebaceous glands (SG), and eccrine sweat glands and ducts.

(d) Micrograph of labia minora. The skin is devoid of hair follicles, but rich in sebaceous glands (SG), which open directly onto the surface. Note that the dermis is highly vascular.

CLITORIS

The clitoris is located below the mons pubis and is the female equivalent of the penis.

The clitoris is composed of two corpora cavernosa of erectile vascular tissue which lie side by side surrounded by a fibrocollagenous sheath; an incomplete central septum partly separates the two corpora (see Fig. 17.1b).

The clitoris is covered by thin epidermis that is devoid of hair follicles, sebaceous glands, eccrine and apocrine glands, but is richly equipped with sensory nerves and a variety of receptors.

Over the superior surface of the clitoris the skin forms an incomplete hood (the clitoral prepuce), and, on the inferior surface, a thin midline frenulum. At the base of the clitoris, the corpora cavernosa diverge to lie along the pubic rami, where they contain fibers of the ischiocavernosus muscle.

The clitoris, which is small before puberty, enlarges to a greater or lesser extent with the onset of sexual maturity. During sexual arousal it becomes engorged in a manner similar to that of the penis.

The urethral meatus opens to the exterior in the midline below the clitoris.

On either side of the meatus are the openings of the para-urethral glands (of Skene). These glands are located around the urethra, mainly posteriorly and laterally, and are lined by pseudostratified columnar epithelium.

VAGINA

The vagina is a fibromuscular tube extending from the vestibule to the uterus.

In the mature female the vagina is 7–9 cm long, but is capable of both marked distension and elongation (see Fig. 17.1). It forms an angle of more than 90° with the normal anteverted uterus (see Fig. 17.2).

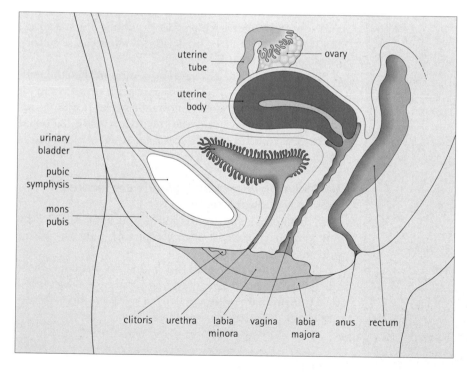

Fig. 17.2 Lateral view of female genitalia.
Note the angle of insertion of the uterus into the vagina.

At its inner end the vagina forms a cuff around the protruding cervix of the uterus, forming anterior, posterior and lateral pouches known as the fornices.

The vagina has four layers (Fig. 17.3) as follows:

- stratified squamous epithelial mucosa;
- lamina propria (subepithelial region), which is rich in elastic fibers and thin-walled blood vessels, mainly veins and venules;
- a fibromuscular layer containing ill-defined bundles of circularly arranged smooth muscle and a more prominent outer layer of longitudinally arranged smooth muscle.
- adventitia, which is composed of fibrocollagenous tissue containing numerous thick elastic fibers, large blood vessels, nerves and clumps of ganglion cells. At the lower end the fibromuscular layer also contains some skeletal muscle, which is found mainly around the vaginal introitus in the hymeneal region.

The rich meshwork of elastic fibers in the vaginal wall is responsible for its elasticity and permits the great temporary distension required during parturition. The extensive submucosal plexus of thin-walled blood vessels is thought to permit the diffusion of watery fluid across the epithelium and contribute to vaginal fluid.

Although structurally a tube, at rest the vagina is collapsed so that the anterior wall is in contact with the posterior wall, and for much of its length there are shallow longitudinal grooves in the midline of both these walls. In addition, the vaginal mucosa is rugose, being thrown up into a series of closely packed transverse mucosal folds or ridges.

The structure of the vagina varies with age and hormonal activity.

Changes occur in the non-keratinizing, stratified squamous epithelium which lines the vagina.

Before puberty, the epithelium is thin, a state to which it reverts after the menopause, but during the reproductive years the epithelium responds to the activity of estrogens and thickens. The basal cells and the distinct parabasal layer show increased mitotic activity, while the more superficial cells increase not only in number but also in size as a result of the accumulation of stored glycogen and some lipid within the cytoplasm.

Glycogen content is maximal at the time of ovulation, and some glycogen-rich surface squames are shed into the vaginal cavity after ovulation, during the secretory phase of the menstrual cycle.

Breakdown of the glycogen by commensal lactobacilli in the vaginal cavity produces lactic acid, resulting in an acid pH. This restricts the vaginal bacterial flora to acid-loving commensals and deters invasion by bacterial pathogens and fungi such as *Candida albicans*, which is the cause of vaginal 'thrush'.

Bartholin's (vulvovaginal) glands are located around the lower vagina.

The Bartholin's glands are composed of acini lined by tall columnar mucus-secreting cells with pale cytoplasm and small basal nuclei.

These glands open into the vagina posterolaterally at the level of the hymeneal remnants through a duct lined by a transitional epithelium with a surface mucin-secreting layer.

Fig. 17.3 Vagina.
Micrograph of vaginal wall showing glycogen-rich stratified squamous epithelial mucosa (M), a highly vascular submucosa (S), and irregular smooth muscle (SM).

UTERUS

The uterus is a muscular organ and receives the right and left uterine (Fallopian) tubes. It is lined by columnar epithelium and at its lower end it opens into the vagina.

The uterus can be divided into three parts: the fundus, the body and the cervix (Fig. 17.4). Whereas the fundus and body have the same histologic structure (see page 335), that of the cervix is different.

CERVIX

The cervix is the lower part of the uterus, part of which protrudes into the vagina.

The junction between the cervix and the uterine body is the internal os, and at this point the nature of the lining epithelium and the uterine wall changes (Fig. 17.5).

The cervical lumen opens into the vaginal cavity at the external os, where again there is an important change in the nature of the lining epithelium. This zone is the site of many important pathologic changes (see Fig. 17.8).

The cervix is cylindrical and symmetrical, being about 3 cm long and 2–2.5 cm in diameter, but becomes more barrel-shaped after pregnancy and parturition. After childbirth, the external os becomes a transverse slit dividing the distal end of the cervix into anterior and posterior lips, whereas the external os of the nulliparous cervix is circular.

The cervical stroma is important in childbirth.

The cervical stroma is composed of smooth muscle fibers embedded in collagen, the proportions of the two components varying with age and parity. Normally the cervix is firm and rubbery, and the cervical lumen is a narrow channel, but the cervix can be dilated under some circumstances, a fact which is used in investigative gynecologic practice to obtain samples of the uterine lining epithelium for histologic examination. A measure of the capacity of the cervix for dilatation is the fact that a cervical lumen which is normally a narrow canal incapable of taking a pencil becomes, at childbirth, capable of allowing the passage of a baby. Furthermore, after delivery the cervix reverts to normal in a very short time.

This capacity depends on radical alterations in the nature of the cervical stroma, attended by a change in texture ('cervical softening')

Fig. 17.4 Uterus.
Section through the uterus of a 35-year-old woman showing the fundus (F), body (B) and cervix (Cx). Note the endometrial cavity (EMC), endocervical canal (ECC) and ectocervix (Ecx). The smooth muscle of the body contains a small tumor, a leiomyoma (L) (See Fig. 17.11).

Fig. 17.5 Cervix.
Low-power micrograph of cervix. The stroma (S) is composed of smooth muscle fibers embedded in collagen, the proportions of muscle and fibrous tissue varying according to age and parity; blood and lymphatic vessels are prominent and numerous. The ectocervix (Ecx) is covered with stratified squamous epithelium, while the endocervical canal (ECC) is lined by tall columnar epithelium.

The junction between the squamous and columnar epithelium is located in the region of the external os. In this example, there is a transformation zone (TZ) (see page 333) of squamous epithelium which has extended into the endocervical canal; note the Nabothian follicles (NF).

The cervix in childbirth

The normally firm and rubbery uterine cervix with a narrow lumen of less than 1 cm in diameter dilates to approximately 10 cm during labour. This is achieved by softening and increased elasticity in the cervical stroma. The changes in the cervix in late pregnancy are complex.

In the glycosaminoglycan matrix, hyaluronic acid concentration between collagen fibers increases, drawing in water molecules which increase the bulk and softness of the matrix and separate the collagen fibers of the cervical stroma. Dermatan sulfate concentration decreases, leading to weakening of the dermatan sulfate bridges holding adjacent collagen and elastin fibers together. This further contributes to the separation of collagen fibers.

There are also changes in collagen and elastin fibers. Type I and type II collagen fibers become separated from each other, lose their strong parallel alignment and become shorter. The separation of collagen fibers, their rearrangement from a compact parallel pattern to a more haphazard arrangement, and the shortening of individual fibers, all lead to a reduction in tensile strength and a decreased resistance to the pressure exerted by the presenting part of the fetus being expelled from the uterine body. Similar changes probably occur in elastin fibers.

THE EPITHELIAL CONTENT OF THE CERVIX

The external surface of the part of the cervix that protrudes into the vagina is the ectocervix and the lining of the lumen is the endocervix.

The ectocervix is covered by epithelium continuous with that of the vagina at the vaginal fornices.

Like vaginal squamous epithelium, the ectocervical epithelium is non-keratinizing, stratified, squamous and rich in glycogen in the sexually mature period (Fig. 17.6). It undergoes cyclical changes during the menstrual cycle under the influence of estrogens and progesterone.

Before the menarche and after the menopause the epithelium is much thinner, with fewer layers and smaller cells containing less glycogen.

The endocervical canal runs between the uterine and vaginal cavities.

The canal is lined by a single layer of tall columnar mucus-secreting epithelium, the endocervical epithelium (Fig. 17.7a).

Longitudinal or transverse histologic sections of the cervix have given the impression that there are glandular structures (endocervical mucus glands) extending into the underlying stroma. Three-dimensional studies indicate, however, that the structures are in fact deep, slit-like invaginations of the surface epithelium, with blind-ended tubules arising from the clefts (Fig. 17.7b). Thus, there is a large surface area for the production of cervical mucus, which fills the endocervical canal. Before puberty and after the menopause, the amount of cervical mucus is greatly reduced.

Fig. 17.6 Ectocervix.
Stratified squamous epithelium (E) covers the ectocervix. Like those of the vagina, the cells are rich in glycogen during the period of sexual maturity.

Fig. 17.7 Endocervix.
ⓐ The endocervical canal is lined by a single layer of tall columnar mucus-secreting epithelium (E).
ⓑ Numerous deep invaginations (I) of the mucus-secreting epithelium extend into the cervical stroma and greatly increase the surface for mucus production.

As well as contributing to vaginal lubrication during sexual intercourse, the mucin in the endocervical canal acts as a protective barrier, preventing bacterial ascent into the endometrial cavity.

Movement of endocervical mucus into the vaginal canal is facilitated by a few ciliated columnar epithelial cells scattered among the mucus-secreting endocervical cells, particularly at the upper end of the canal, close to the junction with the endometrium.

Both the mucin-secreting and ciliated cells have fine microvilli which are only visible ultrastructurally.

The columnar epithelium of the endocervical canal and the squamous epithelium of the ectocervix meet at the squamo–columnar junction of the cervix.

This is the most likely area of the cervical epithelium to be affected by disease.

The original squamous columnar junction is usually located in the region of the external os but its precise location at birth is influenced by maternal hormone exposure in utero.

At about puberty, hormonal influences lead to extension of the columnar epithelium onto the ectocervix forming an ectropion or cervical erosion (Fig. 17.8), which is augmented by a first pregnancy, particularly when this occurs shortly after menarche.

Before puberty the pH of the vagina and cervix is alkaline but afterwards bacterial breakdown of the glycogen in the vaginal and cervical squamous epithelium renders an acidic environment, with a pH of about 3.

Cervical Mucin

During the menstrual cycle, the physiochemical properties of cervical mucin are subject to marked changes, but the endocervical columnar epithelium shows little microscopic variation, although ultrastructural changes in cytoplasmic organelles have been noted.

During the proliferative (follicular, estrin) phase, the mucin is thin, watery and abundant, and has an alkaline pH (features which may facilitate movement of spermatozoa). It is composed of a network of glycoprotein micelles, the spaces in between being occupied by plasma rich in Na^+, K^+ and Cl^-. The high ionic concentration is responsible for its ability to crystallize ('ferning' or 'arborization' pattern) in this ovulatory phase.

After ovulation the mucus becomes viscid and scanty, and has an acidic pH, deterring penetration by spermatozoa, and sealing the uterus in preparation for possible embryo implantation.

Exposure of the sensitive columnar epithelium of the ectropion to the postpubertal acidic environment of the vagina induces squamous metaplasia and a transformation zone between the endocervical columnar epithelium and the ectocervical squamous epithelium.

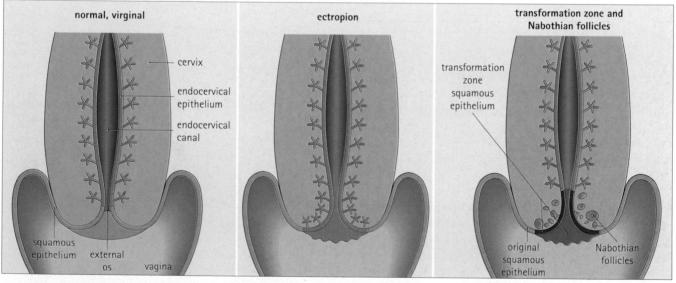

Fig. 17.8 Squamous/columnar junction of the cervix.
Diagram illustrating the mobility of the squamous/columnar junction, the development of ectropion, and the formation of the transformation zone.
ⓐ The squamous/columnar junction is originally situated in the region of the external os.
ⓑ At puberty the endocervical epithelium extends distally into the acid environment of the vagina and forms an ectropion.
ⓒ A transformation zone forms as squamous epithelium regrows over the ectropion. The openings of the crypts may be obliterated in the process, resulting in the formation of mucus-filled Nabothian follicles (see Fig. 17.5).

Thus the squamous columnar junction is of variable size but its site always approximates to the external os. In older women it may retreat into the endocervical canal.

The transformation zone is composed of new squamous epithelium in an area previously occupied by columnar epithelium.

One almost invariable consequence of squamous metaplasia near the external os is that the openings of some of the deep crypts of previously everted endocervical mucous glands become obliterated so that mucin produced deep in the crypts cannot be excreted into the endocervical lumen or vagina. Instead it accumulates within the blocked clefts and produces spherical cystic masses of inspissated mucus lined by flattened endocervical mucus-secreting epithelium; these are called **Nabothian follicles**. Other consequences of this constant change of epithelium include the development of abnormal epithelium, which may progress to cancer.

UTERINE CERVIX

- lower part of uterus, protruding into vagina

- canal is lined by tall columnar mucin-secreting epithelium

- surface protruding into vagina is covered by stratified squamous epithelium

- squamous columnar junction is an important site of disease

- has a stroma of smooth muscle fibers embedded in collagen; proportions of each vary according to age and parity

CARCINOMA OF THE CERVIX

The transformation zone of the cervical epithelium is the most common site of origin of carcinoma of the cervix, the development of which is usually preceded by histologic abnormality of the squamous epithelial cells in this zone. The abnormal cells:
- lose their regular stratified pattern;
- have a high nucleus-to-cytoplasm ratio;
- show variation in shape and size and increased mitotic activity.

These cytologic features are characteristic of malignant tumor cells and are usually associated with evidence of invasive behavior. However, in the cervix, the cytologic changes of malignancy may be present for years before the abnormal epithelium begins to invade the underlying stroma; they are referred to as carcinoma-in-situ or cervical intraepithelial neoplasia (CIN) (Fig. 17.9a).

Eventually the abnormal epithelial cells breach the basement membrane and invade the cervical stroma (Fig. 17.9b), gaining access to blood and lymphatic vessels which are their route for spread to other sites, such as the lymph nodes around the iliac arteries. This is invasive carcinoma. Early diagnosis of CIN can be obtained by cervical cytology (cervical smear); cells are scraped from the epithelial surface in the region of the cervical os and examined microscopically for abnormal cells. Abnormal areas can then be treated, usually by surgical removal, thus preventing the future development of invasive cancer.

Fig. 17.9 Carcinoma of the cervix.
ⓐ The cervical epithelial cells (E) have lost their regular stratified pattern, have high nucleus-cytoplasm ratios and show increased mitotic activity (compare with Fig. 17.6). As the basement membrane (BM) between the epithelium and underlying stroma (S) is intact, this is carcinoma-in-situ or cervical intraepithelial neoplasia (CIN)
ⓑ Some of the abnormal epithelial cells have breached the basement membrane and invaded the cervical stroma (arrow); this is invasive carcinoma.

UTERINE BODY

The body and fundus of the uterus have thick walls composed of smooth muscle (myometrium).

The myometrial smooth muscle is arranged into three ill-defined layers.

Myometrium is hormone-sensitive and undergoes both hypertrophy (an increase in cell size) and hyperplasia (an increase in cell numbers) during pregnancy (Fig. 17.10), progressively returning to its normal size (involution) in the weeks after delivery.

Within the myometrium are prominent blood vessels, both arterial and venous, which undergo marked dilation and thickening of their walls during pregnancy.

With cessation of hormonal stimulation after the menopause, the myometrial cells atrophy and the uterus shrinks. The fibrocollagenous tissue between the muscle bundles, which is comparatively insignificant when the myometrial smooth muscle is prominent during sexual maturity, then becomes obvious.

Fig. 17.10 Myometrium.
ⓐ Normal myometrium from a non-pregnant 35-year-old woman. The muscle cells are small and tightly packed.
ⓑ Myometrium from a 28-year-old woman in the 8th month of pregnancy, photographed at the same magnification as ⓐ. Note the enormous increase in size of the individual muscle fibers, almost entirely due to an increase in cytoplasm. This is an example of physiologic hypertrophy, and is a common response of muscle cells to an increased workload, in this case the need to increase the propulsive power of the uterus to expel the fetus at childbirth.

LEIOMYOMA

The myometrium is the site of one of the most common benign tumors, the leiomyoma or fibroid (Fig. 17.11, see also Fig. 17.4), which is derived from smooth muscle of the uterine wall.

Like normal uterine smooth muscle, leiomyomas are hormone-dependent and progressively enlarge until the menopause, after which time they regress.

Fig. 17.11 Leiomyoma.
Micrograph of a typical small leiomyoma.

The body of the uterus is lined by the endometrium, which is composed of glands and supporting stroma.

Before puberty, the endometrium is simple and composed of low cuboidal epithelium supported by a scanty spindle-celled stroma. Downgrowths of epithelium into the stroma produce a small number of rudimentary tubular glands.

Between the menarche (the first menstrual period) and the menopause the endometrium can be differentiated into two layers, a deep basal layer at the junction with the myometrium, and a superficial functional layer lining the lumen. It is the functional layer which is hormone-responsive and undergoes the monthly cycle of proliferation, secretion, necrosis and shedding. The endometrium is sensitive to the fluctuating levels of estrogen and progesterone secreted by the ovary, and the changes are known as the **menstrual cycle**. The relationships between the histologic changes in the endometrium and the ovarian and pituitary hormone secretions are discussed and illustrated in Fig 17.24, page 346.

If fertilization and successful implantation of an ovum occur, the endometrium remains unshed and forms the decidua (see page 352).

The basal layer, which is not shed at menstruation, provides a cellular reserve from which a new functional layer develops after menstrual shedding. The endometrium does not respond evenly to ovarian hormonal stimulation; functional endometrium in the lower segment close to the junction with the cervix, and patches around the entrances of the uterine tubes, may show little proliferative or secretory activity, and often resembles the basal layer. As the menopause approaches, more and more of the endometrium may fail to respond fully to the hormonal stimulus.

At the menopause, when hormonal stimulation ceases, the endometrium reverts to the simple prepubertal pattern, although the tubular downgrowths may undergo cystic distension and the stroma may become compact (atrophic cystic endometrium).

UTERINE TUBES

The uterine (Fallopian) tubes convey ova from the ovary to the lumen of the body of the uterus (endometrial cavity).

They are also the site of fertilization of the ovum by spermatozoa. After fertilization, the tube transmits the fertilized ovum to the endometrial cavity where implantation can take place.

Each uterine tube is 10–12 cm long and extends from a dilated open end close to the ovary to a narrow portion which passes through the myometrial wall of the uterus before opening into the uterine cavity. There are four recognizable tubal segments (Fig. 17.12), each differing histologically, particularly in their proportions of muscle and epithelium, and the degree of convolution of their epithelium.

Fig. 17.12 Uterine (Fallopian) tube.

ⓐ Diagram of the uterine tube, ovary and uterus.

ⓑ Low-power micrograph of the ampulla, showing its thin muscular wall and large lumen with markedly papillary mucosa.

ⓒ High-power micrograph of tubal epithelium at the ampulla, showing a high proportion of ciliated cells (CC), thin delicate stroma (S) and an occasional intraepithelial lymphocyte (IEL).

ⓓ Scanning electron micrograph of tubal mucosa at the ampulla, showing numerous ciliated cells (CC) and relatively scanty secretory cells (SC).

ⓔ Low-power micrograph of the isthmus, showing its thick muscular wall and small lumen with simpler, non-papillary mucosa.

ⓕ Scanning electron micrograph of tubal mucosa at the isthmus, showing few ciliated cells (CC) and many secretory cells (SC) with abundant microvilli.

The infundibulum is surrounded by a fringe of epithelial-coated **fimbriae**, some of which may become adherent to the nearby ovary. Medial to the infundibulum is a thin-walled zone called the ampulla where ovum fertilization usually takes place.

The ampulla leads into a narrower, thick-walled segment called the isthmus. In turn, the isthmus is continuous with the short intramural segment, which opens into the uterus.

The uterine tube is essentially a muscular tube lined by specialized epithelium which is variably folded and plicate, differing in appearance at different sites.

The smooth muscle wall of the uterine tube is composed of two layers.

The inner layer of smooth muscle in the uterine tube appears to be circular in histologic sections and the outer layer appears to be longitudinal. In reality these layers are almost certainly arranged as a tight spiral (circular) and a loose spiral (longitudinal) as seen in the ureter (see Chapter 15). Close to the uterus, a third muscular layer is also present.

Internal to the muscle layers, a delicate vascular lamina propria supports the tubal epithelial lining.

There are two types of epithelial cell lining the uterine tube: ciliated cells and secretory cells.

The ciliated cells are particularly numerous near the ovarian end of the tube where they form the majority population (about 60–80%), but close to the uterus they are the minority population (about 25%) and secretory cells predominate (see Fig. 17.12).

Two other cell types have been described in the tubal epithelium: the peg cell and the reserve basal cell. The peg cell is currently considered to be an effete secretory cell and the reserve basal cells have been shown to be intraepithelial cells of the lymphoid series.

The ciliated tubal epithelial cell is a columnar cell, the height of which varies during the menstrual cycle.

The ciliated tubal epithelial cell is at its tallest and most ciliated at about the time of ovulation, after which it progressively shortens and loses some cilia until menstruation. The decrease in height and ciliation is presumably a progesterone effect, since similar changes occur and persist throughout the duration of a pregnancy. With the resumption of estrogen secretion after menstruation or delivery, the cells again lengthen and become more ciliated.

The ciliated cells may be responsible for movement of the ovum through the infundibulum and ampulla, though tubal peristalsis probably plays a greater role. They may also have a role in propelling the spermatozoa in the opposite direction.

The secretory cells are columnar cells with surface microvilli.

The secretory cells produce a watery tubal fluid (see Fig. 17.12) which is rich in potassium and chloride ions and also contains normal serum proteins, including immunoglobulins.

The tubal fluid is assumed to have a nutritive function for spermatozoa and fertilized or unfertilized ova.

DISORDERS OF THE UTERINE TUBE (1)

An important disorder of the uterine tube is tubal ectopic pregnancy.

Tubal ectopic pregnancy

Occasionally the fertilized ovum is held up in the tubal lumen and implants in the wall of the uterine tube producing a tubal ectopic pregnancy.

Partial development of the embryo and placenta proceeds for a time, but the thin-walled uterine tube is an unsatisfactory site for implantation and the embryo cannot survive. The vascular placental tissues penetrate into the thin tubal wall (Fig. 17.13a) and often perforate through, producing brisk bleeding into the lumen of the tube and into the peritoneal cavity. This produces lower abdominal pain and, if the blood loss is severe, shock.

Fig. 17.13 Disorders of the fallopian tube.
(a) Micrograph of a tubal ectopic pregnancy; chorionic villi (CV) are developing in the lumen of the tube and trophoblast (T) is eroding into the tubal wall producing bleeding (B).

DISORDERS OF THE UTERINE TUBE (2)

Acute and chronic salpingitis

Bacterial infection of the tube (e.g. by the gonococcus) produces acute inflammation in the papillary folds and muscular wall and pus formation in the lumen (Fig. 17.13b).

Such infections may persist, with abscess formation and chronic inflammation, or may heal with scarring, leaving a blocked or distorted lumen, which may obstruct the passage of the fertilized ovum and predispose to tubal ectopic pregnancy.

Fig. 17.13 ⓑ In this section from an infected tube, the papillary folds and muscular wall are infiltrated by neutrophils and there is pus (P) in the lumen.

OVARY

INTRODUCTION

The paired ovaries are small flattened ovoid organs lying in the right and left lateral pelvic cavities. They have two major functions:

- they are the source of mature ova;
- they are endocrine organs, producing the steroid hormones that prepare the endometrium for conception and maintain pregnancy should fertilization occur.

The surface of the ovary is covered by a single layer of epithelium.

This surface layer is usually cuboidal or low columnar in type (see Fig. 17.16), but commonly flattens with increasing age and when the ovary is enlarged.

The epithelium is continuous with the pelvic peritoneum at the hilum of the ovary (though the cells differ structurally from the peritoneal mesothelial cells). It is called the germinal epithelium, which is however a misnomer because the epithelial cells are not the source of the female gametes.

The surface epithelial cells have prominent surface microvilli and occasional cilia; mitochondria are abundant and small pinocytotic vesicles are associated with the base of some microvilli.

The ovarian surface is usually irregularly fissured, and the fissures are also lined by the surface epithelium. The necks of the fissures may seal over, leaving islands of surface epithelium within the ovarian cortex. Fluid secretion by the cells then converts these islands into cysts (germinal inclusion cysts), which are common.

The surface epithelial cells show little alteration during the menstrual cycle but usually lengthen during pregnancy.

A substantial basement membrane (the tunica albuginea) separates the surface cells from the underlying ovarian tissue in the mature ovary.

The ovary can be divided into three components: hilum, medulla and outer cortex.

The ovarian **hilum** is the route whereby blood vessels, lymphatics and nerves enter and leave the ovary, and is continuous with the medulla, the central core of the ovary (Fig. 17.14).

In addition to the vessels and lymphatics, the medulla and hilum also contain vestigial remnants of the embryonic Wolffian duct and clusters of hilus or hilar cells.

Fig. 17.14 Ovary.
Micrograph of ovary showing the hilum (H), medulla (M) and cortex (C). Gamete formation and maturation occur in the cortex and are responsible for the cystic spaces seen here.

The Wolffian duct remnants persist as irregular tubules lined by flat or cuboidal epithelium (rete ovarii).

The hilus cells are histologically identical to the interstitial (Leydig) cells of the testis (see page 317) and are round or oval, with eosinophilic granular or foamy cytoplasm containing brown lipofuscin-like pigment. They are densely packed (Fig. 17.15).

Occasional hilus cells contain Reinke's crystalloids (see page 317) and some contain round eosinophilic hyaline bodies as well. The small clumps of hilus cells are often found close to nerves and blood vessels.

The ovarian **medulla** often contains clusters of stromal cell identical to those occupying the bulk of the cortex.

The ovarian **cortex** has two components:
• a supporting stroma;
• gamete-producing structures and their derivatives.
The proportions and appearances of these two components in any individual ovary will depend on both age and hormonal stimulation.

The cortical stroma is composed of closely packed, spindle-shaped fibroblast-like cells.

The stromal cells are arranged haphazardly or in a variable whorled pattern (Fig. 17.16). The cytoplasm of these cells is rich in ribosomes and microfilaments; mitochondria are also numerous and tend to collect around the nucleus. Micropinocytotic vesicles are found in association with the cell surface, and there are small numbers of lipid droplets.

Reticulin and collagen fibers between the stromal cells are particularly prominent in the outer part of the cortex. Progressive collagenization of this area begins early in reproductive life and becomes more marked with time, so that by the menopause it is almost universal.

The cellularity of the ovarian stroma, and the amount of lipid the cells contain, are both dependent on hormonal stimulation. An increase in lipid accumulation in the stromal cells is called **luteinization of stromal cells** and is particularly prominent during pregnancy.

The ovarian stroma has three main functions:
• it provides structural support for the developing ova;
• it gives rise to the theca interna and theca externa around the developing follicle (see Fig. 17.19b);
• it secretes steroid hormones.
Although it is probable that all stromal cells have the potential to produce steroid hormones under appropriate circumstances, three types of steroid-secreting stromal cells are recognized:
• the cells that surround the follicle (i.e. theca layers-see Figs 17.19b and 17.21b);
• the scattered lipid-rich luteinized stromal cells;
• a population of stromal cells, called enzymically active stromal cells (EASC), which exhibit marked oxidative and other enzyme activity.

Fig. 17.15 Ovary — hilus cells.
A clump of hilus cells (H) is shown adjacent to a nerve (N) in the ovarian hilum, a characteristic location. These cells have ill-defined borders, foamy eosinophilic cytoplasm, and granules of brown lipofuscin pigment.

Fig. 17.16 Ovarian cortical stroma and surface epithelium.
Note the whorled pattern of the spindle-shaped ovarian stromal cells (S), and the single layer of cuboidal surface epithelial cells (E).

EASC are particularly numerous in postmenopausal women. They are disseminated in clusters in the cortex and medulla, and have been shown to secrete testosterone and other androgenic steroids.

GAMETE PRODUCTION AND MATURATION IN THE OVARY

The number of gametes in an ovary, and their appearance, varies with age. Embryologically they are derived from primordial germ cells which develop in the yolk sac and migrate to the developing ovary (Fig. 17.17).

Mitotic divisions of primordial germ cells produce small oogonia.

Oogonia multiply by further mitotic divisions within the developing fetal ovary.

During the second trimester of pregnancy the mitotic divisions cease, and the large numbers of oogonia increase in size and are called **primary oocytes**. At this stage they number several million in each ovary, but many degenerate, so that by birth each ovary contains about one million oocytes.

The oocytes continue to degenerate throughout life and at the onset of puberty oocyte numbers are reduced to a quarter of a million or so.

The primary oocytes which survive degeneration in the second trimester enter the prophase of the first meiotic division.

Primary oocytes remain in this phase for many years and acquire a single layer of flat surrounding cells (granulosa cells); these structures are called **primordial follicles** (Fig. 17.18a). At birth the ovarian cortex is packed with large numbers of primordial follicles embedded in the cellular cortical stroma, and some of these persist in the ovarian cortex throughout the period of sexual maturity (Fig. 17.18b).

Some primordial follicles develop further at puberty to produce primary follicles.

At puberty, the cyclical secretion of follicle stimulating hormone (FSH) from the pituitary stimulates the further development of a small number (probably 30–40) of the primordial follicles.

The first step is enlargement of the oocyte, which is associated with an increase in size of the surrounding granulosa cells so that they become cuboidal or columnar; at this stage the structure is called a **unilaminar primary follicle**.

Continuing FSH secretion then induces the granulosa cells to divide to produce a multilayered surround to the enlarging oocyte, while a distinct glycoprotein layer of eosinophilic (PAS-positive) material forms between the oocyte and these cells (Fig. 17.19a). This layer is called the **zona pellucida** and is traversed by microvilli protruding outwards from the oocyte and by thin cytoplasmic processes from the inner layer of the granulosa cells. The follicle is now known as a **multilaminar primary follicle**.

Meanwhile ovarian stromal cells come to lie in roughly concentric layers around the enlarging follicle to form a capsule-like arrangement. At about this stage, most follicles then degenerate by a process called **atresia** (see page 344). A small number of follicles however continue to develop, although atretic degeneration still occurs at all subsequent stages; thus only a few follicles reach full maturity.

Continuing maturation leads to the formation of secondary follicles.

With continuing follicle maturation, the granulosa cell layers increase in thickness and the outer capsule of ovarian stromal cells begins to differentiate into two layers.

Fig. 17.17 Ovary in embryo.
ⓐ The developing ovary (O) in a 9-week-old embryo is shown close to the developing kidney (K).
ⓑ At this stage of development the columns of primordial germ cells (G) are embedded in a mesenchymal stroma (S) surrounded by a layer of cuboidal surface cells (E).

The inner layer of stromal cells (the **theca interna**) increases in size as the cells develop prominent smooth endoplasmic reticulum and mitochondria with tubular cristae (features characteristic of cells producing steroid hormones) and begin to secrete estrogens; this layer also acquires a prominent capillary network.

The outer layer of stromal cells (the **theca externa**) remains small and compact and has no known secretory function. The follicle is now known as a **secondary follicle** (Fig. 17.19b).

The fully mature follicle is called the tertiary (Graafian) follicle and is ready for ovulation.

A small fluid-filled split appears in the layers of granulosa cells surrounding the oocyte. It enlarges to form a fluid-filled cavity (the **antrum**) which progressively increases in size; the fluid is slightly viscous and is rich in hyaluronic acid.

The oocyte lies to one side of the by now large follicle and is separated from the follicle fluid by a coat of granulosa cells called the cumulus oophorus. The follicle is

Fig. 17.18 Primordial follicles.
ⓐ Ovarian cortex from a 32-week-fetus; it is packed with primordial follicles, each comprising a large primary oocyte (O) with a single surrounding layer of flat granulosa cells (G). Most primordial follicles undergo continuing atresia throughout infancy, childhood and the years of sexual maturity.

ⓑ Ovarian cortex from a 25-year-old woman showing persistence of some primordial follicles (F).

Fig. 17.19 Follicle maturation.
ⓐ Micrograph of a multilaminar primary follicle. The granulosa cells (G) have divided to produce a layer 3–5 cells thick, and the pink-staining zona pellucida (ZP) becomes apparent between the oocyte (O) and the granulosa cells.
ⓑ Further maturation to a secondary follicle occurs by

continuing proliferation of the granulosa cells (G), the appearance of a fluid-filled cavity (C) within them, and condensation of stromal cells around the follicle to form an inner layer of plump cells (theca interna, TI), and an outer layer of smaller spindle-shaped cells, (theca externa, TE).

now known as a **tertiary** or **Graafian follicle** and is ripe for ovulation (Fig. 17.20a, b).

The first stage of meiosis is then completed to produce a haploid gamete and a small polar body which can sometimes be seen attached to the oocyte (now called a **secondary oocyte**). Follicle maturation takes approximately 15 days, by which time the mature follicle is ready for ovulation.

The theca interna secretes increasing amounts of estrogen to stimulate proliferation of the endometrium (see Fig. 17.24) in preparation for possible implantation of a fertilized ovum.

Ovulation is stimulated by luteinizing hormone from the anterior pituitary.

At ovulation, the Graafian follicle is usually so large that it distorts the surface of the ovary; it appears to the naked eye as a small cystic mass bulging from the ovarian surface, covered only by a thin layer of germinal epithelium and membrane, and an attenuated zone of cortical stromal cells.

The stimulus to ovulation is probably a surge of luteinizing hormone (LH) from the pituitary, which induces completion of the first stage of meiosis, and probably leads to disruption of the structure of the follicle as well.

Before leaving the ovary, the oocyte may break free from its attachment in the follicle wall and float freely in the follicle fluid, surrounded by an irregular ring of granulosa cells which remain attached to it (the **corona radiata**).

The area of follicle wall in intimate contact with the germinal epithelial covering of the ovarian surface breaks down and the follicular fluid containing the oocyte is disgorged into the peritoneal cavity.

The oocyte with its surrounding corona radiata is then drawn into the infundibular opening of the uterine tube, possibly by the waving action of the fimbriae at the infundibular margin.

With rupture of the follicle, there is bleeding from the decompressed lining (particularly from the highly vascular theca interna), filling the follicle antrum with blood clot. Small quantities of blood may pass into the peritoneal cavity.

The disgorgement of blood and follicular fluid onto the pain-sensitive peritoneal surface is thought to be responsible for the transient mid-cycle (day 14–16) lower abdominal pain experienced by some women.

Fig. 17.20 Tertiary (Graafian) follicle.

(a) A mature tertiary follicle. Note the fluid-filled antrum (A), the eccentrically located oocyte (O) and the cumulus oophorus (C) of granulosa cells around the oocyte.

(b) Micrograph of the oocyte (O), cumulus oophorus (C) and granulosa cell layer (G) at higher magnification. The theca layer (T) is highly vascular.

The ruptured follicle becomes a corpus luteum after ovulation.

After ovulation the remains of the follicle change under the influence of continuing LH secretion by the pituitary gland. The clot-filled lumen of the follicle (corpus hemorrhagicum) undergoes progressive organization and fibrosis over the following weeks.

The main changes occur in the granulosa and theca interna cells. In these cells, LH induces changes (luteinization) which convert the follicle remnants into an endocrine structure known as the corpus luteum.

Thus the granulosa cells enlarge, acquire a substantial network of smooth endoplasmic reticulum, become distended with lipid (granulosa lutein cells), and secrete progesterone (Fig. 17.21).

Some of the theca interna cells, already well equipped with smooth endoplasmic reticulum, also accumulate lipid and persist as theca lutein or paralutein cells, continuing to secrete estrogens as they did before ovulation. However, many theca interna and externa cells involute, becoming small, compact and spindle-shaped.

The formed corpus luteum therefore has a central area of fibrosing blood clot surrounded by a broad zone of yellow, lipid-rich granulosa lutein cells, with scantier collections of smaller theca lutein cells scattered around the periphery.

Fibrous septa partly separate the granulosa lutein masses, and clusters of theca lutein cells are particularly prominent in the regions of these septa (Fig. 17.21b).

At its maximum size (usually on about day 20 of the menstrual cycle), a corpus luteum is commonly an ovoid structure up to 2 cm long and 1.5 cm wide; it then begins to involute, unless the cycle has been interrupted by fertilization of the oocyte in the uterine tube (see page 349).

The corpus luteum changes into a corpus albicans.

Normally, involution of the corpus luteum begins by a decrease in the size of the granulosa and theca lutein cells, with the appearance of vacuoles in their previously uniformly eosinophilic cytoplasm. Progression of this change leads to reduced secretion of progesterone and estrogen by the two cell types.

At the same time the spindle-shaped cells of the theca externa and the spindle-shaped fibroblasts forming the fibrous septa rapidly produce collagen, which replaces the involuting lutein cells.

By about the 26th day of the cycle the hormone-secreting cells are completely eliminated, and the progesterone and estrogen levels fall dramatically with a significant impact on the endometrium (see Fig. 17.24g).

The end-result of corpus luteum involution is a small ovoid mass of relatively acellular (hyaline) collagenous

Fig. 17.21 Corpus luteum.

ⓐ Micrograph of an ovary containing two corpora lutea (CL), two follicles having ripened to maturity in the same ovary in the same menstrual cycle, providing the potential for non-identical twins. Each corpus luteum shows central blood clot (BC) surrounded by a thick layer of lipid-rich granulosa lutein cells (GL).

ⓑ Micrograph of the large pale-staining granulosa lutein (GL) cells and the small compact theca lutein (TL) cells, which are mainly concentrated along fibrous septa at the periphery of the corpus luteum.

tissue with the general physical configuration of the corpus luteum. This structure is a corpus albicans (Fig. 17.22) and remains in the ovary, decreasing in size with the passing years, but never disappearing.

Most female gametes do not grow to maturity, but undergo atresia.

Of the vast number of oogonia formed in utero by mitotic division of primitive germ cells, only about 500–600 reach full maturity and ovulation during a woman's reproductive life. Some fail to develop, while others undergo a process called **atresia**.

Atresia can occur at any stage, but is most marked during intrauterine life when primary oocyte numbers are enormously reduced. As atresia continues throughout infancy, childhood, and the reproductive years, degenerating primary and secondary oocytes can be seen on histologic examination of any ovary.

Atresia can supervene at any stage of follicle development. When the follicles are small (primary and secondary stages), the components of the follicle undergo cellular degeneration and complete resorption, leaving no scar (Fig. 17.23a). However larger follicles (tertiary

stage) with a substantial cellular component undergo gradual disintegration and replacement by hyaline fibrous tissue. The oocyte disintegrates and the granulosa cells separate and degenerate, while the zona pellucida collapses and wrinkles but remains identifiable.

Often a glassy membrane develops between the degenerating granulosa cells and the outer thecal layers; this may proliferate transiently, perhaps providing the source of the fibrocollagenous fibrous tissue which ultimately replaces the atretic follicle.

When a large follicle has undergone atresia, a substantial collagenous scar may form, a **corpus fibrosum**, which resembles a small corpus albicans in shape.

Fig. 17.23 Follicle atresia.
(a) Micrograph showing a cluster of four primordial follicles, of which three are undergoing atresia (A); they will leave no scar.
(b) Micrograph showing a primary follicle undergoing atresia which is mainly manifest by a degenerate oocyte (O) and a collapsing zona pellucida (ZP).

Fig. 17.22 Corpus albicans.
The corpus luteum involutes to form a shrunken mass of collagenous tissue, the corpus albicans (CA), which approximately maintains the shape of the original corpus luteum. Incomplete involution of a corpus luteum may produce a luteal cyst, which is a cyst lined by attenuated granulosa and theca lutein cells.

OVARIAN CORTEX

- cortex is composed of stromal cells in which are embedded female gametes

- stromal cells: small compact spindle cells, potentially capable of secreting estrogens

- female gametes in cortex: primordial follicles ➜ primary and secondary follicles ➜ tertiary (Graafian follicles); ripening follicles secrete estrogens

- ovulation: bursting of a mature Graafian follicle with release of oocyte

- after ovulation, ruptured follicle becomes a corpus luteum which secretes progesterone until it involutes at end of menstrual cycle

- most female gametes undergo atresia

- ovarian cycle under control of FSH and LH from anterior pituitary

MENSTRUAL CYCLE

INTRODUCTION

During the reproductive years, the histologic appearance of the superficial functional zone of the endometrial lining varies from day to day on a regular cyclical basis, the **menstrual cycle**.

A complete cycle normally takes about 28 days, but there is considerable variation between women, and also some variation in individual women at different times. For example, the first few cycles after the menarche and after a pregnancy tend to be irregular, and increasing irregularity of the cycle is common prior to the menopause.

At the end of every cycle the superficial functional endometrium undergoes necrosis and is shed via the cervix and vagina with bleeding (**menstruation**), leaving only the basal endometrium to act as a reservoir for the development of a new functional layer during the next cycle.

Menstruation lasts for about 4 days and the day it starts is taken as the first day of the menstrual cycle.

The cyclical changes in the functional endometrium are governed by the changing pattern of hormone secretion by the ovaries, which in turn is influenced by the cyclical secretion of hormones (FSH and LH) by the pituitary gland. The secretion of the gonadotropic hormones is in turn controlled by the secretion of gonadotropin-releasing hormones by the hypothalamus. Thus the histologic appearance of endometrial curettings can be used to stage (within a few days on either side) the endometrial cycle.

The sequence of changes in the menstrual cycle, is repeated throughout the period of sexual maturity, from the menarche to the menopause, and is interrupted only by pregnancy or hormone therapy, for example estrogen and progesterone given as a contraceptive.

The proliferative (estrin or follicular) phase of the menstrual cycle lasts from day 4 to about day 15 or 16.

During menstruation the entire superficial functional zone of endometrium is shed (days 1–4), leaving the compact basal endometrium behind.

At the same time, a new cycle of ovarian follicle maturation begins, the resulting increasing estrogen secretion by the developing follicle stimulating mitotic activity in the basal endometrial glands and stroma (Fig. 17.24a, b). Continued proliferation of these cells over 10–12 days re-establishes a substantial functional endometrial layer comprising straight tubular endometrial glands embedded in stroma.

As the levels of estrogen continue to rise in the latter stages of this phase the glands usually become slightly tortuous and their lumina may distend, while continued mitotic proliferation of endometrial gland columnar cells may produce some heaping up of cells, and therefore a pseudostratified appearance.

Ovulation occurs at about day 14–16.

Ovulation is accompanied by the development of subnuclear vacuolation in the endometrial glands (Fig. 17.24c), which coincides with peak levels of LH secretion by the pituitary gland. Eventually all of the glands show this change.

The secretory (luteal) phase lasts from about day 16 to day 25 or so.

The onset of the next (secretory or luteal) phase in the menstrual cycle is marked by the appearance of supranuclear secretory vacuoles at the apical poles of the endometrial gland cells. Secretory material is shed into the gland lumen by the apocrine method (see Fig. 3.24) and the luminal surfaces of the gland cells become irregular and ill-defined. The glands themselves become tortuous (Fig. 17.24d) and their lumina distend with secretion (Fig. 17.24e).

This phase of gland secretion occurs in response to progesterone secreted by the corpus luteum.

The premenstrual phase lasts from about day 25 to menstruation at day 28.

At about day 22 the secretory activity of the endometrial glands declines and they begin to show involutional changes; the luminal secretion diminishes and that which remains becomes inspissated. The glands become irregular and begin to collapse and there are significant changes in the stroma, including prominent spiral arterioles (Figs. 17.24 f, g) and swelling of the stromal cells, particularly around the arterioles.

These changes are precipitated by the sudden fall in progesterone and estrogen secretion due to involution of the corpus luteum.

At menstruation, the superficial functional layer of the endometrium undergoes necrosis and is shed.

Increased coiling of the spiral arterioles decreases blood flow and further constriction of the arterioles leads to significant ischemia of the functional endometrium. Subsequent dilatation of deeper vessels, combined with necrosis of the walls of the more superficial vessels, then leads to hemorrhage into the stroma.

The necrotic endometrial glands and stroma, together with the stromal accumulations of blood, are then shed as menstrual debris, usually piecemeal, with the most superficial endometrium shed first; the deeper layers are lost over the next 4–5 days until only basal endometrium remains. During this time the endometrium begins to regenerate, with re-epithelialization of the naked surface of remaining basal endometrium. This healing process is not hormone-dependent.

hypothalamus

pituitary

FSH stimulates maturation of one or more follicles

continuing FSH stimulation of ripening Graafian follicle

surge of LH initiates ovulation

continuing LH secretion induces luteinization of granulosa and theca cells of ruptured follicle

LH and FSH secretion ceases, corpus luteum begins to involute

changes in spiral arterioles in stroma produce ischemic necrosis of functional endometrium which is shed (menstruation)

estrogen secretion from follicle granulosa cells initiates proliferation of endometrium

endometrial proliferation maintained by increasing estrogen secretion from enlarging follicle

early progesterone secretion by luteinizing follicle stimulates early secretory changes in endometrium

continued progesterone secretion from granuloma lutein cells maintains secretory change in endometrium; some estrogen from theca lutein cells

involuting granulosa and theca lutein cells suddenly cease to produce progesterone and estrogen; secretory endometrial glands degenerate

Day 1–4   Day 5–14   Day 14–16   Day 16–28

Fig. 17.24 Menstrual cycle.

The combination of artwork, photomicrographs and flow diagram on page 346 shows the interrelationships between pituitary hormones and ovary, and ovarian hormones and the endometrium in the menstrual cycle.

The cycle starts at the first day of menstruation when the functional endometrium from the previous cycle is shed, with bleeding (days 1–4).

Release of pituitary follicle stimulating hormone (FSH) stimulates the maturation of an ovarian follicle, some of the cells of which secrete estrogen which initiates and maintains the proliferation of new functional endometrium.

ⓐ A new layer of functional endometrium (F) in the early proliferative stage arising from the compact basal endometrium (B).

ⓑ High-power detail of one of the proliferating endometrial glands. Nuclei are prominent and some cells are in mitosis (arrow).

The proliferative stage lasts from day 4 to 14, at which time a surge of pituitary luteinizing hormone (LH) initiates ovulation (days 15–16), and luteinization of the wall of the ovarian follicle. The luteinized cells of the follicle begin to secrete progesterone which inititiates early secretory changes in the endometrium.

ⓒ The earliest changes of secretory activity in the endometrial glands. They develop subnuclear vacuoles (V) and the previously straight tubular glands begin to become convoluted.

Continuing secretion of progesterone by the corpus luteum produces further convolution of the endometrial glands, increase in bulk of the stroma and increasing secretory activity of the gland epithelium.

ⓓ A low-power photomicrograph of the endometrium at about day 22 of the cycle. The glands (G) are markedly convoluted and distended by secretion.

ⓔ High-power detail of a late secretory endometrium with secretory vacuoles (V) now in a supranuclear position and secretion (S) in the lumen of the convoluted gland.

At about day 25 of the cycle, the secretion of LH and FSH by the pituitary ceases, causing involution of the corpus luteum in the ovary with consequent abrupt reduction in progesterone and estrogen secretion. This reduction in hormones leads to ischemic necrosis of the late secretory endometrium initiating menstruation. Just before undergoing necrosis, the endometrium is very bulky with early decidual change in the stroma and prominent spiral arterioles.

ⓕ Part of the premenstrual endometrium at low magnification. Note the highly convoluted glands and the very bulky decidualized endometrial stroma (DC), particularly near the surface.

ⓖ A high-power photomicrograph showing the thick-walled and contorted spiral arterioles (SA).

ENDOMETRIAL CHANGES IN NORMAL (28-DAY) MENSTRUAL CYCLE

- Days 1–4: menstrual phase: necrotic endometrium from previous cycle shed

- Days 4–14: proliferative phase: new straight tubular endometrial glands and stroma grow from residual basal endometrium. Much mitotic activity

- Days 14–16: ovulatory phase: earliest sign of secretory activity in endometrial glands in subnuclear vacuolation

- Days 16–25: secretory phase: endometrial glands become tortuous and lumina fill with secretion

- Days 25–28: premenstrual phase: spiral arterioles prominent in stroma; ischemia leads to degeneration, then necrosis, of secretory endometrium

MENSTRUAL IRREGULARITIES

Irregularity and abnormality of menstruation is a common and important complaint in women of reproductive age. There is a normal tendency for menstrual periods to be irregular in interval, duration and intensity at three times in a woman's life: for the first few cycles after puberty, for the first one or two cycles after pregnancy and for a variable number of cycles before the menopause. The following clinical features imply some form of pathology.

Amenorrhoea (absence of menstruation). A complete absence of menstruation in the woman from puberty is termed primary amenorrhoea and the cause is usually an endocrine abnormality. Amenorrhoea where there has previously been normal menstruation is termed secondary amenorrhoea.

Menorrhagia describes excessive bleeding at menstruation, both in intensity and duration of blood loss. There is often an underlying endometrial or myometrial abnormality.

Dysmenorrhoea is excessively painful menstruation often caused by an endometrial or myometrial disorder.

Intermenstrual bleeding is usually caused by an abnormality in the cervix, vagina or vulva.

Postmenopausal bleeding is a most important symptom as it is the way in which most malignant diseases of the uterus present.

ENDOMETRIAL DISORDERS

There are many abnormalities which can occur in endometrium, most resulting from inappropriate ovarian hormone stimulation and causing abnormal patterns of menstruation.

Since the endometrium is largely shed once a month, many abnormalities are transient, but persisting endometrial abnormalities are important.

Benign cystic hyperplasia (Fig.17.25a) of the endometrium is the result of unopposed estrogen secretion and may occur in the presence of an estrogen-secreting ovarian tumor.

Atypical endometrial hyperplasia is marked by hyperplastic endometrial glands, which show disorganization of architectural arrangement, while the epithelial cells show atypical dysplastic features similar to those seen in malignant tumors of endometrial glands. This condition (Fig. 17.25b) is considered capable of conversion into an invasive endometrial tumor.

The typical malignant tumor of the endometrium, the **endometrial adenocarcinoma** (Fig. 17.25c), occurs mainly in post-menopausal women and presents as post-menopausal bleeding.

(c)

Fig. 17.25 Important endometrial growth disorders.
ⓐ Simple cystic hyperplasia of the endometrial glands. Note the cystically dilated glands.
ⓑ Atypical complex hyperplasia. Note the crowded irregular glands composed of tall epithelial cells in which some dysplastic features will be present.
ⓒ Invasive endometrial adenocarcinoma (C) fills the endometrial cavity and is invading into the myometrium (M) and part of the way down the endocervical cavity (EC). Note that near the fundus (arrow), the white malignant tumor has almost infiltrated through the myometrium to the serosal surface of the uterus.

(a)

(b)

PREGNANCY

INTRODUCTION

The cyclical changes in the ovary and endometrium described above are seen either when fertilization of the ovum does not occur or if fertilization is followed by death of the zygote or failure of implantation into the endometrium.

In the event of successful fertilization and implantation, the cyclical changes are suspended until some time after childbirth, and almost all of the tissues of the female genital tract undergo structural changes.

The structural changes in the cervix, myometrium and uterine tube have been described on pages 331, 335 & 337.

Fertilization of the ovum usually occurs in the uterine tube (oviduct).

When the ovum is disgorged from the ovary at ovulation it enters the open infundibular end of the uterine tube and passes into the dilated ampullary portion, which is the most common site for its fertilization.

The second meiotic division of the ovum is only completed once the ovum has been successfully penetrated by a spermatozoon. The nuclear material of the penetrating haploid spermatozoon then joins with that of the haploid ovum, forming a diploid zygote, which immediately begins a series of mitotic divisions to produce a solid ball of cells, the **morula**.

The morula migrates down the uterine tube and arrives in the endometrial cavity about 4–5 days after fertilization.

Further divisions rapidly produce a cystic mass called the **blastocyst**, comprising a fluid-filled cavity (the **blastocoele**) surrounded by a cellular wall (the **trophoblast**). A solid collection of cells, internal to the trophoblast at one pole of the blastocyst, is called the **inner cell mass** and gives rise to the embryo.

After a day or so floating free in the endometrial cavity, the blastocyst must implant in the secretory endometrium if the pregnancy is to continue.

Attempts at implantation begin about 6 days after fertilization.

Fertilization is usually 7–8 days after ovulation, and on day 21–22 of the menstrual cycle. If unsuccessful, the blastocyst degenerates and is expelled with the degenerate

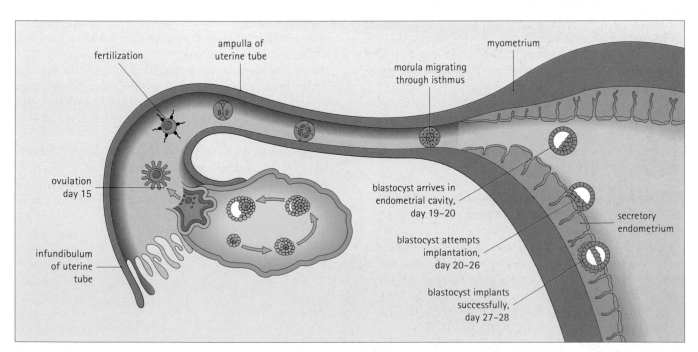

Fig. 17.26 Fertilization and implantation.
Diagram illustrating the main features of fertilization and implantation.

endometrium and blood with the onset of menstruation at 28 days.

Sometimes implantation occurs, but cannot be maintained; menstruation eventually supervenes, often after some delay, and the menstrual loss may be greater than usual.

When implantation is successful, the blastocyst gains access to the endometrial stroma, probably directly across the endometrial surface, and by about 11 days after fertilization (i.e. day 27 of the cycle) is completely embedded in endometrial stroma.

After implantation, the pregnancy is initially maintained by progesterone secreted by the persisting corpus luteum.

From about the time of ovulation, the corpus luteum secretes progesterone. If fertilization and implantation occur it does not regress, but increases in size up to 3–4 cm in diameter (the **corpus luteum of pregnancy**). This persists throughout the first trimester of pregnancy and is a constant source of progesterone, which is necessary to sustain the pregnancy; thereafter the placenta takes over this function and the corpus luteum of pregnancy involutes.

At the time of implantation, the endometrium is in its late secretory phase (see Fig. 17.24e), being characterized by bulky tortuous secretory glands and a stroma which may be demonstrating early decidual change (see Fig. 17.24f).

Implantation stimulates the development of true decidual change under the influence of the continuing progesterone secretion from the **corpus luteum of pregnancy**.

Because of the progesterone secretion, the endometrial glands develop exaggerated secretory appearances, which, taken in conjunction with the stromal decidual change, produce the appearance known as **pregnancy pattern endometrium**.

Further development of the trophoblast and some of the decidual endometrial stroma produce the placenta.

The placenta is responsible for continued nourishment of the developing embryo and also for continued secretion of hormones necessary for maintaining the pregnancy.

Further development of the embryo from the inner cell mass is beyond the scope of this book.

TROPHOBLAST

INTRODUCTION

On implantation the single layer of trophoblast, which forms the outer wall of the blastocyst, becomes a double layer.

The outer layer is characterized by the loss of its lateral cell margins so that it forms a thin syncytial layer, the **syncytiotrophoblast**. The inner layer begins as a continuous monolayer of cuboidal cells with pale staining cytoplasm, the **cytotrophoblast**.

The syncytiotrophoblast has numerous surface microvilli and the ability to erode or invade adjacent tissue.

This ability of the syncytiotrophoblast ensures successful erosion of the endometrial tissues and vessels at implantation. The blastocyst initially attaches to the surface epithelium of the endometrium by adhesion. Individual trophoblast cells then intrude between the epithelial cells so that the blastocyst can insinuate itself through the epithelium and into the endometrial stroma, where erosion of an endometrial capillary ensures it an adequate blood supply (Fig. 17.27a).

The breach in the endometrial surface is covered by a small blood clot and the surface is quickly re-epithelialized.

The presence of the blastocyst within the endometrial stroma induces early decidualization of the stromal cells, which rapidly involves all of the endometrium and leads to marked thickening.

Once the blastocyst is embedded in the endometrial stroma, the trophoblast rapidly proliferates and the outer syncytial layer extends as irregular protrusions into the surrounding stroma, eroding the walls of small blood vessels as it goes.

Lakes of maternal blood form between the protrusions (Fig. 17.27b) and the surface microvilli of the syncytiotrophoblast probably assist in transferring oxygen and nutrients from the maternal blood to the developing blastocyst.

Fig. 17.27 Implantation site.
(a) Low-power micrograph showing an early human implantation site. The blastocyst has infiltrated the superficial endometrium and the trophoblast (T) is beginning to infiltrate the endometrial stroma. Part of the inner cell mass (M) can be seen.
(b) High-power micrograph from the area of trophoblast infiltration. Cords of syncytiotrophoblast (S) have eroded blood vessels and produced lakes of maternal blood (L). Islands of cytotrophoblast (C) are extending into the syncytial masses.

The cytotrophoblast grows into the syncytial protrusions as finger-like extensions.

The solid masses of cytotrophoblast covered by syncytium form the **primary** or **stem chorionic villi**.

With the development of a loose mesenchymal core, the origin of which is uncertain, the villi are known as **secondary villi**, and soon acquire a system of capillaries which become part of the blood circulatory system of the embryo.

Fully vascularized villi are referred to as **tertiary villi** (see Fig. 17.29).

As the villi mature, the mesenchymal core contains interlacing vascular channels, fibroblasts, some smooth muscle cells and large pleomorphic cells with vacuolated cytoplasm (**Hofbauer cells**). These cells have some of the ultrastruc-

tural and immunocytochemical features of macrophages, and are believed to be motile macrophages with a particular facility for protein ingestion and pinocytosis.

The early chorionic villi subdivide in an arborizing pattern to form a complex system which provides an immense surface area for exchange between the maternal and fetal circulations.

After the complex branching of the villi, the terminal villi contain small, thin-walled capillaries, all of which connect with larger vessels in the larger 'twigs', 'branches' and 'trunks' of the tree-like proliferation; these vessels ultimately combine to form the two arteries and single vein that run in the umbilicus to the blood circulation of the embryo (Fig. 17.28).

Fig. 17.28 Placental structure.
This diagram illustrates the basic structure of the placenta and the relationship between the fetal and maternal blood.

The appearances of the chorionic villi change with time.

In early pregnancy the villi contain central capillaries embedded in bulky mesenchyme, but later the capillaries proliferate and come to lie close to the trophoblast surface. As the capillaries become more numerous and dilated, the mesenchyme is reduced in bulk, and its cellular component is reduced; in particular, Hofbauer cells become scarce.

Initially the cytotrophoblast cells predominate and the syncytiotrophoblast is a thin layer (Fig. 17.29a). Division of cytotrophoblast probably maintains the syncytial cell mass throughout gestation. As the pregnancy progresses, the syncytiotrophoblast becomes the predominant layer and the cytotrophoblast appears to partly regress, becoming a discontinuous layer, then collections of scattered cells beneath the syncytiotrophoblast.

At term (Fig. 17.29b), the villi show increasing hyalinization of the mesenchymal stroma, and fibrin is deposited in the blood-filled intervillous spaces, often coating the outer surface of the villi.

The arrangement of complex chorionic villi of fetal origin intruding into a constantly blood-filled intervillous space of maternal origin provides an efficient means of transferring oxygen, nutrients, maternal antibodies and hormones from the mother to the fetus, and waste metabolites from the fetus to the mother (see Fig. 17.28).

Endocrine functions of the placenta

In addition to being a site of exchange, the placenta also acts as an endocrine organ.

- The syncytiotrophoblast secretes human chorionic gonadotropin (HCG) (Fig. 17.30), which is responsible for maintaining the corpus luteum of pregnancy (see page 350) after cessation of the LH stimulus from the pituitary gland.

- The syncytiotrophoblast secretes human chorionic somatomammotropin (HCS), which is believed to stimulate lactogenesis.

- The placenta secretes progesterone and estrogens; estrogen precursors produced by the adrenal cortex and liver of the fetus are converted into active estrogens in the placenta.

Fig. 17.30 Chorionic villi and HCG.
Micrograph showing a chorionic villus from a term placenta demonstrating localization of human chorionic gonadotropin (HCG), stained brown, to the syncytiotrophoblast (S).

Fig. 17.29 Chorionic villi.
(a) Micrograph showing part of an early chorionic villus, which is covered by a layer of cuboidal cytotrophoblast (C) and an outer layer of syncytiotrophoblast (S). Note the villus capillaries (VC) filled with nucleated fetal red cells (FRC).
(b) Micrograph of chorionic villi close to end of pregnancy; note the prominent heaped up syncytiotrophoblast (S), maternal blood in the intervillous space (IVS), and fetal blood in the villous capillaries (VC).

DECIDUA

After implantation, the endometrial stroma undergoes decidualization.

The normally small compact cells of the endometrial stroma undergo remarkable enlargement; this process is known as **decidualization**.

Decidualization begins in the stromal cells around the implanted blastocyst, but soon spreads to involve the rest of the pregnancy endometrium. As the stromal cells enlarge they dominate the endometrium and the glandular component becomes insignificant. The thickened superficial endometrial layers become the decidua as follows (Fig. 17.31):

- the endometrium immediately beneath the implantation site, into which the major trophoblast growth occurs, becomes the **decidua basalis**;
- the thin rim of endometrial stroma overlying the blastocyst becomes the **decidua capsularis**;
- the endometrium lining the rest of the uterine cavity is called the **decidua parietalis**;

Of the decidua, the decidua basalis is the most important since the vessels in this part of the modified endometrium supply maternal arterial blood to the lacunae between the fetal chorionic villi and receive venous blood from the lacunae. The villous trophoblast (from the fetus) and the decidua basalis (from the mother), and the intervillous spaces between them, comprise the placenta.

Decidual stromal cells have prominent pale-staining round or ovoid nuclei, often with finely granular chromatin and one or two nucleoli; their cytoplasm is bulky, and usually eosinophilic, and granular or slightly foamy, although some cells may have a basophilic tinge (Fig. 17.31c).

Ultrastructurally the decidualized stromal cells contain prominent, often long mitochondria, together with variable amounts of rough endoplasmic reticulum.

The eosinophilia or basophilia of the cytoplasm in individual cells depends on the relative proportions of mitochondria (eosinophilic) and rough endoplasmic reticulum (basophilic).

Fig. 17.31 Decidua.
ⓐ Diagram showing the decidua and their relationships with the developing fetus and placenta.
ⓑ Photograph showing the decidua defined in **a** . Note the decidua parietalis (DP), decidua capsularis (DC) and decidua basalis (DB).
ⓒ Micrograph of decidual cells. They are large polygonal cells with pale-staining nuclei and granular eosinophilic cytoplasm

1. THE TRANSFORMATION ZONE OF THE CERVIX

(a) is the site where endometrium changes to endocervix at the internal os

(b) is the result of vaginal acid acting on the lower endocervical epithelium

(c) is an important site for the development of cervical cancer

(d) results in Nabothian follicles

(e) develops shortly after birth

2. THE SEXUALLY MATURE ENDOMETRIUM

(a) is the site of implantation of the fertilized ovary

(b) is shed every month at the time of ovulation

(c) is regenerated every month from its basal portion

(d) undergoes atrophy after the menopause

(e) fails to respond to estrogens and progesterone after the menopause

3. A CORPUS LUTEUM IN THE OVARY

(a) develops from a ruptured tertiary Graafian follicle

(b) secretes progesterone but not estrogens

(c) undergoes involution at the end of each menstrual cycle

(d) converts into a corpus fibrosum after involution

(e) persists as a progesterone secreting source in the first three months of pregnancy

4. IN THE OVARY

(a) the cortex consists of a spindle-cell stroma which surrounds the gamete-producing structures

(b) most primordial follicles undergo atresia

(c) a primary follicle is composed of an oocyte surrounded by granulosa cells and Sertoli cells

(d) a tertiary follicle is also called a Graafian follicle

(e) the thecal cells which surround the secondary follicle are derived from stromal cells

18. Skin and Breast

The skin is an extensive organ covering the exterior of the body. It varies in structure from site to site according to specific functions, which include:
- protection from external damaging agents;
- thermoregulation;
- sensation (touch, heat, pressure, pain);
- secretion of protective lipids, milk, etc.

The breast is a highly modified area of skin with specialized sweat glands to produce nutritious secretions under hormonal influences.

The skin is composed of two main layers, the epidermis and dermis, and a variable third layer, the subcutis.

The **epidermis** is the surface epithelial layer in contact with the external environment. Downgrowths of this layer produce sweat glands, hair follicles and other epidermal appendages.

The **dermis** is a middle supporting layer containing the epidermal appendages, blood vessels, nerves and nerve endings, which are embedded in an elastocollagenous stroma produced by fibroblasts

The **subcutis** is the deepest layer, and varies in size and content, but is usually composed mainly of adipose tissue (Fig. 18.1).

Fig. 18.1 Architecture of the skin.
The most superficial layer of the skin is the epidermis. This varies in thickness from site to site and is covered by acellular keratin, which is thick in thick skin and thin in thin skin.

Beneath the epidermis is the dermis which has two components: a more superficial loose papillary dermis and a denser reticular dermis, which comprises the bulk of the layer. The dermis is mainly composed of collagen with some elastic fibers.

The deepest layer of the skin, the subcutis, has a variable structure; when prominent it is composed largely of adipose tissue intersected by fibrocollagenous septa.

The subcutis contains the main subcutaneous network of arteries and veins from which vessels extend upwards and form a network (the cutaneous plexus) at the dermo-subcutaneous junction. From here, smaller vessels penetrate the dermis, giving branches to the skin appendages and culminating in a superficial network of small venules and arterioles (the subpapillary plexus). Capillary loops from this plexus extend upward into the dermal papillae to lie close to the dermo-epidermal junction.

Blood vessels do not penetrate the epidermis.

EPIDERMIS

The epidermis is the protective skin layer in contact with the external environment.

A stratified epithelium (see page 34), the surface layer of the epidermis is composed of closely packed flat plates of protein (**keratin**) which form a tough, water-repellent layer (**stratum corneum**).

Keratin is produced by the main cell type in epidermis, the keratinocyte. Note that, contrary to traditional teaching, the stratum corneum is not cellular, but composed entirely of intracytoplasmic keratin remnants bound to the skin surface after the death of the keratinocytes that produced them (Fig. 3.27). Each keratin plate conforms roughly to the shape of the keratinocyte shortly before its death.

Although normally thin, the stratum corneum is very thick in skin exposed to constant trauma, such as that on the soles and palms.

Epidermis is traditionally regarded as a stratified squamous epithelium, but in fact only the most superficial two or three living cell layers of the epidermis approach a squamous or flat configuration, most keratinocytes being cuboidal or polyhedral.

The surface plates of keratin, and the flat dying keratinocytes which precede them, are known as squames, and result from the maturation of the other layers of keratinocytes comprising the epidermis. These layers are the basal layer, the prickle cell layer and the granular layer (Fig. 18.2).

Keratinocytes are separated from the underlying support tissues of the dermis by a basement membrane.

The junction between the dermis and epidermis is an important area, tethering the two layers together (Fig. 18.3), and structured to minimize the risk of dermo-epidermal separation by shearing forces as follows;

- Tethering fibers connect the dermis and epidermis to intervening basement membrane.
- The basal cell membrane of individual basal cells, and the underlying basement membrane are convoluted (Fig. 18.6).
- There is a system of **rete ridges** (i.e. downgrowths of epidermis into dermis) which varies markedly from site to site. In protected areas, where the skin is not normally subjected to shearing stress (e.g. the trunk), rete ridges are barely evident and the dermo-epidermal

junction appears flat, but in areas constantly exposed to shearing stress (e.g. tips of fingers, palms and soles), the rete ridge system is highly developed (Figs. 18.1 and 18.19–18.23).

The basement membrane at the dermo-epidermal junction can be seen to consist of three main layers, specifically:

- an electron-lucent lamina lucida on the epidermal side;
- an electron-dense lamina densa in the middle;
- an ill-defined fibroreticular lamina, which contains abundant fibronectin, on the dermal side.

Fig. 18.2 Epidermis.
The three cell layers of the epidermis are most clearly seen in thick skin, as shown here; the basal layer (B) sits on the basement membrane, and is covered by the prickle cell layer (P) and then the granular layer (G) which is characterized by its content of dark-staining keratohyaline granules. In thick skin, there is a thick layer of dense acellular keratin (K).

Two non-keratinocyte cells of the epidermis, a melanocyte (M) and a Langerhans' cell (L) (see page 360), are also evident.

The basal cells are tethered to the lamina densa by hemidesmosomes from which anchoring proteins cross the lamina lucida. On the dermal aspect fine anchoring fibrils of type VII collagen attach the lower surface of the lamina densa to collagen fibers in the papillary dermis, while fibrillin microfibrils attach it to upper dermal elastic fibers. In addition, the zone immediately beneath the lamina densa contains abundant fibronectin (see page 54).

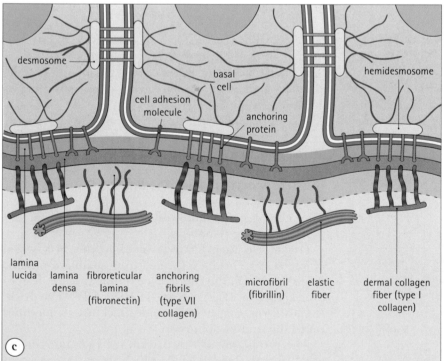

Fig. 18.3 Dermo–epidermal junction.
(a) In this paraffin section, the basement membrane (BM) at the dermo-epidermal junction is demonstrated by the PAS stain.
(b) In this electronmicrograph of dermo-epidermal junction, the basement membrane can be seen to consist of three main layers: a superficial electron-lucent lamina lucida (L) an electron-dense lamina densa (D) and an ill-defined fibroreticular lamina.

The basal cells are tethered to the lamina densa by hemidesmosomes (Hd) from which anchoring proteins (A) cross the lamina lucida. On the dermal aspect fine anchoring fibrils (F) of type VII collagen attach the lower surface of the lamina densa to collagen fibers (C) in the papillary dermis, while fibrillin microfibrils attach it to elastic fibers. In addition, the zone immediately beneath the lamina densa contains abundant fibronectin (see page 56).
(c) Diagram of dermo-epidermal junction showing the components of the basement membrane and its attachments to basal cells and dermal fibers.

BASAL BLISTERS

The dermo-epidermal junction is a site where fluid can accumulate in sufficient quantity to lift the epidermis away from the dermis, thus forming a basal blister. This can result from:

• excessive shearing force;
• structural abnormality.

Excessive shearing forces are the most common cause and are usually due to constant shearing friction, such as occurs with tight-fitting shoes.

Structural abnormalities may be primary or secondary, and the most important primary cause is the rare inherited skin disease **epidermolysis bullosa**, in which the dermo-epidermal junction is intrinsically weak and unable to resist even minimal shearing trauma. There are a number of different types of epidermolysis bullosa, depending on the site of separation, which can be ascertained by electron microscopy.

Secondary causes are more common and usually result from inflammatory skin disease that damages the basal layer and its underlying basement membrane, for example the blistering disease **pemphigoid** and **dermatitis herpetiformis** (Fig. 18.4).

Fig. 18.4 Dermatitis herpetiformis.
Micrograph showing a secondary cause of basal blistering, dermatitis herpetiformis, in which patients develop an intensely itchy blistering eruption.

In dermatitis herpetiformis the immunoglobulin IgA becomes deposited in the tips of the dermal papillae close to the basement membrane. This activates the complement cascade via the alternative pathway, and neutrophil polymorphs are attracted to the site by the release of chemotaxins. As a result the dermis (D) is damaged just below the dermo-epidermal junction, and the epidermis (E) separates, leaving a basal blister containing fluid and some remnants of neutrophil polymorphs. Note the numerous neutrophils in the small early blister shown here.

The basal layer is the deepest cell layer of the epidermis and is responsible for the constant production of keratinocytes.

The basal layer cells are cuboidal or low columnar in shape and are attached to the basement membrane, which separates it from the underlying dermis, by hemidesmosomes, and to adjacent basal cells by true desmosomes.

Fig. 18.5 Basal cells.
The basal cells (B) are smaller than the other keratinocytes and may show a regular, regimented arrangement (palisading). They have rounded or oval nuclei, and rest on the basement membrane marking the junction between epidermis and dermis (D).

Basal cells have round or oval nuclei (Fig. 18.5) with prominent nucleoli, and their cytoplasm is rich in ribosomes and mitochondria; tonofibrils are present in small numbers. In pigmented skin the cytoplasm also contains melanin granules and lysosomes.

It is in the basal layer that cells in mitosis are seen, as well as scattered non-keratinocyte cells, melanocytes and Merkel cells (see page 360).

The keratinocytes above the basal cells form the prickle cell layers.

The cells are polyhedral with central round nuclei and pinkish-staining cytoplasm.

Prickle cells are in contact with each other by a system of intercellular bridges, formed from small cytoplasmic projections from the cell surface terminating in desmosomal junctions (Fig. 18.6, see also Fig. 3.11). The prickle cells form a layer of variable thickness, sometimes called the stratum spinosum.

The cytoplasm of the prickle cells contains many tonofilaments (see Fig. 3.27), which are particularly concentrated in the cytoplasmic projections leading into the desmosomes, and are more numerous in the cell layers closest to the granular layer.

The cells of the upper prickle cell layer are flatter than the polyhedral cells of the deeper layers. The narrow interstices between the prickle cells are partly occupied by the cytoplasmic projections of melanocytes and Langerhans' cells.

The granular cell layer produces the surface keratin and non-wettable substances.

The granular keratinocytes contain small or oval hematoxyphilic round bodies (**keratohyaline granules**) composed of proteinaceous material containing abundant sulfur-rich amino acids (e.g. cysteine). They also contain abundant tonofibrils and small round lamellated **keratinosomes** or **Odland bodies**.

In the upper layer the cytoplasm of granular keratinocytes is largely composed of masses of keratohyaline material and tightly packed tonofibrils, with little cytosol or cytoplasmic organelles, and at this level the cells are flat. Death of the nucleus and cytoplasm leaves the keratohyaline and tonofibrils which combine to form the keratin (see Fig. 3.27) of the acellular surface layer, the stratum corneum (Fig. 18.7).

Keratinosomes produce a complex hydrophobic glycophospholipid which is released when the superficial granular keratinocytes die and probably acts as a glue, cementing together the flakes of keratin. This substance also renders the skin surface relatively non-wettable, although prolonged exposure will wash it away, permitting the keratin to absorb water, swell and soften. This feature is obvious in the skin of the hands after prolonged immersion in water, particularly when the water is hot and contains some form of lipid-dissolving detergent.

Surface keratin is constantly lost due to normal wear and tear from surface friction, washing and scrubbing.

Surface keratin needs to be constantly replenished from the granular layer, which in turn is constantly repopulated by cells from the prickle layer. The prickle cells are produced by proliferation of cells in the basal layer.

Turnover, from basal cell to desquamated keratin, varies from site to site, being faster (i.e. 25–30 days) in traumatized areas (e.g. soles); slow turnovers range from 40–50 days. The turnover period is considerably shortened in some skin diseases, particularly psoriasis.

NON-KERATINIZING EPIDERMAL CELLS.

In addition to keratinocytes, the epidermis also contains melanocytes, Langerhans' cells and Merkel cells.

Melanocytes produce the protective pigment, melanin.

Melanin is largely responsible for skin color, and minimizes tissue damage by ultraviolet radiation.

Melanocytes are derived from neuroectoderm and are located in the basal layer of keratinocytes in contact with

Fig. 18.7 Granular cell layer.
ⓐ Micrograph showing the granular layer (G) of the epidermis with acellular keratin (K) above it. The cytoplasm becomes progressively darker staining near the surface due to its increasing content of keratohyaline granules. The most superficial cells have lost their nuclei and are flat plates of keratohyaline and keratin (KK).
ⓑ Electronmicrograph showing part of the cytoplasm of a cell in the granular layer; it is packed with irregular masses of electron-dense keratohyaline (Kh) and round or oval keratinosomes (Ks) some of which show lamellation.

Fig. 18.6 Prickle cell layer.
A thin epoxy resin section of skin stained with toluidine blue showing the basal layer (B) and the prickle cell layer (P) above it.

Prickle cell cytoplasm stains more intensely than the basal cell cytoplasm because of its high content of tonofilaments. The characteristic intercellular bridges to which the prickle cells owe their name are easily seen and are the site of desmosomal attachments between adjacent prickle cells.

the basement membrane. They are pale-staining, with large ovoid nuclei and abundant cytoplasm from which numerous long cytoplasmic processes extend into the spaces between the keratinocytes. Melanocyte cytoplasm contains characteristic membrane-bound ovoid granules (**premelanosomes** and **melanosomes**), which have a striated electron-dense core and produce melanin (Fig. 18.8). In the production of melanin, tyrosine is converted into an intermediate pigment which polymerizes into melanin.

Melanin binds to proteins to form the active melanoprotein complex, which appears ultrastructurally as spherical masses of homogeneous electron-dense material, and often obscures the premelanosomes.

Melanoprotein complexes pass along the cytoplasmic processes of the melanocyte and are transferred into the cytoplasm of basal and prickle cell layer keratinocytes, the highest concentration being in the basal layers.

Melanocyte numbers remain more or less constant but their degree of activity is genetically variable, accounting for racial and individual variation in skin color.

Langerhans' cells are antigen recognition cells.

Langerhans' cells are located in all layers of the epidermis but are most easily seen in the prickle cell layer. They recognize antigen and are an important component of the immune system (see page 123).

Like melanocytes, Langerhans' cells have an ovoid, pale-staining nucleus surrounded by pale-staining cytoplasm from which cytoplasmic (dendritic) processes extend between the keratinocytes.

Langerhans' cell cytoplasm contains scattered characteristic Birbeck granules, which are rod-like structures with periodic cross-striations, and are most numerous near the Golgi. Sometimes one end of the rod is distended to form a spherical saccule, giving the appearance of a tennis racket (Fig. 18.9).

Although present in small numbers in healthy skin, Langerhans' cells are increased both in number, and in the extent and complexity of their dendritic processes, in many chronic inflammatory skin disorders, particularly those with an allergic or immune etiology, such as chronic atopic dermatitis.

Merkel cells are sensory receptors in the epidermis.

Merkel cells are scanty and difficult to demonstrate in normal skin. They are found in the basal layer and resemble melanocytes by routine light microscopy but electron microscopy reveals rounded membrane-bound cytoplasmic neuroendocrine-type granules.

Merkel cells form synaptic junctions with peripheral nerve endings at the base of the cell and also scanty desmosomal attachments to adjacent keratinocytes (Fig. 18.10). They occur either as scattered solitary cells or as aggregates, when they are associated with a so-called hair disk, located immediately beneath the basement membrane. Such aggregates are thought to be touch receptors and are sometimes called tactile corpuscles.

Fig. 18.8 Melanocyte.

ⓐ Micrograph showing a melanocyte (M) with its pale-staining cytoplasm. In this section of black skin it can be clearly seen against the pigment-laden basal cells.

ⓑ Ultrastructurally melanocytes contain premelanosomes (PM) and melanosomes, and their cytoplasmic processes (CP) extend between keratinocytes of the basal and lower prickle cell layers.

ⓒ High-magnification electronmicrograph showing the characteristic boat shape of premelanosomes; both coarse longitudinal and fine transverse striations can be seen.

Fig. 18.9 Langerhans' cells.

(a) In paraffin or resin sections stained with H&E, Langerhans' cells (L) are irregular, pale-staining cells in the prickle cell layer, with pale-staining oval or reniform nuclei which are often cleft. Their numerous cytoplasmic processes (CP) pass between the keratinocytes.

(b) Langerhans' cells (L) carry CD1 marker and can be clearly visualized by immunoperoxidase techniques.

(c) Ultrastructurally Langerhans' cells have an irregular cleft nucleus and are devoid of tonofilaments. They have prominent mitochondria (M) lysosomes and rough endoplasmic reticulum (RER). Birbeck granules are not seen at this magnification.

(d) High-magnification electron micrograph showing characteristic Birbeck granules, one with a distended vesicle (V) at one end.

Fig. 18.10 Merkel cells.

Merkel cells can be distinguished from melanocytes by their ultrastructural features (compare with Fig. 18.8b,c). They have a convoluted nucleus which occupies much of the cell, and no cytoplasmic processes insinuating between keratinocytes, but may have short protrusions which contact adjacent keratinocytes at occasional desmosomes (D).

Round neuroendocrine vesicles (EV) are present in the cytoplasm, particularly at the base of the cell, close to the basal nerve terminal which communicates with the underlying nerve disk (not shown here). The cytoplasm also contains a prominent Golgi, smooth endoplasmic reticulum and scattered ribosomes.

DERMATITIS (INFLAMMATION OF SKIN)

The skin is exposed to many damaging agents, such as chemicals and ultraviolet irradiation, which produce a wide variety of common rashes. A common type of dermatitis, seborrheic dermatitis, is shown in Fig. 18.11.

In addition, the skin reacts to internal abnormalities, and produces rashes in response to disorders such as viral infections (e.g. measles) and drug allergies (e.g. penicillin rash).

The cause of most skin diseases is not known.

Fig. 18.11 Seborrheic dermatitis.
The epidermis (E) is thickened, and is disrupted by an infiltration of lymphocytes (L) associated with an accumulation of water (clear areas) between keratinocytes. Note that the surface keratin layers still contain remnants of keratinocyte nuclei. This is termed **parakeratosis** (P) and is a manifestation of disordered keratinocyte maturation in areas of epidermal damage. Blood vessels (BV) in the upper dermis are dilated and surrounded by lymphocytes and macrophages. In seborrheic dermatitis the damaging agent is thought to be a fungus.

SKIN APPENDAGES

The skin appendages are the pilosebaceous apparatus, isolated sebaceous glands, eccrine sweat glands and ducts, and apocrine sweat glands and ducts.

The pilosebaceous apparatus produces hair and sebum, which is a non-wettable secretion that protects the hair and augments the non-wettable characteristics of the keratin.

The components of a pilosebaceous apparatus are hair follicle, hair shaft, sebaceous glands and erector pili.

PILOSEBACEOUS APPARATUS

Hair is derived from the epithelium of the follicle.

The **hair follicle** is a tubular epithelial structure opening onto the epidermal surface. At its lower end, a bulbous expansion (the **hair bulb**) with a concave lower surface contains a specialized area of dermis called the **hair papilla**. This is richly supplied with myelinated and non-myelinated nerve endings and abundant small blood vessels.

In the hair bulb numerous small, actively proliferating germinative cells produce the hair shaft and the internal root sheath which lie within the external root sheath.

Germinative hair bulb cells have dark basophilic cytoplasm with a scattering of melanocytes.

The internal root sheath of the hair follicle is composed of three layers:

- Henle's layer, which is a single cell layer;
- a thicker layer characterized by the presence of large eosinophilic trichohyalin granules;
- the cuticle, which consists of overlapping keratin plates.

The cuticle is continuous with the cuticle of the hair shaft (see below) in the lower regions of the hair follicle.

The internal root sheath undergoes keratinization to produce the hair shaft. It extends up from the hair bulb to about the level of the insertion of the sebaceous glands, where it disintegrates, leaving a potential space around the hair shaft into which the sebaceous gland products are secreted.

The external root sheath of the follicle is modified epidermis

Near the opening of the follicle onto the skin surface it consists of all three epidermal layers (basal, prickle cell and granular). In the deeper parts of the hair follicle, below the point of insertion of the sebaceous glands, it is composed of highly modified prickle cells, with large pale-staining cells rich in glycogen.

Outside the external root sheath is a thick basement membrane which is strongly eosinophilic and is known as the glassy membrane (Fig. 18.12).

Fig. 18.12 Pilosebaceous apparatus.

ⓐ Diagram to show the general architecture of the pilosebaceous apparatus. The hair bulb is a collection of compact epithelial cells surrounding a vascularized fibrocollagenous dermal papilla, and produces the various components of the hair shaft (i.e. medulla, cortex and cuticle). In dark-haired people, abundant active melanocytes in the basal layer of the hair bulb supply melanin to the pre-cortex cells; the medulla and cuticle are not pigmented.

The outer cells of the hair bulb epithelium produce the internal root sheath, the middle layer of which contains numerous red-staining trichohyalin granules.

The external root sheath is derived from the epidermis by downgrowth, and is bound externally by a distinct homogeneous membrane, the glassy membrane. This separates it from the fibrocollagenous follicle sheath which surrounds the entire follicle and also encloses the sebaceous glands as a thin, variably distinct layer.

Attached to the fibrocollagenous follicle sheath at, or just below, the level of the sebaceous glands is the erector pili muscle, which extends obliquely upward from this lower attachment to its upper attachment in the papillary dermis.

The lower parts of the hair shaft consist of partly keratinized cells in which the nuclei of the progenitor epithelium can still be seen, but higher up the hair is composed of anuclear hard compact keratin which does not stain with eosin.

ⓑ Transverse section through a hair follicle just below the sebaceous glands. The hair shaft (H) is anuclear and composed of non-staining hard keratin; a central medullary remnant (M) can be seen. The outer fibrocollagenous root sheath (F) and glassy membrane (G) around the external root sheath (E) are well formed, but the internal root sheath (I) is acellular and degenerate.

ⓒ Transverse section through a hair follicle just above the hair bulb. The hair shaft (H) contains nuclear remnants and is strongly eosinophilic. The cellular internal root sheath (I) is well formed and contains eosinophilic trichohyalin granules. Note the external root sheath (E) and the outer fibrocollagenous root sheath (F).

ⓓ Transverse section through a hair bulb showing melanocytes (M) supplying melanin to the pre-cortex epithelium.

ⓔ Longitudinal section through a hair bulb. There are no active melanocytes in this example.

Each hair shaft is composed of two or three layers of highly organized keratin.

Each hair can be divided into an inner medulla, an outer cortex and a superficial cuticle.

The **medulla** is a variable component and is not present in the finer vellus and lanugo hairs. When present it is composed of layers of tightly packed polyhedral cells. The **cortex** is composed of tightly packed keratin, which is produced without the incorporation of keratohyaline granules; it is 'hard' keratin and differs in composition from the soft keratin of the epidermal surface. The **cuticle** consists of a single layer of flat keratinous scales which overlap in a highly organized manner.

Hair shafts contain variable amounts of melanin depending on melanocyte activity in the germinative cells of the hair bulb.

The erector pili muscle positions the hair follicle and hair shaft.

A further component of the pilosebaceous apparatus is a narrow band of smooth muscle, the **erector pili**, which originates in the fibrocollagenous sheath surrounding the hair follicle and runs obliquely upward into the upper dermis. Its contraction makes the hair follicle and shaft more vertical so that the hair appears to stand on end.

Sebaceous glands develop as lateral outgrowths of the external root sheath

Sebaceous glands secrete a mixture of lipids called sebum. They are largely inactive until puberty, after which they enlarge and become secretory.

Sebaceous glands are composed of lobules of large polyhedral pale-staining cells containing abundant lipid droplets and small dark-staining central nuclei. There is a single layer of cuboidal or flattened precursor cells between the basement membrane of each lobule and the central mass of cells. The sebaceous gland lobules are connected to the hair follicle, usually about two-thirds to three-quarters of the way up from the hair bulb, by short ducts lined by stratified squamous epithelium, showing all the layers seen in the normal epidermis.

Sebum is a lipid mixture which includes triglycerides and various complex waxes.

Sebum is produced by large scale death of sebaceous cells, resulting in the release of their lipid content into the ducts (Fig. 18.13), and thus into the space between the formed hair shaft and the external root sheath, following degeneration of the internal root sheath. This pattern of secretion is called holocrine secretion (Fig. 3.24).

The number, size and activity of sebaceous glands varies from site to site within the skin.

Sebaceous glands are particularly abundant on the face, scalp, ears, nostrils and vulva, and around the anus, but are absent from the soles and palms.

In certain areas of the body, the sebaceous glands do not empty into hair follicles, but open directly onto the epidermal surface. This occurs in:

- the labia minora (see page 327);
- areolar skin around the nipple, where they are known as Montgomery's tubercles (see page 370);
- the eyelids, where they are known as Meibomian glands (see page 394);
- the lips and buccal mucosa (Fordyce spots).

ECCRINE SWEAT GLANDS AND DUCTS
Eccrine glands produce sweat and are controlled by the autonomic nervous system.

Sweat is a hypotonic watery solution, with a neutral or slightly acid pH, containing various ions, particularly sodium, potassium and chloride ions.

Fig. 18.13 Sebaceous gland.
ⓐ Micrograph showing a sebaceous gland (G) opening through a narrow duct (D) into the hair follicle (HF). The sebum is formed by necrosis (N) of the lipid-packed cells of the gland.
ⓑ A sebaceous gland at higher magnification showing the single layer of cuboidal or flat precursor cells (P) and the large sebaceous cells (S) distended with lipid droplets.

Eccrine sweat glands and ducts are found everywhere in the skin.

Eccrine glands are particularly numerous on the forehead, scalp, axillae, palms and soles. They arise as downgrowths of the epidermis at about the 16th week of intrauterine life.

The secretory gland component, which is situated deep in the dermis or in the upper subcutis near the dermo-subcutaneous junction, communicates with the exterior by a duct. Proximal to the gland the duct is coiled but thereafter it proceeds in a single direction up to the dermo-epidermal junction. Within the epidermis it again becomes coiled, but this is only seen to any extent where the epidermis is thick, for example in the soles of the feet (Fig. 18.20).

Eccrine sweat glands are composed of two layers of cells, an inner layer of secretory cells and an outer flat layer of contractile myoepithelial cells which is bounded by a distinct, sometimes thick membrane. The dermal ducts consists of two layers of dark-staining cuboidal cells surrounding a distinct lumen, the surface of which is often strongly eosinophilic (Fig. 18.14).

Fig. 18.14 Eccrine gland and duct.
(a) Micrograph showing eccrine glands (G) and ducts (D) in the deep dermis at low magnification.
(b) High-power micrograph showing that the glands (G) are composed of pale-staining secretory cells (S) with an outer layer of indistinct myoepithelial cells (M). The ducts (D) have a more distinct double layer of dark-staining cells.
(c) Thin epoxy resin section stained with toluidine blue showing that the gland (G) is composed of large, pale-staining glycogen-rich cells, some of which contain dark secretory granules (SG) and a smaller number of narrow darker staining cells (DC) which secrete sialomucins. Eccrine glands are surrounded by a thick amorphous membrane (M) and their ducts (D) are lined internally by a homogeneous cuticle which is composed of microvilli covered by an amorphous glycocalyx.
(d) Micrograph showing intraepidermal portion of eccrine duct, which is spiral and is sometimes called the acrosyringium. There is a single layer of cells lining the lumen, and two or three layers of outer cells. The lining cells develop small keratohyaline granules (K) and become keratinized where they emerge through the granular layer of the epidermis.

The spiral course continues through the keratin layer and is most clearly seen in skin with a thick epidermis.

APOCRINE GLANDS
Apocrine glands produce a viscid, slightly milky secretion.

External stimuli such as fear, sexual excitement, etc., cause secretion from apocrine glands, the function of which is not known in man; similar glands in mammals act as scent organs for delineation of territory and sexual attraction by producing scent.

Apocrine glands develop as downgrowths of the epidermis and are scanty in man but well developed in many other mammals. They are small and insignificant in childhood but become more prominent and probably functionally active after puberty.

In man apocrine glands are concentrated mainly in the perineal region, around the anus and genitalia, and in the axillae. Modified apocrine glands are found in the eyelids (**Moll's glands**), in the areolar skin around the nipple, and in the external auditory canal where they form the **ceruminous glands** responsible for the production of ear wax.

Apocrine glands are composed of:
- a secretory glandular unit situated, like the eccrine gland, in the lower dermis or at the dermo-subcutaneous junction;
- a more or less straight duct, which opens into a pilosebaceous unit near the surface, usually above the entrance of the sebaceous duct.

The secretory unit of an apocrine gland is composed of an inner layer of cuboidal epithelial cells and an outer layer of discontinuous flat cells, surrounded by basement membrane. It has a large lumen (Fig. 18.15). The duct resembles the eccrine duct (Fig. 18.14), having a double layer of cuboidal epithelium.

DERMIS
Dermis is the supporting tissue on which epidermis sits.

In the dermis are located the epidermal appendages, blood supply, nerve supply and lymphatic drainage. It is composed of:
- fibroblasts, fibrocytes and their extracellular products (see page 57);
- collagen and elastic fibers;
- glycosaminoglycan-containing matrix;
- blood vessels and nerves;
- small numbers of macrophages, lymphocytes and mast cells.

Two distinct zones of dermis can usually be identified: an upper narrow papillary dermis, which is close to the dermo-epidermal junction, and a thicker reticular dermis, between the papillary dermis and subcutaneous adipose tissue.

Papillary dermis is paler than reticular dermis and contains less collagen and elastin, but more matrix. The thin collagen and elastin fibers are more randomly arranged, with a high proportion perpendicular to the skin surface. It contains small blood vessels of capillary size, fine nerve twigs and nerve endings (Fig. 18.16).

Reticular dermis forms the bulk of the dermis. It is composed of prominent broad bands of dense collagen with intervening long thick fibers of elastin, which usually run parallel to the skin surface. Within this tissue are the blood vessels, lymphatics and nerves of the skin.

Fig. 18.15 Apocrine gland.
(a) Micrograph showing part of an actively secreting apocrine gland (A) from axillary skin, with part of an eccrine gland (E) for comparison. The apocrine gland has an inner layer of cuboidal epithelial cells (C) with markedly eosinophilic cytoplasm and an outer layer of discontinuous flat cells which are thought to be myoepithelial. It is surrounded by a prominent eosinophilic

basement membrane. The lumen is large, and faintly pink homogeneous secretion (S) may be seen within it.
(b) High-power view showing the roughly cuboidal eosinophilic lining cells (C) and the irregular luminal surface resulting from the secretory process, in which fragments of secretion-containing cytoplasm are 'pinched off' into the lumen. Flat myoepithelial cells (M) are present but inconspicuous.

Fig. 18.16 Dermis.

(a) Low-power view of dermis stained with H&E. It is eosinophilic because of its high content of collagen; the papillary dermis (PD), which contains less collagen, is paler. An eccrine unit (E) can be seen in the deeper part of the reticular dermis (RD). Note the concentration of small blood vessels (BV) at the junction between papillary dermis and the densely collagenous reticular dermis.

(b) High-power micrograph showing the different natures of the loose pale-staining papillary dermis (PD) and the more densely collagenous reticular dermis (RD).

(c) Elastic van Gieson-stained section of upper dermis demonstrating elastic (black) and collagen (red) fibers, showing the difference between papillary dermis (PD) in which both collagen and elastin are fine and vertically orientated, and reticular dermis (RD) in which the collagen and elastin fibers are thicker and coarser and are mainly arranged longitudinally.

The dermis contains two vascular plexuses.

The main blood supply to the skin is located within the dermis and arises from larger vessels in the subcutaneous fat. Two distinct plexuses can be identified (Fig. 18.1):

- a deep vascular plexus in the lower reticular dermis close to its border with the subcutis;
- a superficial vascular plexus in the upper reticular dermis close to its junction with the papillary dermis.

Loops of small vessels from the superficial vascular plexus run up into the papillary dermis, with small capillaries lying close to the epidermal basement membrane. No blood vessels penetrate the epidermis.

The dermis contains many arteriovenous anastomotic channels, including highly specialized shunts (**glomus bodies**), which are found mainly in the finger tips. Blood flow variation within the dermis is important to the skin's function as a thermoregulatory organ.

The skin appendages are supplied by branches from vessels connecting the deep and superficial vascular plexuses.

The dermis contains numerous nerves and nerve endings.

The nerve supply of the skin is located in the dermis and comprises:

- a rich, non-myelinated supply derived from the sympathetic autonomic nervous system which controls the skin appendages and vascular flow;
- an afferent myelinated and non-myelinated system, which detects cutaneous sensation.

Detection of cutaneous sensation is by variably specialized nerve endings (Fig. 18.17), the most important of which are:

- **free nerve endings** (myelinated and unmyelinated) which detect pain (and its minor variant, itch) and temperature;
- **Pacinian corpuscles**, encapsulated nerve endings with a characteristic structure, detect pressure and possibly vibration, and are usually found in the deep dermis or subcutaneous fat of the palms and soles;
- **Meissner's corpuscles**, structured nerve endings confined to the dermal papillae, are most numerous on the feet and hands, and detect touch;
- **Merkel cells** and their nerve attachments (see Fig. 18.10), are slowly adapting touch receptors.

SUBCUTANEOUS TISSUE

Subcutaneous tissue is composed largely of adipose tissue.

The adipose tissue in subcutaneous tissue is separated by fibrocollagenous septa and contains the main blood vessels and nerves from which the overlying dermis is supplied (Fig. 18.18). It acts as an effective heat insulator, food store, and shock absorber.

Subcutaneous tissue may contain extensions of skin structures, for example:

- in the scalp it contains the lower parts of the long hair follicles;
- some apocrine and eccrine glands.

Fig. 18.17 Common nerve endings in the skin.
(a) Skin section stained with H&E showing a Meissner's corpuscle, which is an elongated oval body. Meissner's corpuscles are arranged vertically in the dermal papillae of hairless skin, particularly in fingers and toes, but also around lips and nipples. Internally Meissner's corpuscles are composed of spirally arranged cells surrounded by a thin fibrocollagenous capsule. In H&E sections the most commonly seen cells are flattened Schwann cells (see page 83), the axons not being visible.
(b) Meissner's corpuscle stained by an immunoperoxidase method for NFP to demonstrate the spirally arranged axon (A).
(c) Micrograph showing a Pacinian corpuscle in subcutaneous fat from the fingertip demonstrated by an immunoperoxidase method for neurofilament protein NFP. It is a large, loosely laminated structure with a central core (axon, A) surrounded by concentrically arranged lamellae (L) which are modified Schwann cells separated from each other by fluid-filled spaces. The lamellae are more tightly packed peripherally and form a dense pseudocapsule (P).
(d) A Pacinian corpuscle in longitudinal section stained by an immunoperoxidase method for neurofilament protein to show its longitudinally running central axon (A).

Fig. 18.18 Subcutaneous tissue.
Micrograph of subcutaneous tissue from the scalp. It is composed largely of adipose tissue (A) intersected by vertically running bands of fibrocollagenous tissue (F) which extend down from the deep dermis. In this example, the fibrous septa extend through the full thickness of subcutaneous tissues to join the dense fibrocollagenous layer (DF) covering the periosteum of the underlying skull.

Subcutaneous tissue contains the major blood vessels (BV) from which the blood supply of the dermis arises.

FEATURES OF SKIN IN DIFFERENT SITES

The skin shows marked variation in structure at different sites.

Most of the skin covering the body is protected by clothing and is not excessively traumatized; it is not particularly specialized. Thus skin from the back, abdomen, thighs, and arms (Fig. 18.19) has:

- a thin epidermis producing only small amounts of loosely packed keratin;
- a poorly formed rete ridge system;
- small numbers of hair follicles producing fine hairs (large follicles and coarser hairs in men);
- variable numbers of eccrine glands.

SOLE

In contrast to the skin of the back, abdomen, thighs, and arms, the skin of the sole (Fig. 18.20) is modified to withstand constant trauma. It has:

- a thick epidermis which is covered by a thick layer of compact keratin;
- a well developed rete ridge system to prevent epidermal separation from shearing stress;
- no hair follicles;
- abundant eccrine glands and ducts.

SCALP

The characteristic feature of the scalp is the presence of tightly packed hair follicles with their associated sebaceous glands (Fig. 18.21). In straight haired people the follicles are almost vertical, but in curly haired people they are oblique, the degree of curliness depending on the degree of obliquity.

FINGERTIP

Fingertip skin shows two structural modifications: one to minimize damage from shearing stress, the other because of its role as a tactile sensory organ (Fig. 18.22). Thus the skin in this region is characterized by:

- a thick epidermis with thick compact protective keratin;
- a well-developed rete ridge system;
- numerous Meissner's corpuscles in the dermal papillae (see Fig. 18.17);
- Pacinian corpuscles in the dermis and subcutis (Fig. 18.17);
- specialized arteriovenous shunts (glomus bodies);
- abundant eccrine sweat glands and ducts.

AXILLA

Skin in the axilla and groin is similar, possibly because of our quadruped origins. Its most important features are:

- an abundance of highly active apocrine glands;
- numerous oblique hair follicles;
- numerous eccrine glands;
- thin epidermis (Fig. 18.23).

Fig. 18.19 Thin skin.
Micrograph showing the thin epidermal (E) and keratin (K) layers of thin skin, which is also characterized by a poorly developed rete ridge system (RR), small numbers of hair follicles, and variable numbers of eccrine glands.

Fig. 18.20 Thick sole skin.
Micrograph showing the thick epidermal (E) and keratin (K) layers of thick skin, which is also characterized by a well developed rete ridge system (RR) and numerous eccrine glands and ducts (ED).

Fig. 18.21 Scalp skin.
Micrograph showing the tightly packed pilosebaceous units of scalp skin. Note the sebaceous glands (SG) and hair follicles (HF).

Fig. 18.22 Fingertip skin.
Micrograph showing the thick epidermis (E) and well-developed rete ridge system (RR) of fingertip skin, covered by thick compact protective keratin (K). Note the glomus body (G) and the abundant eccrine sweat glands (EG) and their ducts (ED).

Fig. 18.23 Axillary skin.
Micrograph showing the abundant apocrine glands (AG) oblique hair follicles (HF) and thin epidermis (E) of axillary skin.

BREAST

Breasts develop as downgrowths from the epidermis along a line (milk line or streak) which runs obliquely from the axilla toward the groin on each side. In humans only one breast normally develops on each side, but occasionally there is development of an accessory breast though only the nipple component persists after birth.

NIPPLE

Breast secretions emerge to the surface at the nipple.

At the tip of the nipple are the 12–20 small openings of the large nipple ducts (Fig. 18.24) arranged in a ring.

The nipple is a round, raised area of modified skin with a slightly convoluted epidermis which shows increased melanin pigmentation after the first pregnancy.

The nipple is surrounded by the **areola**, which is modified skin containing large sebaceous units forming small nodular elevations (**Montgomery's tubercles**). The areola also shows increased melanin pigmentation after the first pregnancy.

BREAST DEVELOPMENT

Full development of the female breast occurs at puberty.

The nipple and its simple system of ducts is present at birth, but full development of the epithelial downgrowth does not occur until puberty, and then usually only in females.

At puberty, and under the influence of increasing estrogen secretion:
- the breasts increase in bulk, due initially to an increase in adipose tissue;
- the ductular system of the nipple becomes more complex with branches extending into the adipose tissue (Fig. 18.25).

Occasionally the male breast enlarges slightly at puberty, again due to increased adipose tissue and extension of the ductular system. However the enlargement is usually minimal, self-limiting and reversible, though occasionally it can progress.

Normally the male breast remains a rudimentary system of simple nipple ducts and a small amount of fibrocollagenous tissue.

Growth and activity of the female breast are entirely hormone dependent. Continued estrogen secretion after the onset of puberty leads to progressive enlargement and complexity of the duct system.

The parenchyma of the breast is composed of 12–20 distinct lobes.

Each lobe consists of a duct system, with its own separate opening in the nipple, embedded in adipose tissue containing fibrocollagenous septa. Particularly prominent septa separate the individual lobes and are attached to overlying skin by fibrocollagenous bands which are sometimes called Cooper's suspensory ligaments. On their deep surface the septa are attached to the fascia overlying the pectoralis muscle.

Fig. 18.24 Nipple.

ⓐ There are 12–20 openings arranged in a ring on the surface of the nipple, each being lined by keratinized stratified squamous epithelium. In the inactive, non-lactating breast they are normally plugged by keratin. Each opening is the site of emergence of a single lactiferous duct, which is lined by a two-layered epithelium, the basal layer being myoepithelial cells.

Each lactiferous duct receives large mammary ducts, and there is a dilation, the lactiferous sinus, shortly afterward.

The support tissue consists of fibroadipose tissue containing numerous longitudinal and circular smooth muscle bundles.

ⓑ Micrograph of a lactiferous duct (D) of the nipple, with surrounding fibrocollagenous stroma (F) and longitudinal and circular smooth muscle (M).

ⓒ Micrograph of a part of a lactiferous sinus (S) just below the nipple. The sinus contains homogenous proteinaceous fluid (PF) and is surrounded by fibrocollagenous stroma (F) and muscle (M).

Fig. 18.25 Breast development.

ⓐ Micrograph of breast tissue from a 4-month-old female infant. All that is present is a system of scarcely branching nipple ducts (D) embedded in fibrocollagenous tissue (F).
ⓑ Micrograph of breast tissue from an 11-year-old girl at the onset of puberty. The ductular system (D) is beginning to proliferate and produce branches, and the surrounding fibrocollagenous supporting tissue (F) is actively increasing in bulk.

GYNECOMASTIA

Pronounced development of the male breast (Fig. 18.26) is called gynecomastia. It occurs under the influence of excess estrogen secretion, which may be either endogenous (e.g. at puberty) or exogenous (e.g. stilbestrol treatment for prostatic cancer).

Fig. 18.26 Gynecomastia.

Gynecomastia is characterized by proliferation and branching of the mammary duct system, which often dilates (D) and by an increase in the periductal fibrocollagenous tissue (F).

MAMMARY DUCT AND LOBULE SYSTEM

Each lobe of the breast is a system of ever-branching ducts which penetrate deep into the fibroadipose tissue of the breast.

Each duct is lined by columnar or cuboidal epithelium, with a continuous surface layer of epithelial cells with oval nuclei and an outer discontinuous layer of myoepithelial cells which have clear cytoplasm.

Each duct is surrounded by loose fibrocollagenous support tissue containing a rich capillary network. Elastic fibers are present within this fibrous sheath in all but the smallest, most peripheral branches.

The duct system terminates in an ovoid mammary lobule.

The branching duct system ends in a cluster of blind-ending terminal ductules, each cluster and its feeding duct comprising a **mammary lobule**.

The terminal ducts and lobules are embedded in a loose fibrous support tissue which is rich in capillaries and also contains a few lymphocytes, macrophages and mast cells. This tissue is surrounded by a more dense fibrocollagenous support tissue intermingled with adipose tissue (Fig. 18.27).

BREAST CHANGES IN PREGNANCY

Breast structure changes early in pregnancy.

The vascularity and melanin pigmentation of the nipple and areola increase and the mammary lobules enlarge by hyperplastic proliferation of the terminal ductule epithelium, with some vacuolation appearing in the luminal epithelial cells.

By the second trimester, there is evidence of luminal cell secretion, which is copious by the third trimester and accumulates within the hyperplastic terminal ducts (Fig. 18.28).

With this expansion of the lobular units, there is an accompanying increase in the loose lobular support tissue and inflammatory cells. At term and throughout lactation the hyperplastic lobular units are distended by their lipid-rich proteinaceous secretion (milk).

Fig. 18.27 Mammary lobule.
Diagram of a mammary lobule, which consists of a cluster of blind-ending terminal ductules together with the drainage duct system (extralobular and intralobular terminal ducts). Some lobules are located in the dense fibrocollagenous tissue of the breast while others are in adipose tissue.

(b) Micrograph of a typical mammary lobule embedded in fibrocollagenous tissue. Note the difference between the intralobular (IF) and extralobular (EF) fibrocollagenous tissue.

In this inactive lobule the epithelium of the terminal ductules (TD) is identical to that of the intralobular terminal duct (ID). The extralobular terminal duct is not visible.

(c) High-power micrograph showing the epithelium of the intralobular terminal ductules. Essentially two-layered, the inner layer varies between a cuboidal and a low columnar pattern (C) while the outer layer consists of prominent myoepithelial cells (M).

Note the minute amount of secretion (S) in the lumen of the duct resulting from menstrual cycle hormone secretion.

BREAST

- the functional unit of the breast is a lobule surrounded by a specialized stroma

- lobule epithelium is hormone-sensitive and undergoes proliferation in pregnancy

- myoepithelial cells surround each lobule and express secreted milk

- milk is transported along duct systems to the nipple

The breast only reaches its full functional activity during pregnancy and lactation

Functional maturation of the breast in pregnancy is under the influence of pituitary and ovarian hormones which are secreted in high concentrations during pregnancy and throughout breast feeding.

When breast feeding ceases, the breast returns to its normal or resting state by gradual involution over a period of some months. The luminal cells return to their former size without cytoplasmic vacuolation and the lobular support tissue returns to its normal proportions.

Sometimes there is residual increased collagen in the involuting lobular support tissue, and this can lead to progressive distortion of the mammary lobules and persistent cystic dilation of some of the ducts.

Hormone receptors in breast tissue

Steroid hormones can only act on cells which bear receptors specific to the particular hormone; these receptors are binding proteins which link with the hormone and transmit the steroid signal to alter the activity of genes in the nucleus. The function of the breast is dependent on the steroid hormones, estrogen and progesterone, and receptors for both are present in mammary epithelium, particularly in the epithelium of the terminal ductules of the lobule (Fig. 18.29).

In breast cancer, the persistence of estrogen and progestin receptors in the tumor cells indicates likely responsiveness of the tumor to some chemotherapeutic treatments, particularly anti-oestrogens.

Fig. 18.28 Breast in pregnancy.
ⓐ Micrograph showing the hyperplastic breast lobules of pregnancy. The intralobular terminal ductules (D) are increased in size and complexity, and their lumina are distended by secretion (S) from the lining epithelium.
ⓑ Micrograph showing clear vacuoles (V), containing lipid-rich secretion forming on the luminal aspect of terminal ductule lining epithelium.

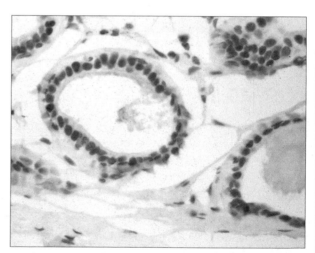

Fig 18.29 Estrogen receptors in lobule epithelium. This photomicrograph demonstrates a brown positive immunocytochemical staining in the nuclei of lobular epithelium, indicating the presence of estrogen receptor.

FIBROADENOSIS

Repeated exposure of the mammary lobules to varying estrogen and progesterone secretions during numerous menstrual cycles can lead to disproportionate growth of various components and distortion of the normal architecture. Common changes are:

• increased duct and ductular tissue (adenosis);
• increased fibrocollagenous support tissues (fibrosis);
• dilation of the larger mammary ducts.

Such changes when they occur are most severe in multigravid women and cause increased nodulation of the breast tissue, which is sometimes associated with cyst formation (Fig. 18.30). This is the most common disorder of the breast and is variably called fibroadenosis, cystic mammary dysplasia, benign mammary dysplasia or fibrocystic disease of the breast.

Fig. 18.30 Fibroadenosis.
Micrograph of section of breast showing the features of fibroadenosis: fibrosis (F) adenosis (A) and cyst formation, (C).

CARCINOMA OF THE BREAST

The epithelial component of the extralobular mammary ducts, the intralobular mammary ducts and the terminal ductules may undergo cancerous change to produce one of the most important and common cancers in women, breast cancer. Cancers originating in the terminal ductules are called lobular carcinomas, those from the ducts are called ductal carcinomas (Fig 18.31).

The breast is well equipped with small blood and lymphatic vessels, so spread of the cancer away from its site of origin in the breast is common and can lead to a poor outlook. Spread along lymphatics is usually to the axillary group of lymph nodes on the side of the affected breast, producing metastatic deposits in the nodes (Fig. 8.13), while spread via the bloodstream usually occurs at a later stage, metastatic carcinoma being deposited in many organs, particularly the lungs and bones.

Fig. 18.31 Mammary carcinoma.
Micrograph showing the features of a typical carcinoma derived from mammary ducts. The cells have broken through into the surrounding fibroadipose tissue to produce an invasive carcinoma.

Fig. 18.32 Breast.

ⓐ Micrograph showing normal breast tissue from a 23-year-old woman. At the centre is a breast lobule in which the system of terminal ducts and ductules is embedded in loose intralobular fibrocollagenous stroma (F). There is a narrow surrounding zone of dense extralobular fibrocollagenous support tissue (DF) outside which is the soft adipose tissue (A) that forms the bulk of the breast.

ⓑ Micrograph showing normal breast tissue from a 43-year-old woman. As women age, the amount of fibrocollagenous tissue, (F) in the breast increases, replacing some of the adipose tissue. The mammary lobules become enclosed in dense collagen.

1. THE BASAL LAYER OF THE EPIDERMIS

(a) is responsible for the constant production of keratinocytes
(b) is composed of cuboidal or columnar keratinocytes
(c) is attached to the basement membrane by desmosomes
(d) contains scattered melanocytes
(e) contains keratinosomes

2. MELANOCYTES

(a) are pigmented because of the melanin they contain
(b) have long cytoplasmic processes which extend between keratinocytes
(c) are greatly increased in number in dark-skinned races
(d) contain characteristic spherical premelanosomes
(e) are neural-derived and also act as mechanoreceptors

3. IN THE SKIN APPENDAGES

(a) sebaceous gland units usually open directly onto the skin surface.
(b) apocrine glands secrete sweat
(c) eccrine glands are particularly frequent on the palms and soles
(d) the internal root sheath of the hair follicle produces the hair shaft
(e) erector pili muscles control the position of the hair shafts

4. THE MAMMARY LOBULE

(a) is embedded in loose fibrous support tissue
(b) contains terminal ductules which are the main secretory component
(c) terminal ductule epithelium cells show vacuolation in the second half of the menstrual cycle
(d) contain myoepithelial cells which lie beneath the terminal ductule epithelium
(e) undergoes structural and functional atrophy after the menopause

19. Special Senses

INTRODUCTION

A vital function of the nervous system is the gathering of sensory information.

Sensory information is derived from a variety of specialized sensory nerve endings. These include:

- sensory endings in the skin to detect touch (fine touch, pressure), pain and temperature (see Chapter 18);
- tendon endings and muscle spindles to detect movement and position of the limbs;
- chemoreceptive organs such as the carotid body;
- sensory endings on the tongue to detect taste;
- sensory endings in the olfactory mucosa to detect smell.

In addition, information is obtained by the specialized sensory organs, the eye and the ear; the ear and the vestibular system detect sound, acceleration and position, and the eye perceives light.

EAR

The ear is divided into external ear, middle ear and inner ear.

The external ear comprises the **pinna** and **external auditory canal.** The pinna is composed of elastic cartilage covered by hair-bearing skin. The external auditory canal is lined by hair-bearing skin. Within its subcutaneous tissues are wax-secreting **ceruminous glands** which are modified sebaceous glands. The outer two-thirds of the canal is surrounded by elastic cartilage in continuity with the pinna; the inner third is surrounded by the temporal bone of the skull.

The middle ear is separated from the external ear by the tympanic membrane.

The **tympanic membrane** marks the boundary between the external ear and the cavity of the middle ear, which is also termed the **tympanic cavity** (Fig. 19.1).

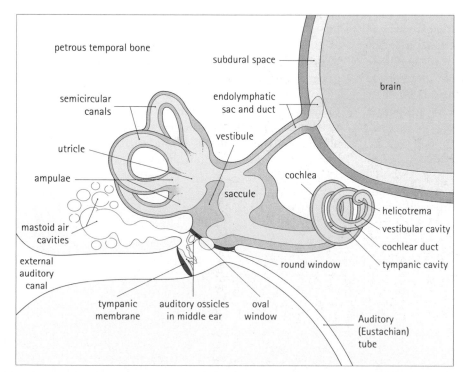

Fig. 19.1 Anatomy of the ear.
The ear consists of the external ear, middle ear and inner ear. The inner third of the external auditory canal of the external ear is surrounded by the temporal bone, while the middle ear and inner ear are contained within cavities in the temporal bone.

The middle ear is an air-filled cavity containing the auditory ossicles. It is connected to the nasopharynx by the auditory (Eustachian) tube and is in direct continuity with the mastoid air cells.

The inner ear is a fluid-filled cavity divided into three main spaces (semicircular canal space, vestibule and cochlea). Within the inner ear are a series of interconnecting fluid-filled sacs (semicircular canals, utricle, saccule and cochlear duct).

The endolymphatic duct runs from the membranous sacs to the subdural space around the brain.

The tympanic membrane is a three-layered structure:
- the outer aspect is covered by stratified squamous epithelium;
- the central portion is composed of fibrocollagenous support tissue containing numerous elastic fibers to provide mechanical strength;
- the inner portion is lined by a low cuboidal epithelium which is continuous with that lining the rest of the middle ear.

The middle ear transmits sound vibrations to the inner ear.

The middle ear cavity is lined by a low cuboidal epithelium and contains three auditory ossicles, the **incus**, **malleus** and **stapes**. These are:
- composed of compact bone;
- articulated by synovial joints (see Chapter 13);
- covered externally by the same low cuboidal epithelium that lines the inner ear.

Two small skeletal muscles, the stapedius and the tensor tympani, are associated with the ossicles and dampen motion between the bones, which occurs in response to loud noise.

The middle ear cavity communicates directly with air-filled spaces in the mastoid bone (**mastoid sinuses**), which are lined by low cuboidal or flattened squamous epithelium.

The auditory (Eustachian) tube equalizes pressure in the middle ear cavity.

The **auditory tube** extends from the middle ear cavity to the nasopharynx and is lined by ciliated epithelium similar to that of the respiratory tract. Its function is to equilibrate pressure between the middle ear cavity and the atmosphere.

Normally the auditory tube is collapsed, but it is opened by movement of muscles in the nasopharynx such as occurs with swallowing or yawning.

The inner ear is a series of fluid-filled sacs encased in bone.

The inner ear consists of fluid-filled sacs (**membranous labyrinth**) lying within cavities in the temporal bone of the skull (**bony or osseous labyrinth**).

The membranous labyrinth comprises the **cochlear duct**, the **saccule**, the **utricle** and **semicircular canals**, and the **endolymphatic sac and duct**, the walls of which are composed of sheets of fibrocollagenous support tissue lined by a flat epithelium. These sacs are filled with a fluid called **endolymph** and have epithelial and sensory specializations to detect position and sound.

The osseous labyrinth is composed of three cavities, the vestibule, the semicircular canals and the cochlea, which are lined by periosteum and filled with fluid called **perilymph**.

Movement is detected in the inner ear by mechanoreceptors.

Mechanoreceptors or **hair cells** are specialized epithelial cells bearing a highly organized system of microvilli (**stereocilia**) on their apical surface. Deflection of the microvilli causes electrical depolarization of the hair cell membrane which is transmitted to the central nervous system by the connecting axons of sensory nerve cells (Fig. 19.2).

Patches of hair cells are located in three sites:
- within the vestibular apparatus in the ampullae of the semicircular canals to detect acceleration;
- within the macula of the utricle and saccule to perceive the direction of gravity and static position;
- within the organ of Corti of the cochlea to detect sound vibration.

At each site the hair cell microvilli are embedded in a gelatinous matrix which moves according to the stimulus it is detecting. Movement of the microvilli toward the tallest row excites (depolarizes) the hair cell membrane, while movement towards the shortest row inhibits (hyperpolarizes) it.

Hair cells are arranged in different parts of the membranous labyrinth (Fig. 19.3) in order to sense movement generated by different causes.

Support cells surround the hair cells and are anchored to them at their apex by occluding junctions. These junctions maintain ionic gradients between the endolymph and the extracellular fluid around the cells, the gradients being reversed on depolarization.

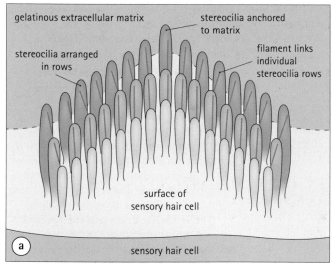

gelatinous extracellular matrix

stereocilia anchored to matrix

stereocilia arranged in rows

filament links individual stereocilia rows

surface of sensory hair cell

a

sensory hair cell

gelatinous extracellular matrix

endolymph

stereocilia

hair cell

tight junction

support cell

extracellular fluid

sensory axon

b

gelatinous extracellular matrix moves within endolymph

stereocilia bend causing membrane depolarization

axon fibers

signal passes to sensory neurons of sensory ganglion

c

Fig. 19.2 Hair cell microvilli.

(a) The apical surface of each hair cell bears a highly organized system of microvilli (stereocilia), which are arranged as three parallel rows in a V- or W-shaped pattern.

The height of the microvilli progressively decreases from the back to the front of the hair cell to form a so-called 'organ pipe' arrangement.

Fine filaments link individual microvilli from each row, with the tips of the shorter microvilli being coupled to the shafts of the taller microvilli behind.

While the hair cell is rigidly fixed in place by support cells, the tips of the tallest row of microvilli are embedded in a gelatinous extracellular matrix which is free to move within the fluid cavities of the inner ear or vestibular system.

(b) Hair cells are supported by adjacent cells and are in contact with the axon of a sensory nerve. The support cells are anchored to the hair cells by occluding junctions. The stereocillia are embedded in a gelatinous matrix.

(c) Movement of the gelatinous matrix deflects the stereocilia causing membrane depolarization of the hair cell, which is relayed to the central nervous system via the axon of a sensory nerve.

Hair cells are arranged in different patterns in the cochlea and vestibular apparatus to detect acceleration (movement), gravity (position), or sound (hearing).

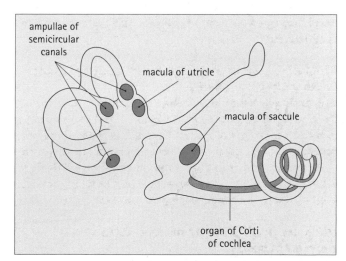

ampullae of semicircular canals

macula of utricle

macula of saccule

organ of Corti of cochlea

Fig. 19.3 Distribution of hair cells in the membranous labyrinth.

The hair cells are arranged in patches in the ampullae of the semicircular canals to detect acceleration, in the macula of the utricle and saccule to perceive gravity direction and static position, and in the organ of Corti of the cochlea to detect sound vibration.

Sound is detected in the inner ear by the organ of Corti in the cochlear duct.

The **cochlear duct** is a blind-ended tubular diverticulum filled with endolymph. It makes $2^3/_4$ turns within the spiral-shaped bony cochlea in the temporal bone, and is compressed between two other tubular spaces, the **vestibular** and **tympanic cavities**, which are filled with perilymph (Fig. 19.4a–b).

Within the cochlear duct is the **organ of Corti**, which is a special adaptation of the epithelial cells lining the cochlear duct and detects sound vibration (Fig. 19.5a–b).

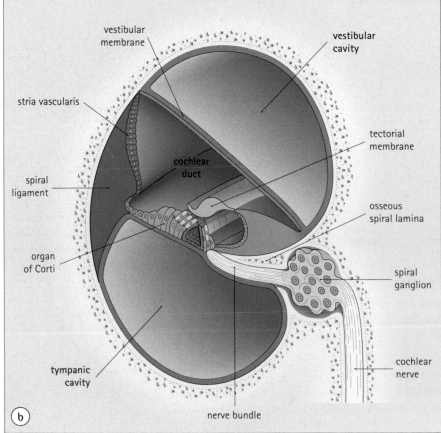

Fig. 19.4 Cochlea

(a) The cochlea of the osseous labyrinth contains three spaces, the vestibular cavity, the cochlear duct, and the tympanic cavity. These spaces are wound in a spiral within the temporal bone. The central spiral of bone within the cochlea is called the **modiolus**.

The vestibular cavity and the tympanic cavity contain perilymph continuous with that in the vestibule (see Fig. 19.1), while the cochlear duct, which is continuous with and part of the membranous labyrinth, is filled with endolymph.

At the apex of the cochlea the vestibular and tympanic cavities connect at an opening termed the **helicotrema**. The cochlear nerve emerges from the base of the cochlea and carries signals to the brain.

(b) Shown here is one section through the cochlea. The **vestibular membrane (Reissner's membrane)** consists of two layers of flattened epithelium separated by a basement membrane, one cell layer being in continuity with the cells lining the vestibular cavity and the other in continuity with the cells lining the cochlear duct. The cells are held together by well developed occluding junctions to maintain different electrolyte concentrations between the endolymph and perilymph.

The **stria vascularis** is a specialized area of epithelium with a rich vascular supply in the lateral wall of the cochlear duct. Many of the cells here have ultrastructural features indicating an ion transport function, and it is thought that they secrete endolymph.

The basilar membrane is thicker than the vestibular membrane and consists of collagen fibers as well as a basement membrane. On one side it is covered by cells lining the tympanic cavity, and on the other by specialized cells lining the cochlear duct.

Medially, the basilar membrane is continuous with the organ of Corti, which is a specialized area of support cells and sensory hair cells subserving hearing (see Fig. 19.5). The organ of Corti is supported by a spur of bone called the osseous spiral lamina.

Laterally the basilar membrane is attached to the spiral ligament which is a mass of tissue developed from the endosteum of the surrounding bone.

Neurons of the spiral ganglion are present adjacent to the osseous spiral lamina.

Fig. 19.5 Organ of Corti

(a) The organ of Corti is composed of epithelial support cells and sensory hair cells. Medially it rests on the rigid bony osseous spiral lamina; laterally it is located on the deformable basilar membrane.

There are two groups of hair cells, an **inner group** and an **outer group**, which are separated by a small opening at the end of the osseous spiral lamina termed the **inner tunnel (tunnel of Corti).** The inner group are smaller and rounder than the outer group and arranged as a single row along the cochlea. the outer group are tall and thin and arranged in 3 to 5 parallel rows, depending on the position in the length of the cochlea.

The hair cells are surrounded by epithelial support cells, the inner hair cells being completely surrounded, while the outer hair cells are enclosed only at their extreme apex and basal portions, leaving a bare mid-zone in contact with extracellular fluid.

The microvilli of the outer hair cells are attached to a sheet of gelatinous extracellular matrix braced by filamentous proteins (tectorial membrane), while those of the inner hair cells are free. Axons make synaptic contact with the hair cells and run to the spiral ganglion. The tectorial membrane is secreted by epithelial cells (**interdental cells**).

There are several classes of support cell in the organ of Corti. **Pillar cells** contain abundant scaffolding microtubules, and surround and support the triangular cavity (inner tunnel) at the level of the lip of the osseous spiral lamina. In contrast, **phalangeal cells** support the hair cells and are attached to them by occluding junctions at their apices, thus isolating the basal membrane of hair cells from the endolymph and maintaining electrochemical gradients.

(b) Micrograph of the organ of Corti. Note the tectorial membrane (T), the mass of phalangeal cells bearing the hair cells (P), and the stria vascularis (S) on the spiral ligament (SL) within the cochlea duct (C).

Detection of sound in the inner ear

Sound waves cause vibration of the tympanic membrane which is then transmitted to the oval window membrane via the auditory ossicles.

Pressure waves are thence transmitted to the perilymph of the vestibular cavity, causing the vestibular and basilar membranes to bow inward toward the tympanic cavity, and to the round window, which bows outward.

Because the tectorial membrane remains relatively rigid, bowing of the vestibular and basilar membranes causes relative movement of the hair cell sterocilia, which results in membrane depolarization.

The signal is transmitted to the sensory nerves of the spiral ganglion, and then through the cochlear cranial nerve to the brain, where it is perceived as sound.

Low-frequency sound is detected by stereocilia towards the apex of the cochlea, while high-frequency sounds are detected at the base.

HEARING LOSS

Many diseases of the ear are associated with temporary or permanent hearing loss. Deafness can be divided into conductive and sensorineural types.

Conductive loss occurs when sound waves cannot be transmitted to the inner ear; common causes include blockage of the external auditory meatus (e.g. wax) or damage to the middle ear by infection ('otitis media').

Sensorineural loss is the result of damage to the inner ear, the nerves linking the cochlea with the brain, or in the brain itself. The most common type is called **presbyacusis** which occurs in elderly people; it results from reduction in hair cells, atrophy of the stria vascularis and neuron loss in the spiral ganglia.

Recently, it has been possible to place electronic implants into the cochlea to treat deafness. Sound is detected by an external device and this causes direct stimulation of the cochlear nerve, allowing hearing.

Gravity and static position are detected by hair cells in the macula of the utricle and the macula of the saccule.

The macula of the utricle lies in the horizontal plane, while the macula of the saccule lies in the vertical plane at right angles to the macula of the utricle (see Fig. 19.3).

Each macula is histologically identical, and is composed of the following three cell types (Fig. 19.6):

- support cells (sustentacular cells), which are columnar cells with short apical microvilli;
- type I hair cells, which are polygonal in shape and surrounded by a network of afferent and efferent nerve endings;
- type II hair cells, which are cylindrical in shape, with basal synaptic afferent and efferent nerve endings.

In addition to an organ-pipe arrangement of tall microvilli stereocilia on their apical surface (see Fig. 19.2), these hair cells possess a single true cilium termed a **kinocilium**, which is located just behind the tallest row of sterocilia.

The stereocilia and kinocilium of each new hair cell are embedded in a gelatinous plaque of extracellular matrix called the **otolithic membrane**, which is suspended in the endolymph. This membrane is covered by numerous small particles composed of protein and calcium carbonate, the **otoconia** (**otoliths**).

The macula can detect the direction of gravity by sensing the direction of pull of the otolithic membrane and otoconia on the mass of hair cells that results from head movement either backward and forward (macula of utricle) or from side to side (macula of saccule).

Fig. 19.6 Macula.
In this micrograph, the sterocilia of the hair cells of the macula are embedded in the otolithic membrane. The otoconia (O) are visible as numerous purple-stained particles. The stereocilia appear as pink tufts (T) arising from the cell surface, but neither individual microvilli nor type of hair cell can be identified at this magnification. The support cells (SC) appear as an epithelial sheet.

Acceleration and motion are detected by hair cells in the ampullae at the end of the semicircular canals.

There are three semicircular canals, which assume posterior, superior and horizontal positions.

Each ampulla is a 1 mm long dilated region of the membranous labyrinth and contains a patch of hair cells arranged in a tall finger-like structure (an **ampullary crista**). The sterocilia of the sensory hair cells are attached to a dome-shaped gelatinous matrix termed a cupola (Fig. 19.7).

With rotary motion of the head endolymph moves within the membranous labyrinth because of the static inertia of the fluid relative to the rest of the vestibular apparatus. Such movement causes displacement of the cupola, and the direction of this displacement is detected by the hair cells.

When integrated, perception from the three semicircular canals arranged in planes perpendicular to each other provides information on the direction and rate of acceleration of head movement.

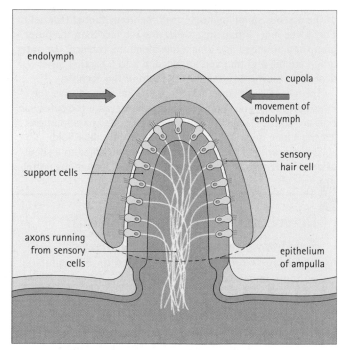

Fig. 19.7 Ampullary region of semicircular canal.
Within the ampullae of the semicircular canals, hair cells are arranged over a finger-like protrusion of the lining called the ampullary crista. The hair cells are both type I and type II and are associated with adjacent support cells.

The axons innervating the cells emerge from the base of the ampullary crista, being derived from sensory nerve cells in the ganglion of the vestibular nerve (Scarpa's ganglion), which connect with the vestibular nucleus in the brain stem.

The hair cell stereocilia and kinocilium are embedded in the gelatinous matrix of the cupola which, unlike the tectorial membrane of the maculae, does not contain otoconia.

THE EAR

- the ear is divided into external, middle and inner ear

- the middle ear cavity is lined by cuboidal epithelium, contains the auditory ossicles, and communicates with the pharynx via the auditory tube

- the tympanic membrane is composed of fibrocollagenous tissue covered on one side by squamous epithelium and by cuboidal epithelium on the other

- sound is detected in the organ of Corti in the cochlear duct

- gravity and static position are detected by the maculae

- acceleration and movement are detected by the ampullae of the semicircular canals

EYE

The eye is designed to focus light onto specialized receptors that respond to light. It is composed of sclera, cornea, uvea and retina arranged around three chambers (Fig. 19.8).

The sclera proper is the outer fibrocollagenous coat of the globe of the eye.

The sclera varies in thickness from 1 mm posteriorly to 0.5 mm anteriorly, and is composed of flat plates of collagen oriented in different directions, but parallel to the surface.

The sclera is composed of three layers:
- the episclera, an external layer of loose fibrocollagenous tissue running adjacent to the periorbital fat;
- the stroma, the middle layer, which is composed of bundles of collagen thicker than those of the episclera;
- the inner part of the sclera, adjacent to the choroid layer.

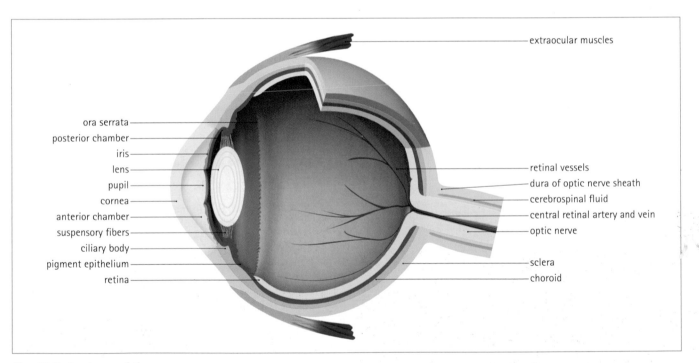

Fig. 19.8 Anatomy of the eye.

The eye is a spherical structure with a translucent disc-shaped area (**cornea**) on its anterior surface. This merges at its margins with a tough fibrocollagenous outer coat (**sclera**) at the limbus. The sclera surrounds the globe and is attached to a series of skeletal muscles (**extraocular muscles**) responsible for eye movement.

The choroid is composed of blood vessels, support cells and melanocytes posteriorly and is continuous with the ciliary body and iris anteriorly, the iris being a disc-shaped membrane containing smooth muscle, with a central aperture (the pupil) to allow the passage of light.

A special epithelial layer (**retinal pigment epithelium**) lies inside the choroid and inside this is the receptor and nerve cell layer of the eye (**retina**). The **ora serrata** marks the end of the specialized sensory layer of the retina anteriorly.

Nerves from the retina emerge from the posterior aspect of the globe in the **optic nerve**, which is surrounded by a covering layer of fibrocollagenous tissue and cerebrospinal fluid, in continuity with that surrounding the brain.

Blood is supplied to the retina by the central artery of the retina, which runs with the optic nerve.

The transparent biconvex **lens** is suspended by a series of fine filaments from the ciliary body. The **ciliary body** contains smooth muscle and its contraction regulates the lens shape.

The globe is divided into three chambers: the **anterior chamber** in front of the iris, the **posterior chamber** behind the iris, and the **vitreous** behind the lens. The anterior and posterior chambers contain a clear fluid called the **aqueous**. The vitreous is a gelatinous transparent extracellular matrix material.

The collagen bundles of the stroma run in sweeping branching patterns mainly looping from front to back, within the stroma. The lamina fusca contains small numbers of elastic fibers.

The blood vessels and nerves (including the optic nerve) running to and from the eye pass through the periscleral and scleral layers. The scleral stroma itself is avascular. Anteriorly, the sclera blends with the cornea in a transition zone (the limbus) which is 1 mm wide.

The cornea is covered on both surfaces by epithelium.

The cornea is the transparent disc-like anterior portion of the globe, and in the adult typically measures 10.5 mm from top to bottom and 11.5 mm from side to side. It is more curved than the globe and protrudes anteriorly. The cornea has five layers (Fig. 19.9).

CORNEAL EPITHELIUM The non-keratinizing squamous epithelium with a basal cell layer gives rise to 5 to 6 superficial layers with a total thickness of about 50 µm. Numerous free nerve endings terminate in this epithelium, and are the afferent part of the blink (ciliary) reflex, which is mediated through the sensory part of the fifth cranial nerve.

BOWMAN'S MEMBRANE This is composed of fine collagen fibrils embedded in an extracellular matrix and is 8–10 µm thick. It is limited anteriorly by the basement membrane of the corneal epithelium, and blends posteriorly with the cornea stroma.

CORNEAL STROMA The the main layer of the cornea is composed of 60–70 broad sheets of tightly bound, parallel collagen fibers (corneal lamellae) embedded in an extracellular matrix composed mainly of sulphated glycosaminolgycans. To provide maximum mechanical strength the direction of the collagen fibers differs in each layer. Between the lamellae are sparse inactive spindle-shaped fibrocytes, (**keratocytes**).

As there are no blood vessels in the cornea, the regular parallel arrangement of the collagen and the paucity of cells render the cornea translucent and allows it to transmit light.

DESCEMET'S MEMBRANE This 7–10 µm thick hyaline layer on the posterior aspect of the corneal stroma is produced by the corneal endothelial cells and is a true basement membrane.

CORNEAL ENDOTHELIUM This consists of a single layer of polygonal, plate-like cells which line the inner surface of the cornea. They are adapted for ion-pumping and therefore possess numerous mitochondria, and are linked together by both desmosomal and occluding junctions (see Figs 3.6 & 3.11).

The corneal endothelial cells pump fluid from the corneal stroma, thereby preventing excessive hydration of the extracellular matrix which would result in opacification of the cornea.

Fig. 19.9 Cornea.
(a) Micrograph of the five layers of the cornea showing epithelium (E), Bowman's membrane (B), stroma (S), Descemet's membrane (D), endothelium (End). Bowman's membrane and Descemet's membrane appear as homogeneous hyaline layers, which stain bright pink with H&E. In paraffin-processed material, as here, artefactual splitting of the collagen plates forming the corneal stroma is common and gives rise to small spaces.
(b) Electronmicrograph showing the base of a corneal epithelial basal cell (E) and its basement membrane (BM) resting on Bowman's membrane (B), in which a felt-like arrangement of fine collagen fibrils can just be discerned. Beneath this are the collagen lamellae of the corneal stroma (S) and a corneal fibrocyte (keratocyte, K).
(c) Electronmicrograph showing endothelium (End) resting on Descemet's membrane (D). Above are the collagen lamellae of the corneal stroma (S) and a corneal fibrocyte (keratocyte, K). Below is the anterior chamber (A).

The uvea is a specialized support tissue within the globe.

The uvea is an intermediate layer in the eye between the dense support tissue of the sclera and the functional neural tissue of the retina. It contains blood vessels, nerves, support cells, contractile cells and melanocytes, and is divided into three specialized areas: the choroid, ciliary body and iris.

The choroid has three layers and supports the retina.

The choroid extends from the ora serrata to the optic nerve and contains the blood vessels and lymphatics supporting the retina (Fig. 19.10). It is a dark brown sheet and blends with the lamina fusca of the sclera in its outer portion, while in its inner portion it is attached to the retina. Next to the sclera is the **choroidal stroma**, which is a loose fibrocollagenous support tissue interspersed with melanocytes, lymphocytes and mast cells, and through which the main arteries and veins run. Inside this is the **choriocapillary layer**, which is a capillary layer supporting the deep layers of the retina and arises from the larger vessels in the stroma. Finally, at the interface between the choroid and the retinal pigment epithelium is **Bruch's membrane** which consists of:

*   the basement membrane of the choriocapillary endothelial cells;
*   an outer collagen fiber layer 0.5 μm thick;
*   an elastic fiber layer 2 μm thick;
*   an inner collagen fiber layer;
*   the basement membrane of the retinal pigment epithelium (part of the retina).

Fig. 19.10 Choroid.
Micrograph showing the vascular choroid layer posterior to the retinal pigment epithelium.

CORNEAL DISEASE

The cornea contributes to the refraction of light into the eye, and damage resulting in corneal opacity may impair vision.

Although loss of corneal epithelium (corneal abrasion) is exquisitely painful, it is soon repaired by regeneration of new cells. Damage to Bowman's membrane, however, results in the formation of an opaque corneal scar because repair is by the haphazard deposition of collagen. If such scarring occurs in the visual axis, it causes loss of visual acuity.

The corneal endothelial cells are not replaced during life, and in some instances become depleted with age. They may also be damaged by disease processes in the anterior chamber of the eye. When the corneal endothelial cells are sufficiently depleted, fluid accumulates in the corneal stroma, which then becomes less transparent. Such waterlogging of the corneal stroma (corneal edema) may cause the overlying epithelium to separate and this is intensely painful.

Diseases of the cornea, including endothelial failure, may be treated by corneal transplantation.

The iris is part of the uvea which forms a diaphragm in front of the lens.

The **iris** delineates the anterior and posterior chambers of the eye. It had a circular aperture (**pupil**), which can be opened and closed by the action of groups of smooth muscle. Contraction of the pupil reduces the amount of light entering the eye and thereby reduces glare from light scattered from the periphery of the lens.

The iris contains pigmented cells and muscle and is composed of four layers: the **anterior limiting membrane**, the **stroma**, the **dilator muscle layer** and the **posterior epithelium** (Fig. 19.11).

The anterior limiting layer is an incomplete, fenestrated layer formed from stellate fibroblastic cells and stellate melanocytes.

The **stroma** is a loose fibrocollagenous support tissue associated with spindle-shaped fibroblasts (stromal cells), blood vessels, nerves and macrophages containing phagocytosed melanin pigment; at the pupil margin is the circumferentially arranged smooth muscle of the sphincter muscle of the pupil.

The blood vessels of the iris generally run in a radial direction with frequent anastomotic channels forming circumferential vascular plexuses.

The dilator muscle layer is composed of the contractile processes of the myoepithelial cells of the inner layer of the posterior epithelium; it extends from the base of the iris to the sphincter muscle.

The **posterior epithelium** is composed of two layers of cells which are densely pigmented with melanin. The inner layer of cells are more correctly myoepithelial in type with a basal zone around the nucleus containing melanin granules and an apical portion, which is melanin-free, constituting the dilator muscle layer. This inner layer is bound by desmosomal junctions to the outer layer cells, which contain numerous melanin granules and are continuous with the retinal pigment epithelial layer. The pigmented cells eliminate light from the eye and reduce glare.

Eye color is determined by the relative number of melanocytes in the stroma. Few cells give a blue color, while many melanin-containing cells produce a dark brown color; gray and green are the intermediate colors.

Fig. 19.11 Iris.
(a) Diagram of the free margin of the iris at the pupil showing its four constituent layers. An incomplete and fenestrated anterior limiting layer containing stellate fibroblasts and melanocytes lies on a loose fibrocollagenous stroma containing the sphincter muscle of the pupil, as well as radially orientated collagen fibers, which give the iris its ribbed and trabeculated surface. Behind the stroma is the dilator muscle, which is backed posteriorly by two layers of melanin-pigmented cells.
(b) Micrograph showing the histologic appearance of the iris. The four layers are not well defined. The anterior limiting layer (L) merges with the stroma (S). The pigmented posterior epithelium cannot be resolved into two layers because of the density of melanin pigment. The dilator muscle (M) is visible as a pink band.

The ciliary body contains the muscle which relaxes the lens.

The **ciliary body** extends from the base of the iris to the ora serrata, where it is continuous with the choroid (see Fig. 19.8). In section (Fig. 19.12) the ciliary body is roughly triangular in shape and is composed of a vascular stroma, smooth muscle, and covering epithelium; it has two anatomically recognizable regions, the **pars plica** and **pars plana**.

The ciliary body contains the **ciliary muscle**, which is a form of smooth muscle. Contraction of the ciliary muscle lessens tension on the suspensory fibers of the lens and allow the lens to assume a more spherical shape.

The pars plica contains the ciliary processes, which are ridges or folds 2 mm long, each with a core of stroma and blood vessels and covered by two layers of columnar epithelium. The outer layer of epithelium is pigmented, but the inner layer, which is in contact with the aqueous, is not.

The non-pigmented epithelial cells in the grooves between the ciliary processes give rise to the suspensory fibers of the lens which are composed mainly of the protein fibrillin. The ultrastructural features of these non-pigmented cells are those of ion-pumping cells; they secrete the aqueous.

The pars plana is a posterior flat area 4 mm long. Its stroma is continuous with the choroid, while the outer pigmented epithelium of the ciliary body is continuous with that of the retina at the ora serrata.

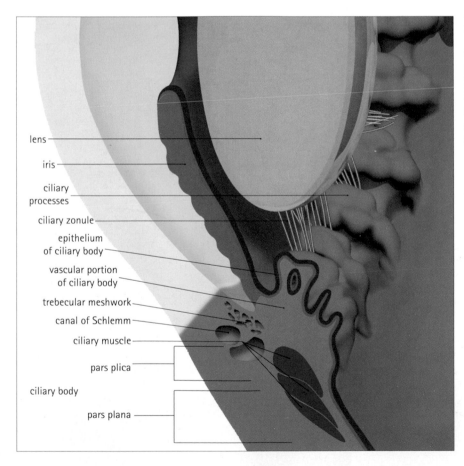

lens
iris
ciliary processes
ciliary zonule
epithelium of ciliary body
vascular portion of ciliary body
trebecular meshwork
canal of Schlemm
ciliary muscle
pars plica
ciliary body
pars plana

Fig. 19.12 Ciliary body.
The ciliary body is continuous with the base of iris and is divided anatomically into the pars plica and pars plana. The ciliary processes give rise to the suspensory fibers of the lens (ciliary zonule), while the ciliary muscle controls the tension on the suspensory fibers, and thereby controls the shape of the lens. The epithelium of the pars plana secretes the aqueous.

The retina contains photoreceptors along with support cells and nerve cells.

The retina is the innermost layer of the eye and is derived embryonically from an outgrowth of the developing brain (the optic cup). It is composed of pigment epithelial cells, photoreceptor cells, retinal support cells and nerve cells.

Retinal pigment epithelial cells maintain and support photoreceptor cells.

The retinal pigment epithelium is a single layer of melanin-containing polygonal cells extending from the optic nerve to the ora serrata. Internally it lies adjacent to the photoreceptor layer of the retina; externally its basement membrane is a component of Bruch's membrane.

The apical surfaces of the pigmented epithelial cells are covered with large microvilli which extend upward and surround the photoreceptors of the retina. Retinal pigment epithelial cells phagocytose worn-out components of the photoreceptor cells.

The two types of photoreceptor cells of the retina are termed rods and cones.

The light-sensitive structures (**photoreceptor discs**) in the photoreceptor cell form huge stacks 600–1000 deep in the outer segment of the cell and originate as deep infolds of the cell membrane (Fig. 19.13).

In rods, photoreceptor discs are formed constantly and pinch off to form free discs, which are shed from the cell

Fig. 19.13 Photoreceptors.
Diagram and ultrastructural details of a photoreceptor cell. Light is detected by its outer segment (OS), which contains flat plates of membrane (photoreceptor discs, D).

The outer segment is connected to the inner segment (IS) by a connecting cilium (C). The inner segment contains numerous mitochondria. The cell body (CB) connects to the inner segment (IS) by a microtubule-rich outer fiber (OF). The synaptic body (SB) is cup-shaped and connects to axons (A) from other retinal neurons.

when old (Fig. 19.14). In cones, however photoreceptor discs remain as deep infolds of cell membrane and do not form free discs. The turnover of cone photoreceptor discs is not clear, but it does not appear to be the same as rods.

Rods are about 2 μm thick and average 50 μm in length, possessing a roughly cylindrical outer segment. The tips of these cells are embedded in the microvilli of pigment epithelial cells, which phagocytose the old photoreceptor discs.

Cones are thicker and slightly shorter than rods being 3–5 μm thick and about 40 μm long; their outer segment is conical in shape. Like rods, cones are also located close to the microvilli of the retinal pigment epithelial cells.

The distribution of rods and cones varies within the retina. Cones, which perceive color, are concentrated in the optical center of the retina in a small pit (the **fovea**). Rods, which perceive light intensity, but not color, are concentrated at the periphery of the retina.

Between the fovea and the periphery of the retina there is a mixture of rods and cones (Fig. 19.15).

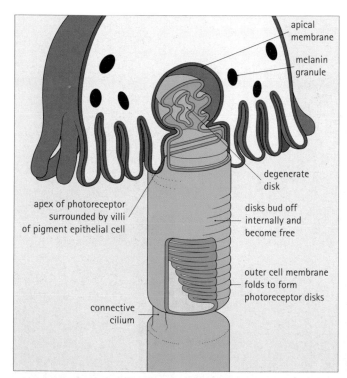

Fig. 19.14 Turnover of photoreceptor discs in rods.
In the rod photoreceptor cell, photoreceptor discs originate at the cilial pole of the outer segment as deep infoldings of the cell membrane. These migrate up through the cell and eventually bud off internally to form free discs within the outer segment.

At the rod apex, effete and aged discs are eliminated and extruded into the extracellular space where they are phagocytosed by the retinal pigment epithelial cell, into which the rod outer segment is buried. There is a constant flow of new photoreceptor discs along the rod outer segment.

Mechanism of light detection

In the dark, the photoreceptor cell is strongly depolarized and this holds voltage-gated Ca^{++} ion channels open in the synaptic region, resulting in a constant release of an inhibitory transmitter substance at the synaptic terminal. This inhibitor prevents firing of nerve cells connected to the photoreceptor.

When stimulated by light, the photoreceptor becomes hyperpolarized and release of the inhibitory transmitter substance at the synaptic terminal is reduced. This reduction allows the axons of nerve cells connected to the photoreceptors to fire.

Photoreceptor cells detect light through its interaction with **rhodopsin** molecules. These are membrane-associated glycoproteins in the photoreceptor discs, and are composed of a protein (opsin) and a light sensitive group (cis-retinal).

When cis-retinal interacts with a photon it undergoes a conformational change to the trans form, which causes a fall in the concentration of a secondary messenger (cyclic GMP) within the cytosol of the photoreceptor. This results in closure of sodium channels in the cell membrane and hence hyperpolarization.

The retina contains two main types of support cell: Müller's cells and astrocytes.

Müller's cells are tall retinal support cells. They extend from the base of the inner segment of the photoreceptor cells, where they link to each other by adherent junctions (see Fig. 3.9) to form the structure known as the outer limiting membrane, up to the retinal surface, where they rest on the internal limiting membrane.

Fig. 19.15 Rods and cones.
Micrograph of a resin section taken tangentially through the retina at the level of the inner segment of the photoreceptors. Rods (R) are identified as thin circular profiles, while cones (C) are larger. There is a mosaic of rods and cones in this retinal area 6 mm temporal to the fovea.

Astrocytes (see page 86) act as support cells to the nerve cells throughout the retina and are characterized by long dendritic processes which form a scaffold for the delicate processes of nerve cells.

Nerve cells of the retina interconnect to integrate the signals from photoreceptors.

The retina contains several classes of nerve cell: bipolar cells, ganglion cells, horizontal cells, amacrine cells and interplexiform cells.

Bipolar cells connect with the synaptic end of the photoreceptor cells and transmit signals to ganglion cells. **Ganglion cells** send axons from the eye to the brain in the optic nerve.

Horizontal cells, amacrine cells and **interplexiform cells** are neurons that act as 'gates' to modulate the passage of impulses from the photoreceptors to the ganglion cells. Their processes interpose the connections between bipolar cells and photoreceptors, and between bipolar cells and ganglion cells. This group of gate cells allows integration of signals from adjacent groups of photoreceptors.

The sensory retina is composed of nine layers made up of different cell types.

- the **photoreceptor layer** of rods and cones, which extends from the retinal pigment epithelium and consists of outer and inner segments of the photoreceptor cells (Fig. 19.16);
- the **external limiting membrane**, which is not a true membrane, but a line marking the zone of adherent junctions between Müller's cells;
- the **outer nuclear layer** consisting of the nuclei and cell bodies of the photoreceptor cells which form 8–9 rows of nuclei;
- the **outer plexiform layer**, which contains the cell processes and synaptic connections between the photoreceptor cells, bipolar neurons and horizontal cells;
- the **inner nuclear layer**, which is composed of the nuclei and cells bodies of bipolar cells, horizontal cells, interplexiform cells and amacrine cells, as well as the nuclei of the Müller's cells;
- the **inner plexiform layer** containing the cell processes and synapses of bipolar cells, amacrine cells, interplexiform cells and ganglion cells;

Fig. 19.16 Sensory retina.
(a) Micrograph of silver stained sensory retina showing its nine constituent layers.
(b) Diagram of the sensory retina showing its nine layers.
(c) Micrograph of H&E-stained sensory retina.

- the **ganglion cell layer** consisting of a row of ganglion cells which have large nuclei with visible nucleoli, and prominent rough ER visible as Nissl substance;
- the **nerve fiber layer**, composed of the axons of the ganglion cells en route to the central nervous system via the optic nerve with supporting astrocytic cells;
- the **internal limiting membrane**, a barely visible basement membrane at the interface between the vitreous and the retina.

The nuclei of rods are small and densely stained, while those of cones are larger and pale stained.

In the outer plexiform layer, the synaptic connections to rods are termed spherals while those to cones are termed pedicles. For both cell types the terminal of a horizontal cell is interposed between the photoreceptor and the bipolar cell to form a structure termed a triad. The horizontal cell can therefore modulate the impulse from the photoreceptors to the bipolar cells and allows integration of signals from adjacent photoreceptors.

The amacrine cells of the inner plexiform layer interpose processes between the processes of bipolar cells and ganglion cells and thereby modify the transmission of impulses from the bipolar cells. The interplexiform cells are similar to amacrine cells but also send a process to synapse in the outer plexiform layer. The ganglion cells of the ganglion layer are separated by the cytoplasm of Müller's cells.

RETINAL DETACHMENT

The term retinal detachment is used to describe splitting of the retina through the photoreceptor layer to leave the attached pigment epithelium. Retinal detachment usually follows a tear in the retina caused either by retinal degeneration or by traction by the vitreous.

The vitreous is normally in contact with the whole of the retina and rotational shearing forces generated by pulling of the extraocular muscles are transmitted uniformly to the whole globe. If the vitreous becomes detached from the retina posteriorly, rotational shearing forces are focally concentrated and cause tearing of the retina.

If the retina does not re-attach, the cell bodies of the rods and cones in the detached area degenerate, with loss of visual function.

The retinal structure is modified in specialized areas.

OPTIC DISC The axons of the nerve fiber layer converge at the optic disc, which is visible in the retina and gives rise to the optic nerve. This area is devoid of photoreceptors and therefore produces a blind spot in the visual field.

MACULA The macula is a small yellow area located 2.5 mm lateral (temporal) to the optic disc. At its center there is a thin zone of retina composed exclusively of cones (the **fovea**), each cone synapsing with a single bipolar cell and thence linking with a single ganglion cell, thus producing a high degree of resolution. This area is at the center of the visual axis and provides high detail color vision.

The yellow color of the surrounding macula is due to the presence of yellow xanthophil pigment in ganglion cells from the fovea, which are displaced laterally so that light can impinge on the cones of the fovea without being dispersed by an overlying neural layer.

PERIPHERAL RETINA In the peripheral retina, many photoreceptors are mapped onto one ganglion cell and form a receptive field with low visual resolution. Electrophysiology has shown that these receptive fields are triggered by different visual stimuli, for example some ganglion cells only fire in response to a bright light, while others only respond to a moving edge.

The retinal blood supply enters with the optic nerve at the back of the globe.

The central artery and vein of the retina enter the back of the eye in the optic nerve and branch in the plane between the vitreous and the inner limiting membrane.

The capillaries, which form a dense plexus within the retina and supply all cells apart from the rods and cones, are characterized by tight junctions between their constituent endothelial cells to prevent diffusion of substances into the neural retina (i.e. they form a **blood–retinal barrier**). The rods and cones are supplied by choroidal vessels.

The retinal vessels are visible by ophthalmoscopic examination and may be damaged in disease, for example high blood pressure (hypertension) causes visible thickening of the arterial walls.

DIABETIC RETINOPATHY

Ophthalmoscopic examination of the retina (fundoscopy) is an important part of a general medical examination because it provides a direct view of blood vessels in a critical area of the circulation. Retinal blood vessels are frequently affected in disease, particularly diabetes mellitus.

In diabetes mellitus, the basement membrane of small blood vessels in the retina thickens and the vessels show dilatations termed microaneurysms.

The abnormal vessels become leaky and exude fluid into the retina, which is visible as white spots. Hemorrhages may also occur. This particularly affects the macula, leading to loss of visual acuity.

If these changes become severe the blood supply to the retina is reduced (ischemia) and this stimulates abnormal growth of new retinal blood vessels (proliferative retinopathy). The newly formed vessels may bleed and also result in retinal detachment.

The severity of diabetic retinopathy, which is the most common cause of blindness in the developed world, is greatly reduced by the careful control of blood-sugar levels. Laser coagulation of leaking vessels delays or prevents development of severe visual loss.

The optic nerve takes axons from the retina to the brain.

The optic nerve contains the axons from the retinal ganglion cells en route to the central nervous system, as well as the central artery and vein of the retina.

The optic nerve leaves the retina at the optic disc and penetrates the collagen of the sclera through a sieve-like plate of channels in an area termed the **lamina cribosa**. Within the orbit the optic nerve is surrounded by a sheath of dura and an extension of the subarachnoid space (Fig. 19.17).

The optic nerve is invested in the pia arachnoid layers (see Chapter 6) and septa from this layer enter the optic nerve and divide the axons into fascicles.

PAPILLEDEMA

If pressure of the cerebrospinal fluid (CSF) within the skull increases (raised intracranial pressure), pressure of the CSF around the optic nerve increases. Initially this impairs cytoplasmic flow along the optic nerve axons, which swell and cause engorgement of the central artery and vein.

Ophthalmoscopic examination of a normal optic disc reveals that it is a cup-shaped depression, but in cases of raised intracranial pressure, the disc is swollen (papilledema) with loss of the cup-shaped depression. Papilledema is an important physical sign and usually denotes abnormal brain swelling caused by disease.

Fig. 19.17 Optic nerve and sheath.
Micrograph showing the optic nerve (N) in longitudinal section. The central artery and vein of the retina run along its center. Around the optic nerve is the optic nerve sheath, which is composed of an extension of the dura (D) and subarachnoid space (S) and is filled with cerebrospinal fluid.

The lens, a soft transparent biconvex structure composed of crystallins, is encased in a capsule.

In the adult the lens is 9 mm in diameter and 3.5 mm thick. It has:

- an outer capsule 10–20 μm thick of hyaline material containing type IV collagen;
- a layer of large cuboidal epithelial cells, (the lens epithelium) beneath the capsule;
- a center composed of tightly packed cells, which have lost their nuclei and become packed by special transparent proteins (crystallins) to form so-called lens fibers (Fig. 19.18).

New lens cells are added to the margin of the lens throughout life from the lens epithelium, but the cells at the center of the lens do not undergo turnover or replacement and are therefore the oldest cells in the body of an adult.

The lens is avascular and is nourished by diffusion from the aqueous and vitreous.

The lens is suspended by suspensory fibers to the ciliary body, the radial arrangement of suspensory fibers being termed the **ciliary zonule**. These fibers are composed mainly of the fibrillar protein fibrillin (see Chapter 4).

The eye is divided into three chambers.

The **vitreous body** is a transparent gelatinous structure located behind the lens and occupying the space bounded by the inner surface of the retina. The vitreous has a volume of 4 ml and is a specialized support tissue, being composed of a few scattered spindle-shaped cells (hyalo-

Fig. 19.18 Lens.
Micrograph showing the lens capsule (C) as a pink-staining hyaline layer, and the subcapsular lens epithelium (E). The center of the lens (L) is composed of cells devoid of organelles (lens fibers) packed with crystalline proteins.

cytes), fine highly dispersed collagen fibers, and an abundant extracellular matrix rich in hyaluronic acid.

The **anterior** and **posterior aqueous chambers** lie anterior to the lens, are delineated by the iris and communicate with each other via the aperture of the pupil (see Fig. 19.8).

The **aqueous humor** is a watery fluid resembling cerebrospinal fluid and is secreted at a rate of about 2 ml/minute by the epithelial cells of the ciliary body in the posterior chamber. It provides nutrients to the structures it bathes and flows from the posterior chamber through the pupil into the anterior chamber.

The aqueous then filters through a network of spaces lined by endothelium, the **trabecular meshwork** (see Fig. 19.12), which runs around the circumference of the root of the iris, at the periphery of the anterior chamber, and enters the **canal of Schlemm** (Fig. 19.19). This canal runs around the whole circumference of the limbus within the sclera. From the canal of Schlemm, the aqueous enters venous vessels.

The angle between the margin of the cornea and the iris root where the trabecular meshwork lies is the **iridocorneal drainage angle**.

There is a normal resistance to the flow of aqueous at the level of the trabecular meshwork such that continued secretion and resorption of the aqueous results in a normal intrinsic resting pressure within the globe (intraocular pressure) of 10–22 mm Hg.

Fig. 19.19 Canal of Schlemm and trabecular meshwork.
ⓐ The canal of Schlemm runs around the circumference of the cornea at the limbus and communicates with the trabecular meshwork, which runs around the circumference of the root of the iris. The aqueous from the anterior chamber of the eye filters through the trabecular meshwork into the canal of Schlemm, and thence drains into venous vessels.
ⓑ Micrograph showing the trabecular meshwork (T) as an area of slit-like spaces with the canal of Schlemm (CS) within the sclera. The aqueous filters from the anterior chamber (A) just above the iris (I).

GLAUCOMA

Abnormalities in the drainage pathway of aqueous humor result in a rise in the intraocular pressure (glaucoma), which if untreated damages the nerve cells of the retina and causes blindness.

ACCESSORY COMPONENTS OF THE EYE

The conjunctiva is composed of a mucin-secreting columnar epithelium.

The normal conjunctiva is a translucent membrane that lines the inner surface of the eyelids (palpebral conjunctiva) and reflects onto the globe (bulbar conjunctiva) to cover its anterior surface up to the margin of the cornea (limbus).

The conjunctiva is covered by two layers of stratified columnar epithelium which give way to a flattened squamous epithelium toward the limbus. Goblet cells (see page 43) are present in this epithelium but mainly in the medial portion, being scarce in the temporal bulbar conjunctiva (Fig. 19.20).

Beneath the epithelium the conjunctival stroma is composed of loose fibrocollagenous support tissue with small blood vessels and lymphatics running through it. With aging there is loss of collagen in this tissue.

The eyelids contain many different secretory glands.

The structure of both upper and lower eyelids is similar and comprises the following four layers:
- skin;
- orbicularis muscle (a layer of skeletal muscle);
- tarsal plate (a plate of dense fibroelastic tissue);
- conjunctiva.

Within these layers are various types of glands (Fig. 19.21):
- Meibomian glands, sebaceous in type and secrete a lipid-rich substance that delays evaporation of the tear film which lubricates and protects the cornea;

THE EYE

- aqueous humor is produced by the ciliary body, goes through the pupil and drains through the trabecular meshwork into the canal of Schlemm

- the cornea is kept translucent by the action of the ion-pumping endothelial cells on its inner surface

- the uvea contains melanocytes and comprises the choroid, ciliary body and iris

- the photoreceptor layer of the retina is maintained by its close contact with the retinal pigment epithelium

- the retina is supplied by a single artery which runs through the optic nerve

- the nerve fibers in the optic nerve originate from the retinal ganglion cells

- cones are concentrated in an area of the macula termed the fovea which is responsible for high-resolution color vision

- glands of Zeis, small sebaceous glands associated with the eyelashes;
- glands of Moll, apocrine sweat glands at the margin of the eyelid;
- glands of Krause, accessory lacrimal glands in the fornix of the conjunctiva;
- glands of Wolfring, accessory lacrimal glands just above the tarsal plate.

The lacrimal glands produce tears which drain via a duct system into the nose.

Tears are produced by the main lacrimal gland, which is located beneath the conjunctiva on the upper lateral margin of the orbit, and by the accessory glands of Krause and Wolfring (see Fig. 19.21). The glands secrete a serous fluid and have a complex branched structure with secretory acini and ducts (see Fig. 3.25).

The main lacrimal gland drains into the upper fornix of the conjunctiva via a series of about 10 small ducts. Tears then wash over the surface of the eye and drain via two ducts located at the medial end of the eyelids. These ducts, the superior and inferior lacrimal ducts, merge into a common lacrimal duct and drain into the lacrimal sac; this empties, via the nasolacrimal duct, into the nasal cavity through an opening beneath the inferior turbinate bone (see Chapter 10).

The superior and inferior lacrimal ducts are lined by stratified squamous epithelium, whereas the lacrimal sac and nasolacrimal duct are lined by respiratory-type pseudostratified ciliated columnar epithelium.

Fig. 19.20 Conjunctiva. Micrograph showing conjunctival epithelium with goblet cells (G) containing mucin overlying the subepithelial support tissues (S), which contain vessels and lymphoid cells.

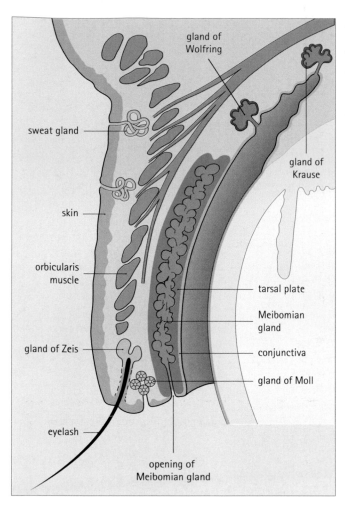

Fig. 19.21 Structure of the eyelid.
Diagram of eyelid, which is composed of skin, orbicularis muscle, tarsal plate and conjunctiva and contains various types of glands.

Labels on figure:
- gland of Wolfring
- sweat gland
- skin
- orbicularis muscle
- gland of Zeis
- eyelash
- opening of Meibomian gland
- gland of Krause
- tarsal plate
- Meibomian gland
- conjunctiva
- gland of Moll

1. IN THE EAR

(a) the pinna is composed of elastic cartilage
(b) the ceruminous glands are modified apocrine glands
(c) the tympanic membrane is lined on one side by cuboidal epithelium
(d) the middle ear cavity is lined by ciliated pseudostratified epithelium
(e) the auditory ossicles articulate by syndesmoses

2. IN THE INNER EAR

(a) hair cells have cilia on their surface to detect movement
(b) the ampullae of the semicircular canals detect acceleration
(c) the macula of the saccule detects sound
(d) the vestibular and tympanic cavities contain perilymph
(e) the basilar membrane is continuous with the organ of corti

3. IN THE EYE

(a) the posterior chamber lies behind the lens
(b) the lens is suspended from the ciliary body
(c) the inner part of the cornea is lined by endothelium
(d) the aqueous drains through the trabecular meshwork
(e) aqueous is produced by the epithelium of the ciliary body

4. IN THE RETINA

(a) retinal pigment epithelial cells are responsible for phagocytosis of photoreceptor membranes
(b) cones are concentrated at the periphery of the retina
(c) the photoreceptor layer is isolated from the rest of the retina by a belt of adherent junctions forming the external limiting membrane
(d) the macula contains the fovea
(e) the optic disc is devoid of photoreceptors

Answers

2. The Cell
1. a) T b) F c) F d) F e) T
2. a) T b) T c) T d) T e) T
3. a) T b) F c) T d) T e) T
4. a) T b) T c) F d) T e) T

3. Epithelial Cells
1. a) T b) T c) T d) F e) T
2. a) T b) T c) F d) T e) T
3. a) T b) T c) F d) F e) T
4. a) F b) T c) F d) T e) F

4. Support Cells and the Extracellular Matrix
1. a) T b) F c) T d) T e) T
2. a) T b) F c) T d) F e) F
3. a) F b) T c) T d) T e) T
4. a) T b) T c) F d) F e) T

5. Contractile Cells
1. a) T b) F c) T d) T e) T
2. a) T b) T c) F d) T e) T
3. a) T b) T c) T d) T e) T
4. a) T b) T c) T d) T e) T

6. Nervous Tissue
1. a) F b) F c) F d) F e) T
2. a) F b) T c) F d) F e) T
3. a) F b) F c) T d) F e) T
4. a) T b) F c) F d) T e) T

7. Blood Cells
1. a) T b) T c) T d) F e) T
2. a) F b) F c) T d) F e) T
3. a) F b) T c) T d) T e) F
4. a) T b) T c) F d) F e) F

8. Immune System
1. a) T b) T c) F d) T e) T
2. a) T b) T c) F d) T e) T
3. a) F b) T c) F d) T e) T
4. a) T b) T c) F d) T e) T

9. Blood and Lymphatic Circulatory Systems and Heart
1. a) T b) T c) T d) F e) T
2. a) F b) T c) F d) T e) T
3. a) T b) F c) F d) T e) F
4. a) T b) T c) T d) T e) T

10. Respiratory System
1. a) F b) F c) F d) T e) T
2. b → d → a → e → c
3. a) F b) T c) F d) F e) F
4. a) T b) F c) T d) F e) T

11. Alimentary Tract
1. a) T b) T c) F d) T e) T
2. a) T b) T c) F d) T e) T
3. a) F b) T c) T d) T e) F
4. a) F b) T c) F d) F e) T

12. Liver
1. a) F b) T c) T d) T e) F
2. a) F b) T c) T d) T e) T
3. a) T b) T c) T d) T e) F
4. a) T b) T c) F d) T e) T

13. Musculoskeletal System
1. a) F b) T c) T d) T e) F
2. a) F b) T c) T d) T e) F
3. a) T b) F c) F d) T e) T
4. a) T b) T c) T d) T e) T

14. Endocrine System
1. a) F b) T c) T d) F e) T
2. a) F b) F c) T d) T e) T
3. a) a=iii b) b=iv c) c=i d) d=ii
4. a) F b) T c) F d) T e) T

15. Urinary System
1. a) T b) T c) F d) T e) T
2. a) T b) T c) T d) F e) F
3. a) F b) T c) F d) T e) T
4. a) T b) T c) F d) F e) T

16. Male Reproductive System
1. a) F b) T c) T d) T e) T
2. a) T b) T c) F d) T e) F
3. a) F b) T c) T d) F e) T
4. a) F b) T c) T d) T e) T

17. Female Reproductive System
1. a) F b) T c) T d) T e) F
2. a) T b) T c) T d) T e) T
3. a) T b) F c) T d) F e) T
4. a) T b) T c) F d) T e) T

18. Skin and Breast
1. a) T b) T c) F d) T e) F
2. a) F b) T c) F d) F e) F
3. a) F b) F c) T d) T e) T
4. a) T b) T c) T d) T e) T

19. Special Senses
1. a) T b) T c) T d) F e) F
2. a) F b) T c) F d) T e) T
3. a) F b) T c) T d) T e) T
4. a) T b) F c) T d) T e) T

Index